Healthy Heart Sourcebook for Women

Heart Diseases & Disorders Sourcebook, 2nd Edition

Household Safety Sourcebook

Immune System Disorders Sourcebook

Infant & Toddler Health Sourcebook

Infectious Diseases Sourcebook

Injury & Trauma Sourcebook

Kidney & Urinary Tract Diseases & Disorders Sourcebook

Learning Disabilities Sourcebook, 2nd Edition

Leukemia Sourcebook

Liver Disorders Sourcebook

Lung Disorders Sourcebook

Medical Tests Sourcebook, 2nd Edition

Men's Health Concerns Sourcebook, 2nd Edition

Mental Health Disorders Sourcebook, 2nd Edition

Mental Retardation Sourcebook

Movement Disorders Sourcebook

Obesity Sourcebook

Osteoporosis Sourcebook

Pain Sourcebook, 2nd Edition

Pediatric Cancer Sourcebook

Physical & Mental Issues in Aging Sourcebook

Podiatry Sourcebook

Pregnancy & Birth Sourcebook, 2nd Edition

Prostate Cancer

Public Health Sourcebook

Reconstructive & Cosmetic Surgery Sourcebook

Rehabilitation Sourcebook

Respiratory Diseases & Disorders Sourcebook

Sexually Transmitted Diseases Sourcebook, 2nd Edition

Skin Disorders Sourcebook

Sleep Disorders Sourcebook

Sports Injuries Sourcebook, 2nd Edition

Stress-Related Disorders Sourcebook

Stroke Sourcebook

Substance Abuse Sourcebook

Surgery Sourcebook

Transplantation Sourcebook

Traveler's Health Sourcebook

Vegetarian Sourcebook

Women's Health Concerns Sourcebook, 2nd Edition

Workplace Health & Safety Sourcebook

Worldwide Health Sourcebook

Teen Health Series

Cancer Information for Teens

Diet Information for Teens

Drug Information for Teens

Fitness Information for Teens

Mental Health Information for Teens

Sexual Health Information for Teens

Skin Health Information for Teens

Sports Injuries Information for Teens

Breast Cancer SOURCEBOOK

Second Edition

Health Reference Series

Second Edition

Breast Cancer
SOURCEBOOK

*Basic Consumer Health Information
about Breast Cancer, Including Facts about
Risk Factors, Prevention, Screening and
Diagnostic Methods, Treatment Options,
Complementary and Alternative Therapies,
Post-Treatment Concerns, Clinical Trials,
Special Risk Populations, and New
Developments in Breast Cancer Research*

*Along with Breast Cancer Statistics, a Glossary
of Related Terms, and a Directory of Resources
for Additional Help and Information*

Edited by
Sandra J. Judd

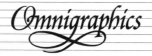
Omnigraphics

615 Griswold Street • Detroit, MI 48226

Bibliographic Note

Because this page cannot legibly accommodate all the copyright notices, the Bibliographic Note portion of the Preface constitutes an extension of the copyright notice.

Edited by Sandra J. Judd

Health Reference Series

Karen Bellenir, *Managing Editor*
David A. Cooke, M.D., *Medical Consultant*
Elizabeth Barbour, *Permissions Associate*
Dawn Matthews, *Verification Assistant*
Laura Pleva Nielsen, *Index Editor*
EdIndex, Services for Publishers, *Indexers*

* * *

Omnigraphics, Inc.

Matthew P. Barbour, *Senior Vice President*
Kay Gill, *Vice President—Directories*
Kevin Hayes, *Operations Manager*
Leif Gruenberg, *Development Manager*
David P. Bianco, *Marketing Director*

* * *

Peter E. Ruffner, *Publisher*

Frederick G. Ruffner, Jr., *Chairman*

Copyright © 2004 Omnigraphics, Inc.

ISBN 0-7808-0668-9

Library of Congress Cataloging-in-Publication Data

Breast cancer sourcebook : basic consumer health information about breast cancer, including facts about risk factors, prevention, screening and diagnostic methods, treatment options, complementary and alternative therapies, post-treatment concerns, clinical trials, special risk populations, and new developments in breast cancer research; along with breast cancer statistics, a glossary of related terms, and a directory of resources for additional help and information / edited by Sandra J. Judd.-- 2nd ed.
    p. cm. -- (Health reference series)
  Includes index.
  ISBN 0-7808-0668-9 (hardcover : alk. paper)
  1. Breast--Cancer--Popular works. I. Judd, Sandra J. II. Series.
  RC280.B8B6887 2004
  616.99'449--dc22

                                                                    2004015399

Table of Contents

Visit www.healthreferenceseries.com to view *A Contents Guide to the Health Reference Series*, a listing of more than 10,000 topics and the volumes in which they are covered.

Part III: Breast Cancer Risk Factors

Part IV: Prevention of Breast Cancer

Part VII: Post-Treatment Concerns

Part VIII: Additional Help and Information

Preface

About This Book

Every year more than 200,000 women in the United States are diagnosed with breast cancer. According to statistics compiled by the National Cancer Institute, one in every eight woman will develop breast cancer at some point during her life. Other than nonmelanoma skin cancers, breast cancer is the most common type of cancer found among American women, and for women between the ages of forty and fifty-five, breast cancer is the leading cause of death. Men are not immune. An estimated 1,300 cases of breast cancer are diagnosed in men each year. Although breast cancer claims 40,000 lives per year in the United States, early detection and improved treatment methods have led to significant declines in the death rate. In fact, when breast cancer is detected in its early stages, the five-year survival rate is 96 percent.

Breast Cancer Sourcebook, Second Edition provides basic consumer health information about breast cancer, including risk factors, methods of prevention, screening and diagnostic methods, treatment options, complementary and alternative therapies, post-treatment concerns, clinical trials, special risk populations, and new developments in breast cancer research. Statistical data, a glossary, and a directory of resources for additional help and information are also included.

How to Use This Book

This book is divided into parts and chapters. Parts focus on broad areas of interest. Chapters are devoted to single topics within a part.

ix

Part I: Breast Health and Breast Cancer Fundamentals describes the anatomy and physiology of the healthy breast and illustrates the procedures women should follow when performing a breast self-examination. It also explains facts about breast cancer, including the biology of breast cancer, types and stages of the disease, and the histologic grades of breast cancer.

Part II: Breast Cancer Statistics and Special Cases provides information about current statistics and trends in breast cancer incidence and mortality rates. It also looks at how breast cancer affects a variety of different populations, including young women, the elderly, pregnant women, men, and people of different ethnic and racial backgrounds.

Part III: Breast Cancer Risk Factors offers an in-depth look at the factors known and believed to affect one's risk of being diagnosed with breast cancer. These factors include family and genetic history, reproductive history, hormone treatments, dietary fat, smoking, environmental chemicals, and alcohol consumption.

Part IV: Prevention of Breast Cancer focuses on factors believed to play a role in preventing breast cancer, including genetic testing, breast-feeding, physical activity, phytoestrogens, chemoprevention, use of tamoxifen and raloxifene, and prophylactic mastectomy.

Part V: Breast Cancer Screening outlines guidelines for the early detection of breast cancer and provides information about methods of screening for breast cancer, including clinical breast exams, mammography, and emerging technologies.

Part VI: Diagnosis and Treatment Options describes diagnostic mammography, biopsy, lumpectomy, mastectomy, chemotherapy, radiation therapy, hormone therapy, clinical trials, and other methods used to diagnose and treat breast cancer. An in-depth guide to pathology reports is also included.

Part VII: Post-Treatment Concerns focuses on factors of concern to recovering breast cancer patients, including cancer recurrence, breast reconstruction, lymphedema, osteoporosis, sexuality, and how to talk to children, family, and friends about breast cancer.

Part VIII: Additional Help and Information offers a glossary of terms related to breast cancer and a directory of organizational resources that can provide further information and help in specific areas.

Bibliographic Note

This volume contains documents and excerpts from publications issued by the following U.S. government agencies: Centers for Disease Control and Prevention (CDC); National Cancer Institute (NCI); National Women's Health Information Center (NWHIC), Osteoporosis and Related Bone Diseases-National Resource Center; and the U.S. Food and Drug Administration (FDA).

In addition, this volume contains copyrighted documents from the following organizations: American College of Physicians; American Council on Science and Health; American Institute for Cancer Research; Breastcancer.org; California Department of Health Services-Cancer Detection Section; CancerNews.com; Cancer Research UK; Cleveland Clinic Foundation; Cornell University Program on Breast Cancer and Environmental Risk Factors in New York State (BCERF); Department of Defense Health Services Region IV Breast Health Program; Imaginis Corporation; John W. Nick Foundation; Lange Productions; Lippincott Williams and Wilkins; National Lymphedema Network; OncoLink; Susan G. Komen Breast Cancer Foundation; Tennessee Breast Center; University at Buffalo/State University of New York; Women's Information Network Against Breast Cancer (WINABC); University of Texas, M. D. Anderson Cancer Center; and Y-ME National Breast Cancer Organization.

Full citation information is provided on the first page of each chapter. Every effort has been made to secure all necessary rights to reprint the copyrighted material. If any omissions have been made, please contact Omnigraphics to make corrections for future editions.

Acknowledgements

Thanks go to the many organizations, agencies, and individuals who have contributed materials for this *Sourcebook* and to medical consultant Dr. David Cooke, verification assistant Dawn Matthews, and document engineer Bruce Bellenir. Special thanks go to managing editor Karen Bellenir and permissions specialist Liz Barbour for their help and support.

About the Health Reference Series

The *Health Reference Series* is designed to provide basic medical information for patients, families, caregivers, and the general public. Each volume takes a particular topic and provides comprehensive coverage. This is especially important for people who may be dealing with a newly diagnosed disease or a chronic disorder in themselves or in a family member. People looking for preventive guidance, information about disease warning signs, medical statistics, and risk factors for health problems will also find answers to their questions in the *Health Reference Series*. The *Series*, however, is not intended to serve as a tool for diagnosing illness, in prescribing treatments, or as a substitute for the physician/patient relationship. All people concerned about medical symptoms or the possibility of disease are encouraged to seek professional care from an appropriate health care provider.

Locating Information within the Health Reference Series

The *Health Reference Series* contains a wealth of information about a wide variety of medical topics. Ensuring easy access to all the fact sheets, research reports, in-depth discussions, and other material contained within the individual books of the series remains one of our highest priorities. As the *Series* continues to grow in size and scope, however, locating the precise information needed by a reader may become more challenging.

A Contents Guide to the Health Reference Series was developed to direct readers to the specific volumes that address their concerns. It presents an extensive list of diseases, treatments, and other topics of general interest compiled from the Tables of Contents and major index headings. To access *A Contents Guide to the Health Reference Series*, visit www.healthreferenceseries.com.

Medical Consultant

Medical consultation services are provided to the *Health Reference Series* editors by David A. Cooke, M.D. Dr. Cooke is a graduate of Brandeis University, and he received his M.D. degree from the University of Michigan. He completed residency training at the University of Wisconsin Hospital and Clinics. He is board-certified in Internal Medicine. Dr. Cooke currently works as part of the University of Michigan Health System and practices in Brighton, MI. In his free time, he enjoys writing, science fiction, and spending time with his family.

Our Advisory Board

We would like to thank the following board members for providing guidance to the development of this series:

Dr. Lynda Baker,
Associate Professor of Library and Information Science,
Wayne State University, Detroit, MI

Nancy Bulgarelli,
William Beaumont Hospital Library, Royal Oak, MI

Karen Imarisio,
Bloomfield Township Public Library, Bloomfield Township, MI

Karen Morgan,
Mardigian Library, University of Michigan-Dearborn, Dearborn, MI

Rosemary Orlando,
St. Clair Shores Public Library, St. Clair Shores, MI

Health Reference Series *Update Policy*

The inaugural book in the *Health Reference Series* was the first edition of *Cancer Sourcebook* published in 1989. Since then, the *Series* has been enthusiastically received by librarians and in the medical community. In order to maintain the standard of providing high-quality health information for the layperson the editorial staff at Omnigraphics felt it was necessary to implement a policy of updating volumes when warranted.

Medical researchers have been making tremendous strides, and it is the purpose of the *Health Reference Series* to stay current with the most recent advances. Each decision to update a volume is made on an individual basis. Some of the considerations include how much new information is available and the feedback we receive from people who use the books. If there is a topic you would like to see added to the update list, or an area of medical concern you feel has not been adequately addressed, please write to:

Editor
Health Reference Series
Omnigraphics, Inc.
615 Griswold Street
Detroit, MI 48226
E-mail: editorial@omnigraphics.com

Part One

Breast Health and Breast Cancer Fundamentals

Chapter 1

Breast Anatomy and Physiology

Although the general shape of a breast is circular or tear-drop, breast tissue can be found from the collar bone to the bra line, and from the breast bone to the armpit. That is why it is important for you to examine that entire area during breast self-examination, and for the surgeon to make a wide enough incision during a mastectomy.

Breasts are made up of milk-producing glands and milk-carrying ducts, imbedded in fatty tissue and fibrous supportive tissue. The glands are grouped in sections, called lobes. Each lobe has many smaller lobules which end in dozens of tiny grape-like bulbs where milk is produced. That is why breasts usually feel lumpy to the touch. Slender tubes called ducts carry the milk from the lobes to the nipple.

Two muscles, the pectorals major and the pectorals minor, are attached to the ribs under the breast. There are no muscles within the breast itself.

Arteries and veins carry blood to and from the breast, supplying it with nutrients and oxygen. Lymph ducts collect lymph (the fluid that leaks out of the blood vessels and accumulates between cells) and bring it back into the main circulation. Along the way, lymphatic fluid is filtered through small bean-shaped organs called lymph nodes.

Most of the lymphatic fluid from the breast drains toward the armpit area(the maxilla), where it is filtered through the maxillary lymph nodes.

How Breasts Grow and Change

From birth to old age, breasts go through more changes than almost any other organ in the body.

One to two years before menarche (the first menstrual period) breasts begin to grow under the influence of the female hormones estrogen and progesterone.

During reproductive years, variations in the levels of these hormones cause the breasts to go through monthly cycles: milk glands become engorged and the breasts swell, as if getting ready for a pregnancy, then return to their inactive state again.

At menopause, levels of hormones drop, many milk-producing glands shrink and disappear, and some of the breast tissue is replaced with fat.

All these changes sometimes damage the cells' DNA—the genetic material that tells the cell how to divide and grow. This damage may lead to cancer.

Vladimir Lange is a physician and the founder and CEO of Lange Productions, a leading producer of medical communications focusing on breast health and other health topics.

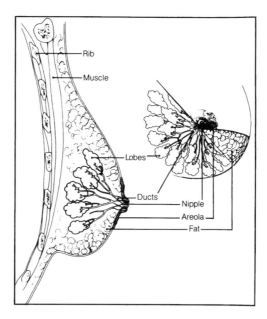

Figure 1.1. *Anatomy of the breast. (Source: NCI Visuals Online, National Cancer Institute.)*

Chapter 2

Breast Lumps and Other Changes

Over her lifetime, a woman can encounter a broad variety of breast conditions. These include normal changes that occur during the menstrual cycle as well as several types of benign lumps. What they have in common is that they are not cancer. Even for breast lumps that require a biopsy, some 80 percent prove to be benign.

Each breast has fifteen to twenty sections, called lobes, each with many smaller lobules. The lobules end in dozens of tiny bulbs that can produce milk. Lobes, lobules, and bulbs are all linked by thin tubes called ducts. These ducts lead to the nipple, which is centered in a dark area of skin called the areola. The spaces between the lobules and ducts are filled with fat. There are no muscles in the breast, but muscles lie under each breast and cover the ribs.

These normal features can sometimes make the breasts feel lumpy, especially in women who are thin or who have small breasts.

In addition, from the time a girl begins to menstruate, her breasts undergo regular changes each month. Many doctors believe that nearly all breasts develop some lasting changes, beginning when the woman is about thirty years old. Eventually, about half of all women will experience symptoms such as lumps, pain, or nipple discharge. Generally these disappear with menopause.

Excerpted from "Understanding Breast Changes: A Health Guide for All Women," National Institutes of Health, National Cancer Institute, NIH Pub. No. 98-3536, September 1998. Reviewed by David A. Cooke, M.D., on February 18, 2004.

Some studies show that the chances of developing benign breast changes are higher for a woman who has never had children, has irregular menstrual cycles, or has a family history of breast cancer. Benign breast conditions are less common among women who take birth control pills or who are overweight. Because they generally involve the glandular tissues of the breast, benign breast conditions are more of a problem for women of childbearing age, who have more glandular breasts.

Types of Benign Breast Changes

Common benign breast changes fall into several broad categories. These include generalized breast changes, solitary lumps, nipple discharge, and infection or inflammation.

Generalized Breast Changes

Generalized breast lumpiness is known by several names, including fibrocystic disease changes and benign breast disease. Such lumpiness, which is sometimes described as "ropy" or "granular," can often be felt in the area around the nipple and areola and in the upper-outer part of the breast. Such lumpiness may become more obvious as a woman approaches middle age and the milk-producing glandular tissue of her breasts increasingly gives way to soft, fatty tissue. Unless she is taking replacement hormones, this type of lumpiness generally disappears for good after menopause.

The menstrual cycle also brings cyclic breast changes. Many women experience swelling, tenderness, and pain before and sometimes during their periods. At the same time, one or more lumps or a feeling of increased lumpiness may develop because of extra fluid collecting in the breast tissue. These lumps normally go away by the end of the period.

During pregnancy, the milk-producing glands become swollen and the breasts may feel lumpier than usual. Although very uncommon, breast cancer has been diagnosed during pregnancy. If you have any questions about how your breasts feel or look, talk to your doctor.

Solitary Lumps

Benign breast conditions also include several types of distinct, solitary lumps. Such lumps, which can appear at any time, may be large or small, soft or rubbery, fluid-filled or solid.

Cysts are fluid-filled sacs. They occur most often in women ages thirty-five to fifty, and they often enlarge and become tender and painful just before the menstrual period. They are usually found in both breasts. Some cysts are so small they cannot be felt; rarely, cysts may be several inches across. Cysts are usually treated by observation or by fine needle aspiration. They show up clearly on ultrasound.

Fibroadenomas are solid and round benign tumors that are made up of both structural (fibro) and glandular (adenoma) tissues. Usually, these lumps are painless and found by the woman herself. They feel rubbery and can easily be moved around. Fibroadenomas are the most common type of tumors in women in their late teens and early twenties, and they occur twice as often in African-American women as in other American women.

Fibroadenomas have a typically benign appearance on mammography (smooth, round masses with a clearly defined edge), and they can sometimes be diagnosed with fine needle aspiration. Although fibroadenomas do not become malignant, they can enlarge with pregnancy and breast-feeding. Most surgeons believe that it is a good idea to remove fibroadenomas to make sure they are benign.

Fat necrosis is the name given to painless, round, and firm lumps formed by damaged and disintegrating fatty tissues. This condition typically occurs in obese women with very large breasts. It often develops in response to a bruise or blow to the breast, even though the woman may not remember the specific injury. Sometimes the skin around the lumps looks red or bruised. Fat necrosis can easily be mistaken for cancer, so such lumps are removed in a surgical biopsy.

Sclerosing adenosis is a benign condition involving the excessive growth of tissues in the breast's lobules. It frequently causes breast pain. Usually the changes are microscopic, but adenosis can produce lumps, and it can show up on a mammogram, often as calcifications. Short of biopsy, adenosis can be difficult to distinguish from cancer. The usual approach is surgical biopsy, which furnishes both diagnosis and treatment.

Nipple Discharge

Nipple discharge accompanies some benign breast conditions. Since the breast is a gland, secretions from the nipple of a mature woman are not unusual, nor even necessarily a sign of disease. For example, small amounts of discharge commonly occur in women taking birth control pills or certain other medications, including sedatives and tranquilizers. If the discharge is caused by a disease, that disease is more likely to be benign than cancerous.

Nipple discharges come in a variety of colors and textures. A milky discharge can be traced to many causes, including thyroid malfunction and oral contraceptives or other drugs. Women with generalized breast lumpiness may have a sticky discharge that is brown or green.

The doctor will take a sample of the discharge and send it to a laboratory to be analyzed. Benign sticky discharges are treated chiefly by keeping the nipple clean. A discharge caused by infection may require antibiotics.

One of the most common sources of a bloody or sticky discharge is an intraductal papilloma, a small, wartlike growth that projects into breast ducts near the nipple. Any slight bump or bruise in the area of the nipple can cause the papilloma to bleed. Single (solitary) intraductal papillomas usually affect women nearing menopause. If the discharge becomes bothersome, the diseased duct can be removed surgically without damaging the appearance of the breast. Multiple intraductal papillomas, in contrast, are more common in younger women. They often occur in both breasts and are more likely to be associated with a lump than with nipple discharge. Multiple intraductal papillomas, or any papillomas associated with a lump, need to be removed.

Infection or Inflammation

Infection or inflammation, including mastitis and mammary duct ectasia, are characteristic of some benign breast conditions.

Mastitis (sometimes called "postpartum mastitis") is an infection most often seen in women who are breast-feeding. A duct may become blocked, allowing milk to pool, causing inflammation and setting the stage for infection by bacteria. The breast appears red and feels warm, tender, and lumpy.

In its earlier stages, mastitis can be cured by antibiotics. If a pus-containing abscess forms, it will need to be drained or surgically removed.

Mammary duct ectasia is a disease found in women nearing menopause. Ducts beneath the nipple become inflamed and can become clogged. Mammary duct ectasia can become painful, and it can produce a thick and sticky discharge that is gray to green in color.

Treatment consists of warm compresses, antibiotics, and, if necessary, surgery to remove the duct.

A word of caution: If you find a lump or other change in your breast, don't use this text to try to diagnose it yourself. There is no substitute for a doctor's evaluation.

Benign Breast Conditions and the Risk for Breast Cancer

Most benign breast changes do not increase a woman's risk of getting cancer. Recent studies show that only certain very specific types of microscopic changes put a woman at higher risk. These changes feature excessive cell growth, or hyperplasia.

About 70 percent of the women who have a biopsy showing a benign condition have no evidence of hyperplasia. These women are at no increased risk for breast cancer.

About 25 percent of benign breast biopsies show signs of hyperplasia, including conditions such as intraductal papilloma and sclerosing adenosis. Hyperplasia slightly increases the risk of developing breast cancer.

The remaining 5 percent of benign breast biopsies reveal both excessive cell growth (hyperplasia) and cells that are abnormal (atypia). A diagnosis of atypical hyperplasia, as it is called, moderately increases breast cancer risk.

Chapter 3

Fibrocystic Breasts

Questions and Answers about Fibrocystic Breasts

What are fibrocystic breasts?

Fibrocystic breast condition is a common, noncancerous condition that affects more than 50 percent of women at some point in their lives. The most common signs of fibrocystic breasts include lumpiness, tenderness, cysts (packets of fluid), areas of thickening, fibrosis (scar-like connective tissue), and breast pain. Having fibrocystic breasts, in and of itself, is not a risk factor for breast cancer. However, fibrocystic breast condition can sometimes make it more difficult to detect a hidden breast cancer with standard examination and imaging techniques.

Fibrocystic breast condition is most common among women between the ages of thirty and fifty, although women younger than thirty may also have fibrocystic breasts. Because the condition is related to the menstrual cycle, the symptoms will usually cease after menopause unless a woman is taking hormone replacement therapy. In some cases, fibrocystic breast symptoms may continue past menopause.

Fibrocystic breast condition is the most common cause of noncancerous breast lumps in women between thirty and fifty years of age. More than 50 percent of women have fibrocystic breast symptoms at some point in their lives.

The information in this chapter is reprinted with permission from www
.imaginis.com. © 2004 Imaginis Corporation. All rights reserved. Complete information about Imaginis is included at the end of this chapter.

11

Symptoms of fibrocystic breasts include:

- cysts (fluid-filled sacs)
- fibrosis (formation of scar-like connective tissue)
- lumpiness
- areas of thickening
- tenderness
- pain

The degree to which women experience these symptoms varies significantly. Some women with fibrocystic breasts experience only mild breast pain and may not be able to feel any breast lumps when performing breast self-exams. Other women with fibrocystic breasts may experience more severe breast pain or tenderness and may feel multiple lumps in their breasts. Most fibrocystic breast lumps are found in the upper, outer quadrant of the breasts (near the axilla, armpit, region), although these lumps can occur anywhere in the breasts. Fibrocystic breast lumps tend to be smooth, rounded, and mobile (not attached to other breast tissue), though some fibrocystic tissue may have a thickened, irregular feel. The lumps or irregularities associated with fibrocystic breasts are often tender to touch and may increase or decrease in size during the menstrual cycle.

What is fibrocystic breast disease?

In the past, many physicians have referred to fibrocystic breasts, or lumpy breasts, as "fibrocystic breast disease." This term is misleading because fibrocystic breast condition is not a disease at all. Rather, it is a common, noncancerous breast condition that affects over half of all women at some point in their lives. Today, most physicians refer to this condition as "fibrocystic breast condition" or "fibrocystic breast change." Other terms that may be used to describe the condition include "cystic disease," "chronic cystic mastitis," or "mammary dysplasia."

In fact, since fibrocystic breasts are so common among women during their reproductive years, some physicians do not even like to label the symptoms as a "condition." They believe that these women simply have lumpier and more tender breasts than others.

What causes fibrocystic breasts?

Fibrocystic breasts occur as a result of changes in the glandular and stromal (connective) tissues of the breast. These changes are related

to a woman's menstrual cycle and the hormones estrogen and progesterone. Women with fibrocystic breasts often have bilateral cyclic
breast pain or tenderness that coincides with their menstrual cycles.

During each menstrual cycle, normal hormonal stimulation causes
the breasts' milk glands and ducts to enlarge, and in turn, the breasts
may retain water. Before or during menstruation, the breasts may feel
swollen, painful, tender, or lumpy. The severity of these symptoms
varies significantly from woman to woman. Some women experience
only mild breast swelling during menstruation, while others experience constant breast tenderness. Because the condition is hormone-
related, it will usually affect both breasts (bilaterally). Symptoms of
fibrocystic breasts usually stop after menopause but may be prolonged
if a woman takes hormone replacement therapy.

How are fibrocystic breasts diagnosed?

Fibrocystic breasts are often first noticed by the woman and further investigated by her physician. Breast tenderness, pain, and
lumpiness are common indicators of fibrocystic breasts, especially
when they coincide with menstruation. Often, fibrocystic breasts will
be diagnosed with a physician-performed clinical breast exam alone.

While having fibrocystic breasts is usually not a risk factor for
breast cancer, the condition can sometimes make breast cancer more
difficult to detect. Therefore, in some cases, breast imaging exams,
such as mammography or ultrasound, will need to be performed on
women who show symptoms of fibrocystic breasts. However, screening mammography may be more difficult to perform on women with
fibrocystic breasts because the breast density associated with
fibrocystic breasts may eclipse breast cancer on the mammogram film.
In some cases, additional mammography or ultrasound imaging, followed by fine-needle aspiration or biopsy, will need to be performed
on women with fibrocystic breasts to determine whether breast cancer is present. Fine-needle aspiration (to drain large, painful cysts)
may also be performed by a physician in order to help relieve some of
the more severe symptoms of fibrocystic breast condition.

How are fibrocystic breasts treated?

Often, physicians may recommend that the symptoms of fibrocystic
breasts be treated with self-care. Depending on the individual situation, several measures may be recommended to relieve the symptoms
of fibrocystic breasts. For instance, women may wish to wear extra
support (athletic-type) bras to help hold the breasts closer to the chest

wall, which may provide some symptomatic relief. Extra support bras are especially important for large-breasted women and may provide relief when breasts are full and tense with fluid. Physicians will often recommend that a support bra be worn both during the day and at night, especially during times of the woman's menstrual cycle when the breasts are most tender.

In addition, certain vitamins (particularly vitamin E, vitamin B$_6$, or niacin) or herbal supplements such as evening primrose oil may help alleviate the symptoms of fibrocystic breasts by reducing inflammation and fluid retention. It is important that these supplements be used according to directions and that women avoid megadoses, since serious side effects may occur with incorrect use.

Some women also find that reducing their caffeine intake by avoiding coffee, tea, chocolate, and soft drinks decreases water retention and breast discomfort. However, this is a controversial topic among healthcare professionals because studies linking breast pain and caffeine have been inconsistent.

In 1978, a study revealed that patients who took oral contraceptives were less likely to have fibrocystic breasts. The study has since been reconfirmed several times, though some health care professionals (and women) do not believe oral contraception has any significant effect on the occurrence of fibrocystic breasts.

If fibrocystic breast pain is severe and interferes with a woman's daily activities, further treatment may be necessary. Diuretics, substances that encourage the excretion of excess fluid from the body in the form of urine (which may, in turn, reduce tissue swelling and pain) are usually reserved for women who experience noncyclical breast pain, but may be used to alleviate the symptoms of fibrocystic breast condition in some cases. The release of fluid in the body can help decrease breast pain and swelling.

Additional drug treatments for severe breast pain include:

- bromocriptine (brand name, Parlodel)
- danazol (brand name, Danocrine)

Bromocriptine and danazol both relieve cyclical breast pain by blocking estrogen and progesterone. However, these drugs may cause serious side effects in some women. Bromocriptine is poorly tolerated by many patients; side effects include nausea, dizziness, and fertility problems. Side effects of danazol may include weight gain, amenorrhea (absence of menstruation), and masculinization (such as extra facial hair) when given high doses. Other drugs, such as tamoxifen (brand name, Nolvadex) or goserelin (brand name, Zoladex) have been shown to have some effect on cyclical breast pain; however, these drugs are currently approved for use only in the United Kingdom for treating severe fibrocystic breast pain.

Treatment of fibrocystic breasts may include:

- Wearing extra support bras
- Avoiding caffeine (controversial recommendation)
- Taking oral contraceptives (controversial recommendation)
- Taking over-the-counter medications such as aspirin, acetaminophen, or Motrin
- Maintaining a low-fat diet rich in fruits, vegetables, and grains
- Applying heat to the breasts
- Reducing salt intake
- Taking diuretics
- Taking vitamin E, vitamin B_6, niacin, or other vitamins
- Taking prescription drugs such as bromocriptine or danazol
- Surgically removing breast lumps

Breast Health Guidelines for Women with Fibrocystic Breasts

The earlier breast cancer is detected, the greater the chances of survival. Women with fibrocystic breasts should follow the same breast health guidelines as other women. These guidelines include breast self-exams, clinical breast exams, and screening mammography (beginning at age forty). Having fibrocystic breasts is not a risk factor for breast cancer. However, fibrocystic breasts can sometimes mask the appearance of breast cancer on a mammogram. Therefore, it is very important that women with fibrocystic breasts become familiar with the normal lumpiness and tenderness associated with the condition so that they can readily identify atypical symptoms that may indicate breast cancer.

Guidelines for the Early Detection of Breast Cancer

- All women between twenty and thirty-nine years of age should practice monthly breast self-exams and have a physician-performed clinical breast exam at least every three years.

- All women forty years of age and older should have annual screening mammograms, practice monthly breast self-exams, and have yearly clinical breast exams.

- Women with a family history of breast cancer or those who test positive for the BRCA1 (breast cancer gene 1) or BRCA2 (breast cancer gene 2) mutations may want to talk to their physicians about beginning annual screening mammograms earlier than age forty, as early as age twenty-five in some cases.

In some cases, density associated with fibrocystic breasts can mask breast cancer on a mammogram film. Therefore, some women with fibrocystic breasts may be referred for additional breast imaging with ultrasound or may be referred for breast biopsies if breast cancer is suspected.

About Imaginis

Imaginis.com is an independent, award-winning, comprehensive resource for news and information on breast cancer prevention, screening, diagnosis, and treatment and related women's health topics such as hormone replacement therapy (HRT), multiple sclerosis, osteoporosis, and ovarian cancer. Imaginis.com also contains extensive information about medical procedures such as angiography, biopsy, CT, MR, nuclear medicine, ultrasound, x-ray imaging, and radiotherapy.

The goal of Imaginis.com is to provide women and their physicians with the most comprehensive and relevant information on breast health and related women's health issues. Imaginis content is created by an independent team of breast health specialists to ensure that it is up-to-date and accurate. Complicated medical terms are explained in everyday language to help individuals understand their options, make informed decisions, and achieve optimal health.

Chapter 4

How to Do a Breast Self-Examination

Breast Self-Examination

Breast self-examination (BSE) should be done once a month so you become familiar with the usual appearance and feel of your breasts. Familiarity makes it easier to notice any changes. Early discovery of a change from what is normal for you is the main purpose of BSE.

The best time to do BSE is one week after your period ends, when your breasts are least likely to be tender and swollen. After menopause, or if you have had a hysterectomy, perform your BSE on the first day of each month.

How to Do a Breast Self-Examination

1. Stand before a mirror with your arms at your sides. Look at both breasts for anything unusual, such as puckering, dimpling, scaling of the skin, or fluid leaking from the nipples.

The next two steps are designed to emphasize any change in the shape or contour of your breasts. As you do them you should be able to feel your chest muscles tighten.

This information is excerpted with permission from the American Institute for Cancer Research brochure "Questions and Answers about Breast Health and Breast Cancer." © 2001 American Institute for Cancer Research. For additional information about cancer prevention, visit www.aicr.org.

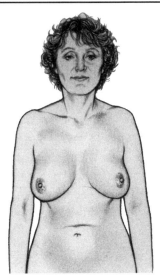

Figure 4.1. Breast self-exam: Step one. (Source: NCI Visuals Online, National Cancer Institute.)

2. Clasp your hands behind your head and press your hands forward. Look closely at your breasts in the mirror.

3. Press your hands firmly on your hips and bow slightly toward the mirror as you pull your shoulders and elbows forward. Once again, look closely at your breasts in the mirror.

Figure 4.2. Breast self-exam: Step two. (Source: NCI Visuals Online, National Cancer Institute.)

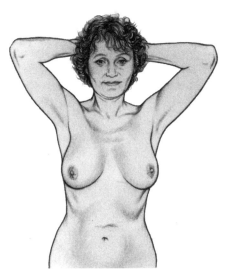

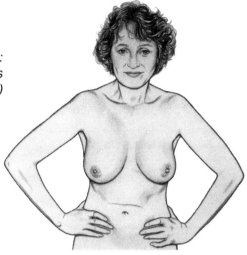

Figure 4.3. Breast self-exam: Step three. (Source: NCI Visuals Online, National Cancer Institute.)

Some women do the next part of the exam in the shower. Fingers glide over soapy skin, making it easy to concentrate on the texture underneath.

4.   Raise your left arm. Use three or four fingers of your right hand to explore your left breast carefully. Beginning at the

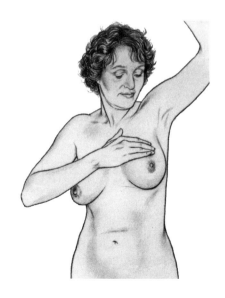

Figure 4.4. Breast self-exam: Step four. (Source: NCI Visuals Online, National Cancer Institute.)

outer edge, firmly press the flat part of your fingers in small circles, moving the circles slowly around the breast. Gradually work toward the nipple. Be sure to cover the entire breast. Pay special attention to the area between the breast and armpit, including the armpit itself. Feel for any unusual lumps or masses under the skin.

5. Gently squeeze the nipple and look for any fluid discharge. Repeat steps 4 and 5 on your right breast. The last part of the exam should be done while lying down.

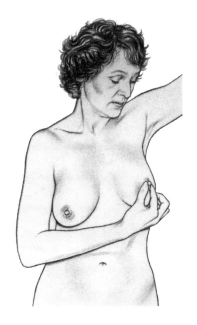

Figure 4.5. Breast self-exam: Step five. (Source: NCI Visuals Online, National Cancer Institute.)

6. Lie flat on your back with your left arm over your head and a pillow or folded towel under your left shoulder. This position flattens the breast and makes it easier to examine. Using the same motions described in steps 4 and 5, examine your left breast, underarm area, and nipple. Repeat on your right side.

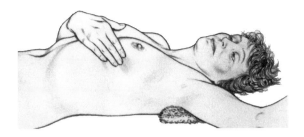

Figure 4.6. Breast self-exam: Step six. (Source: NCI Visuals Online, National Cancer Institute.)

Chapter 5

The Biology of Breast Cancer

To reduce cancer risk, we first need to understand how cancer develops in the body. Understanding how cancer develops can help us find ways to slow down its progress or perhaps stop it from occurring in the first place. For example, understanding that breast tissue of girls and young women is especially sensitive to cancer-causing agents can help direct risk reduction efforts to these groups. Making sense of cancer means taking a step toward more informed decisions about our bodies, our selves, and our environment.

How Does Cancer Develop?

Cancer develops through a multistep process in which normal, healthy cells in the body go through stages that eventually change them to abnormal cells that multiply out of control. In most cases, cancer takes many years to develop.

Normal cells in the body communicate with each other and regulate each other's proliferation (division). Cells proliferate to replace worn-out cells. When cancer occurs, cells escape the normal controls on their growth and proliferation. This escape from control can happen through a variety of pathways.

"The Biology of Breast Cancer," by Rachel Ann Clark, M.S. Science Writer, Cornell University, Roy Levine, Ph.D., Department of Pathology College of Veterinary Medicine, Cornell University, and Suzanne Snedeker, Ph.D., Associate Director for Translational Research, Program on Breast Cancer and Environmental Risk Factors in New York State (BCERF), Fact Sheet #5, updated November 2001, © 2001 Cornell University, reprinted with permission.

Part of the multistep process to cancer includes acquiring damage (mutations) to genes that normally regulate cell proliferation. A series of permanent mutations in tumor suppressor genes and proto-oncogenes (see following) are needed before cancer develops. Buildup of damage in these genes can result in uncontrolled cell proliferation. In some cases, further damage can lead to cells that can break away from the primary tumor and form cancers at other sites in the body (metastasis).

Breast tissue is particularly sensitive to developing cancer for several reasons. The female hormone estrogen stimulates breast cell division. This division can increase the risk of making damage to DNA permanent. Furthermore, breast cells are not fully matured in girls and young women who have not had their first full-term pregnancy. Breast cells that are not fully mature bind carcinogens (cancer-causing agents) more strongly and are not as efficient at repairing DNA damage as mature breast cells.

How Do Things Go Wrong?

When cancer develops it is because things go wrong in the cells of the body. In the breast tissue of young women and girls, cells are especially sensitive to DNA damage from cancer-causing agents.

Mutations in DNA

In every one of the trillions of cells in the body, there is an "operations manual" made up of DNA molecules. The information in the manual is separated into chapters, called genes, which are made up of small units of DNA. Genes are written in a DNA code that must be transcribed and translated in order for the cell to make the protein signals specified in each gene. These proteins are signals that tell the cell how to function.

A change in the genetic code is a mutation. Mutations can happen by subtracting from, adding to, or rearranging the original code. Mutations can happen randomly within the cell's DNA, but they can also be induced. A substance that causes mutations in DNA is called a mutagen. Mutations in a gene may interfere with its ability to make a functional signal, or cause it to code for a protein that sends an incorrect signal to the cell.

Most mutations are repaired by the cell, but in rare cases mutations do not get repaired. If a mutation is not repaired before a cell copies its DNA and divides into two cells, then the mutation is passed on to the two new daughter cells and becomes permanent. Rare genetic disorders (e.g., Ataxia Telangiectasia) are one way that cells are deprived of the ability to repair DNA, and may experience buildup of mutations in cells.

Mutations in most of a cell's DNA have no effect on whether the cell will become cancerous. However, the protein signals coded by a very small proportion of the total genes in each cell regulate cell growth and division. These regulatory genes include the two groups of genes called proto-oncogenes and tumor suppressor genes. A series of mutations in the DNA of either or both groups of these growth-controlling genes can eventually lead to cancer. Buildup of these mutations may take years to develop.

Breast Biology and Susceptibility to Cancer

Cells that divide are at a higher risk of acquiring mutations than cells that don't divide. Cancer is generally rare in tissues in which cells don't divide, like nerve tissue. Alternatively, cancer is more common in tissues in which cells divide frequently, such as with breast, skin, colon, and uterine tissues.

Young women and girls have breast tissue that is especially sensitive to cancer-causing agents (carcinogens). Unlike other tissues in the body like the liver and heart that are formed at birth, breast tissue in newborns consists only of a tiny duct. At puberty, in response to hormones (like estrogen that is secreted by the ovary), the breast duct grows rapidly into a tree-like structure composed of many ducts. Most breast development occurs between puberty and a woman's first pregnancy. The immature breast cells, called "stem cells," divide rapidly during puberty. The cells in the immature, developing breast are not very efficient at repairing mutations, and they are more likely to bind carcinogens. Therefore it is important to reduce the exposure of young women and girls to carcinogens that might damage DNA during this phase of rapid breast development. For example, Japanese infants and young women exposed to ionizing radiation from atomic bombing during WWII have high rates of breast cancer as adults. It is also important to reduce exposure to environmental estrogens during these critical times. Environmental estrogens (estrogen "mimics") are synthetic chemicals that can act like human estrogen in a woman's body, and may stimulate cell division in the breast.

After a woman's first full-term pregnancy, hormonal influences transform a high proportion of her breast cells into mature, differentiated cells that make milk. Milk-producing cells are fully mature and less sensitive to DNA damage than immature undifferentiated cells. Therefore, susceptibility to mutations declines in the breast cells of women who have had an early full-term pregnancy. Some evidence also suggests that breastfeeding further reduces the breast cells' sensitivity to mutations.

Though much of what we know about the biology of breast tissue susceptibility to cancer is based on research in animals, it is believed that most of this knowledge can be applied to human biology.

The Stages to Tumor Development

Cancer develops through different stages. These stages may or may not eventually lead to invasive and metastatic cancer. In most cases it takes many years for cancer to develop. Early detection of any tumor is important because it increases the chances of removing the cancer before it becomes life threatening.

Normal: There are trillions of cells in the healthy human body. Even though adults stop growing, the body constantly replaces worn-out cells with new ones to stay healthy. Cells must communicate and respond to each other's checks and balances to maintain the correct number of healthy cells.

Genetically altered cell(s): Tumor development begins when at least one cell has a genetic mutation (mistake in DNA) that causes it to divide and proliferate when it normally would not. This leads to more cells with the same mistake.

Hyperplasia: Cells look normal but grow too much. Further damage can lead to "dysplasia."

Dysplasia: Cells proliferate too much *and* look abnormal in shape and orientation. Cells are less responsive to surrounding cells and the body's signals to stop proliferating. Further damage or cell changes can lead to "in situ" (pronounced "in-SIGH-two") cancer.

Atypia: Cells look abnormal. Atypia is a general term describing how cells look. For example, one cell can appear atypical, but a group of cells display "dysplasia."

Benign tumor (not life-threatening): Although cells are not normal, they do not have the ability to travel to other parts of the body.

Cells in benign tumors are typically more differentiated (mature) and organized than cells in cancerous tumors. In some cases a benign tumor may eventually become an invasive or metastatic tumor.

In situ carcinoma (cancer): Cells become even more abnormal in growth and appearance but the tumor cells have not broken through the boundary around the tumor that separates it from surrounding tissues. This boundary is like a capsule that contains the tumor. Cells may acquire additional damage or changes that can lead to invasive cancer.

Invasive cancer (can be life threatening—primary tumor): The uncontrolled growth of cells in the tumor allows some cells to break through the capsule-like boundary and invade nearby tissues. Generally, invasive tumors are life-threatening if the cancer cells are present within a vital organ like the kidneys, lungs, or liver. Invasive tumors in nonvital organs like the breasts are not necessarily life threatening unless they become malignant and migrate to a vital organ. Therefore, early detection of any tumor is important because it increases the chances of removing the cancer before it becomes life threatening.

Malignant: Cells from the invasive (primary) tumor gain the ability to enter the blood stream or lymphatic system and to travel to distant areas in the body (metastasize).

Metastatic cancer (life threatening—secondary tumors that come from the primary invasive tumor): Cells from the malignant primary tumor gain the ability to re-establish somewhere else in the body, where they form new cancerous tumors. The secondary tumors are called metastases. Metastatic tumors can become fatal because they may disrupt the function of vital organs.

Where Can Things Go Wrong?

Cells in the body are regulated through the cell cycle. Damaged cells may eventually become deaf to normal regulation and multiply out of control.

Cell Cycle

Even though adults are no longer growing, many cells in an adult's body continue to divide to replace worn-out cells. To divide, a cell must enter a "highway" called the cell cycle. There are specific signals that tell a cell when to enter the cell cycle and how long to stay there and divide. For example, cyclins are molecules that help control the cell cycle. There are also signals that tell the cell when to exit the cell cycle. When a cell divides, it copies its DNA and produces two new daughter cells. If any of the signals controlling the cell cycle fail, cell division may go unchecked.

The female hormone estrogen is one signal that tells certain kinds of breast cells to enter the cell cycle. This leads to increased cell division. In addition, researchers suspect an interaction between estrogen and certain cyclins (e.g., cyclin-D1) that stimulates the cell cycle.

Factors that are locally produced by breast cells can also affect cell division. One example is the growth factor TGF-alpha (transforming growth factor alpha). Researchers have shown that overexpression of TGF-alpha is associated with increased cell division in breast cells, and hence may be associated with breast tumor progression (see Stages to Tumor Development). Overexpression of growth factors may be related to damage in proto-oncogenes (see following).

Proto-Oncogenes and Oncogenes: "Go" Genes

Proto-oncogenes are normal genes that code for the "go" signals controlling the cell cycle. These signals tell a cell to enter the cell cycle and code for how long it should stay there and divide. If a proto-oncogene loses the ability to regulate the cell cycle, the cell may reproduce uncontrollably because it stays in the cell cycle and continues to divide. A mutated proto-oncogene that has lost control of its "go" signal is called an oncogene.

Oncogenes code for protein signals that stimulate the cell to enter or continue in the cell cycle. This leads to inappropriate cell division and growth of a developing tumor. For example, a mutation in a proto-oncogene may cause the overexpression of certain growth factors and lead to inappropriate division of cells. That is why some growth factors are seen at higher levels in many breast tumors.

Another example is the erb-B2 receptor gene, an oncogene that codes for a receptor protein. The receptor in normal cells must be bound to a certain growth factor before it can stimulate the cell to enter the cell cycle and divide. But in faulty versions of the erb-B2 receptor gene, the receptors specified by this gene can release a flood of signals to stimulate increased cell division without being bound to the growth factor. Researchers have shown that up to 30 percent of primary breast cancers have too many copies of the erb-B2 gene.

Other oncogenes that researchers have found to be related to breast cancer include the tyrosine kinase family of growth factor receptors, the c-myc oncogene, cyclin D-1, and the cyclin regulator, CDK-1.

Tumor Suppressor Genes: "Stop" Genes

Just as the cell has "go" signals that tell it when to enter the cell cycle, it also has genes that control the "brakes." Cells with tumor suppressor genes that are mutated or inactivated lose control over their brakes. Brakes are important in the cell cycle. Putting on brakes at certain "checkpoints" allows the cell to check for any damage in its DNA. Repairs must be made before the cell is allowed to go on in the cycle. Without these brakes, cells with damaged DNA copy the mutations, divide, and pass on the damage to daughter cells. The damage is then established as a permanent mutation in subsequent generations of new cells. Therefore, an important function of tumor suppressor genes is to maintain the integrity of the DNA in cells. An example of a vital tumor suppressor ("stop") gene is the p53 gene. A mutation in the p53 gene is the most common genetic change found in breast cancer. One function of this gene is to keep cells with damaged DNA from entering the cell cycle. The p53 gene can tell a normal cell with DNA damage to stop proliferating and repair the damage. In cancer cells, p53 recognizes damaged DNA and tells the cell to "commit suicide" (apoptosis). If the p53 gene is damaged and loses its function, cells with damaged DNA continue to reproduce when normally they would have been removed through apoptosis. This is why the p53 gene has been termed "The Guardian of the Genome."

A small proportion of breast cancer cases (5 percent) are related to the inheritance of susceptibility genes. Alterations of the recently discovered "breast cancer susceptibility genes," BRCA 1 & 2, are involved in some inherited cases of breast cancer. If inactivated, these tumor suppressor genes can act indirectly in the cell by disrupting DNA repair. This allows the cell to accumulate DNA damage, including mutations that can encourage cancer development.

Other tumor suppressor genes that researchers have found may be related to breast cancer include the Retino blastoma, Brush-1, Maspin, nm23, and TSG101 genes.

Cell Adhesion Proteins

Healthy cells in the body are contained in a very orderly arrangement, like cobblestones in a street. Cobblestones are cemented in position and are contained by a curb. Like cobblestones, cells are cemented in position by cell adhesion proteins and are contained in their proper location by a curb called the basement membrane. In order for cells that have become cancerous to metastasize, the cells have to "break through" the basement membrane and enter the blood stream or lymphatic system.

Certain genes code for molecules that signal the cell to make cell adhesion proteins. If these genes are damaged by mutations, the resulting adhesion protein may no longer function properly. Without the cell adhesion proteins, cells do not stick as strongly to each other and to the basement membrane. The cells themselves may no longer stay in their orderly arrangement and may escape the boundaries of the basement membrane. Researchers have shown that expression of normally functioning adhesion molecules is progressively reduced in more advanced tumors. Two types of cell adhesion protein that researchers have found to be related to breast cancer are the cadherins and integrins.

Early detection of tumors is vitally important because damage to the genes governing cell adhesion molecules can be one of the life-threatening stages of tumor progression. Removing a tumor when it is still contained and before cells have escaped the confines of the original tumor reduces the chance that cells may have metastasized and generated new tumors in other areas of the body.

Summary

- Cancer is a multistep process in which normal, healthy cells in the body go through stages that eventually change them to abnormal cells that multiply out of control. In most cases, cancer takes many years to develop.

- Breast tissue can be sensitive to developing cancer. The female hormone estrogen stimulates breast cell division, which can increase the risk of breast cancer. Furthermore, breast cells are not fully mature in girls and young women who have not had their first full-term pregnancy. Breast cells that are not fully mature bind carcinogens more strongly than and are not as efficient at repairing DNA damage as mature breast cells. Therefore, it is very important to reduce exposure to cancer-causing agents during the critical periods in a woman's life.

- Part of the multistep process to cancer includes buildup of mutations to genes that normally regulate cell division. Damage to tumor suppressor genes or proto-oncogenes can eventually cause cancer. Damage to genes that code for cell adhesion proteins can lead to cells that can break away from the primary tumor and form cancers at other sites in the body.

- Development of invasive and metastatic cancer is a multistep process. Early detection of tumors is vitally important. Removing a tumor before cells can escape the confines of the original tumor reduces the chance that cells will metastasize and generate new tumors in other areas of the body.

- Taking steps to reduce risk includes understanding cancer and making more informed decisions about our bodies, our selves, and our environment.

Key References

Breast Cancer Dictionary. 1996. American Cancer Society, Inc.

Dairkee, S. H., and H. S. Smith. 1996. "The Genetic Analysis of Breast Cancer Progression." *Journal of Mammary Gland Biology and Neoplasia* 1, no. 2: 139–49.

Cavenee, W. K., and R.L. White. March 1995. "The Genetic Basis of Cancer." *Scientific American*, 72–79.

Putta, M. 1997. "Tumor Suppressor Genes: Guardians of Our Cells." BCERF *Fact Sheet* #6

Russo, J., and I. H. Russo. 1987. "Biology of Disease: Biological and Molecular Bases of Mammary Carcinogenesis." *Laboratory Investigation* 57, no. 2: 112–37.

Weinberg, R. A. September 1996. "How Cancer Arises." *Scientific American*, 62–70.

*—Prepared by Rachel Ann Clark, M.S., Science Writer, BCERF,
Cornell University; Roy Levine, Ph.D., Department of Pathology,
College of Veterinary Medicine, Cornell University; and Suzanne
Snedeker, Ph.D., Research Project Leader, BCERF, Cornell University*

For More Information

Program on Breast Cancer and Environmental Risk Factors
Sprecher Institute for Comparative Cancer Research
Cornell University
Box 31
Ithaca, NY 14853
Phone: (607) 254-2893
Internet: http://envirocancer.cornell.edu
E-mail: breastcancer@cornell.edu

Chapter 6

Types and Staging of Breast Cancer

Breast cancer is the most common malignancy in women and the second leading cause of cancer death (exceeded by lung cancer). Breast cancer is three times more common than all gynecologic malignancies put together. The incidence of breast cancer has been increasing steadily, from an incidence of one in twenty in 1960 to one in eight women today.

The American Cancer Society estimates that 182,800 new cases of invasive breast cancer will be diagnosed this year and 40,800 patients will die from the disease. Breast cancer is truly an epidemic among women and we don't know why.

Breast cancer is not exclusively a disease of women. For every one hundred women with breast cancer, one male will develop the disease. The American Cancer society estimates that fifteen hundred men will develop the disease this year. The evaluation of men with breast masses is similar to that in women, including mammography.

The incidence of breast cancer is very low before age thirty, gradually increases and plateaus at the age of forty-five, and increases dramatically after age fifty. Fifty percent of breast cancer is diagnosed in women over age sixty-five, indicating the necessity of yearly screening throughout a woman's life.

The information in this chapter is reprinted with permission from the Tennessee Breast Center, http://www.tennesseebreastcenter.com. © 2004 Tennessee Breast Center, Inc. and Melissa E. Trekell, M.D., FACS, M. B.A. All rights reserved. The section "Stages of Breast Cancer" is reprinted from "What You Need to Know about Breast Cancer," National Cancer Institute, NIH Publication Number 03-1556, September 30, 2003.

31

Breast cancer is considered a heterogeneous disease, meaning that it is a different disease in different women, it is a different disease in different age groups, and it has different cell populations within the tumor itself. Generally, breast cancer is a much more aggressive disease in younger women. Autopsy studies show that 2 percent of the population has undiagnosed breast cancer at the time of death. Older women typically have much less aggressive disease than younger women.

Risk Factors for the Development of Breast Cancer

Early onset of menses and late menopause: onset of the menstrual cycle prior to the age of twelve and menopause after age fifty causes increased risk of developing breast cancer.

Diets high in saturated fat: The types of fat are important. Monounsaturated fats such as canola oil and olive oil do not appear to increase the risk of developing breast cancer like polyunsaturated fats, such as corn oil and meat, do.

Family history of breast cancer: Patients with a positive family history of breast cancer are at increased risk for developing the disease. However, 85 percent of women with breast cancer have a negative family history.

Family history includes only immediate relatives—mother, sisters, and daughters. If a family member was postmenopausal (fifty or older) when she was diagnosed with breast cancer, the lifetime risk is increased by only 5 percent. If the family member was premenopausal, the lifetime risk is 18.6 percent. If the family member was premenopausal and had bilateral breast cancer, the lifetime risk is 50 percent.

Women with a significantly positive family history of premenopausal breast cancer should begin screening mammography a decade sooner than that at which their family member was diagnosed. BRCA-1 and BRCA-2 gene testing can identify those patients at increased risk, genetically, for developing not only breast cancer but also a variety of epithelial tumors, including ovarian and colon cancer.

At this time genetic testing is investigational. If a woman is determined to have these genetic markers, should we recommend bilateral mastectomy and oophorectomy? Further, if her insurance company knows that she has these genetic markers of increased risk, she may lose her insurance coverage. If a woman decides to proceed with genetic testing, we recommend that this test be paid for by the individual to keep the results confidential.

Late or no pregnancies: Pregnancies prior to the age of twenty-six are somewhat protective. Nuns have a higher incidence of breast cancer.

Moderate alcohol intake: More than two alcoholic beverages per day.

Estrogen replacement therapy: Most studies indicate that taking estrogen for more than ten years may lead to a slight increase in risk for developing breast cancer. However, these studies indicate that the positive benefits of taking estrogen as far as reducing the risk for osteoporosis, heart disease, and now more recently Alzheimer's disease and colon cancer, far outweigh the slight increase in risk that may be associated with estrogen replacement therapy.

Caution should be exercised in those women with a significantly positive family history of breast cancer or atypical intraductal hyperplasia. Women with breast cancer are not currently given estrogen replacement. There are no scientific studies currently justifying this practice. However, until those studies are available, by convention, women are taken off estrogen.

History of prior breast cancer: Patients with a prior history of breast cancer are at increased risk for developing breast cancer in the other breast. This risk is 1 percent per year or a lifetime risk of 10 percent. The reason for close clinical follow-up after the diagnosis of breast cancer is not only to detect recurrence of the disease, but also to detect breast cancer in the opposite breast.

Female: The mere fact of being female increases the risk of developing breast cancer. However, for every one hundred women with breast cancer, one male will develop the disease.

Therapeutic irradiation to chest wall, such as for Hodgkin Disease (cancer of the lymph nodes): Patients who have had therapeutic irradiation to the chest are at increased risk for developing breast cancer approximately ten years later, and consideration should be given to earlier screening in this population.

Moderate obesity: The relationship of breast cancer to obesity is more complex but associated with an increased risk.

Breast Cancer Types

Ductal carcinoma in-situ: Generally divided into comedo (blackhead, the cut surface of the tumor demonstrates extrusion of dead and necrotic tumor cells similar to a blackhead) and non-comedo types. DCIS is early breast cancer confined to the inside of the ductal system. The distinction between comedo and non-comedo types is important, as comedocarcinoma in-situ generally behaves more aggressively and may show areas of microinvasion (small areas of invasion through the ductal wall into surrounding tissue).

The surgical management is the same as for other types of breast cancer, except axillary node sampling is not done, as only 1 percent of these lesions will have axillary metastasis. We recommend, however, that irradiation be given if treated with conservative breast surgery to reduce the recurrence rate, from 21 percent without irradiation, to 5 percent to 10 percent with irradiation. This is a controversial area of the treatment of breast cancer.

Infiltrating ductal: The most common type of breast cancer, representing 78 percent of all malignancies. These lesions can be stellate (starlike in appearance on mammography) in appearance or well circumscribed (rounded). The stellate lesions generally have a poorer prognosis.

Medullary carcinoma: Comprise 15 percent of breast cancers. These lesions are generally well circumscribed and may be difficult to distinguish from fibroadenoma by mammography or sonography. Medullary carcinoma is estrogen and progesterone receptor (prognostic indicator) negative 90 percent of the time. Medullary carcinoma usually has a better prognosis than ordinary breast cancer.

Infiltrating lobular: Representing 15 percent of breast cancer, these lesions generally present in the upper outer quadrant of the breast as a subtle thickening and are difficult to diagnose by mammography. Infiltrating lobular can be bilateral (involve both breasts). Microscopically, these tumors exhibit a linear array of cells (Indian filing) and grow around the ducts and lobules (targeting).

Tubular carcinoma: Orderly or well-differentiated carcinoma of the breast. These lesions make up about 2 percent of breast cancer. They have a favorable prognosis, with nearly a 95 percent ten-year survival rate.

Mucinous carcinoma: Represents 1 percent to 2 percent of carcinoma of the breast and has a favorable prognosis. These lesions are usually well circumscribed (rounded).

Inflammatory carcinoma: A particularly aggressive type of breast cancer; the presentation is usually noted in changes in the skin of the breast, including redness (erythema), thickening of the skin, and prominence of the hair follicles resembling an orange peel (peau d' orange). The diagnosis is made by a skin biopsy, which reveals tumor in the lymphatic and vascular channels 50 percent of the time.

Stages of Breast Cancer

Doctors describe breast cancer by the following stages.

Stage 0

Stage 0 is called *carcinoma in situ.*

- **Lobular carcinoma in situ (LCIS)** refers to abnormal cells in the lining of a lobule. These abnormal cells are a marker of increased risk. That means a woman with LCIS has an increased risk of developing invasive cancer in either breast sometime in the future. (Both breasts are at risk.)

- **Ductal carcinoma in situ (DCIS)** is a precancerous condition in the lining of a duct. DCIS is also called intraductal carcinoma. The abnormal cells have not spread outside the duct to invade the surrounding breast tissue. However, if not treated, DCIS sometimes becomes invasive cancer.

Stage I

Stage I is an early stage of invasive breast cancer. Stage I means that the tumor is no more than two centimeters (less than three-quarters of an inch) across, and cancer cells have not spread beyond the breast.

Stage II

Stage II is one of the following:

- The tumor in the breast is no more than two centimeters (less than three-quarters of an inch) across, and the cancer has spread to the lymph nodes under the arm; or

- The tumor is between two and five centimeters (three-quarters of an inch to two inches), and the cancer may have spread to the lymph nodes under the arm; or

- The tumor is larger than five centimeters (two inches) but has not spread to the lymph nodes under the arm.

Stage III

Stage III may be a large tumor, but the cancer has not spread beyond the breast and nearby lymph nodes. It is locally advanced cancer.

- Stage IIIA means the tumor in the breast is smaller than five centimeters, the cancer has spread to the underarm lymph nodes, and the lymph nodes are attached to each other or to other structures; or the tumor is large (more than five centimeters across) and the cancer has spread to the underarm lymph nodes.

- Stage IIIB means the tumor may have grown into the chest wall or the skin of the breast; or the cancer has spread to lymph nodes under the breastbone.

- Inflammatory breast cancer is a type of Stage IIIB breast cancer. It is rare. The breast looks red and swollen (or inflamed) because cancer cells block the lymph vessels in the skin of the breast.

- Stage IIIC means the cancer has spread to the lymph nodes under the breastbone and under the arm, or to the lymph nodes under or above the collarbone. The primary breast tumor may be of any size.

Stage IV

Stage IV is distant metastatic cancer. The cancer has spread to other parts of the body.

Recurrent Cancer

Recurrent cancer is cancer that has come back (recurred) after treatment. It may recur locally (in the breast or chest wall) or in any other part of the body (such as bone, liver, or lungs).

Prognostic Indicators

Tumor size: As the size of the tumor increases, the risk of axillary and systemic metastasis increases.

Histologic grade: the appearance of the tumor cells under the microscope; graded as (1) well differentiated, (2) moderately differentiated, or (3) poorly differentiated. The likelihood of survival diminishes with increasing histologic grade.

Estrogen and progesterone receptors: Protein plugs on the surface of the tumor cells to which estrogen and progesterone bind. This complex moves inside the cell, causing cellular division. The presence of estrogen and progesterone receptors is a good prognostic indicator. Tumors displaying these receptors will respond to hormonal manipulation, that is, Tamoxifen.

Axillary nodes: The most important prognostic indicator. Patients with negative axillary nodes (microscopically) have improved disease-free and long-term survival rates.

DNA flow cytometry: Test that determines the genetic material within the cell. Tumors with a normal amount of DNA (diploid) have a better disease-free and long-term survival rate than those with an abnormal amount of DNA (aneuploid). This study also determines the percentage of cells in active division. Tumors with active cellular division of less than 10 percent have a better prognosis.

Her-2/neu: Protein product secreted by the tumor indicating a decreased disease-free and long-term survival rate.

Breast Cancer Staging

Tumor Size or Characteristics

TX = Primary tumor cannot be assessed
TIS = Carcinoma in-situ
T0 = No evidence of primary tumor
TIS = Paget's Disease without a tumor, Carcinoma in-situ
T1 = Tumor less than 2 cm. in greatest dimension
T2 = Tumor larger than 2 cm. in size but less than 5cm.
T3 = Tumor larger than 5 cm. in size
T4 = Tumor of any size extending to the chest wall or skin

Lymph Nodes

N0 = no metastasis to axillary nodes
N1 = Metastasis to moveable axillary nodes

N2 = Metastasis to fixed or matted axillary nodes

N3 = Metastasis to supraclavicular, infraclavicular, or internal mammary nodes

Metastasis

M0 = no distant metastasis

M1 = distant metastasis

Table 6.1. Stages of Breast Cancer

Stage	Tumor (T)	Nodes (N)	Metastasis (M)
Stage 0	TIS	N/A	M0
Stage I	T1	N0	M0
Stage II	T0	N1	M0
	T1	N1	M0
	T2	N0, N1	M0
Stage IIIA	T0	N2	M0
	T1	N2	M0
	T2	N2	M0
	T3	N0, N1, N2	M0
Stage IIIB	Any T	N3	M0
	T4	Any N	M0
Stage IV	Any T	Any N	M1

Table 6.2. Five Year Survival Rate by Stage

Stage	Survival Rate
Stage 0	100%
Stage I	98%
Stage II	88%
Stage IIIA	56%
Stage IIIB	49%
Stage IV	16%

Chapter 7

Histologic Grades of Breast Cancer: Helping Determine a Patient's Outcome

What Is a Histologic Grade System?

Histology is the study of tissues, including cellular structure and function. Pathologists (physicians who conduct laboratory studies of tissues and cells) often assign a histologic grade to a patient's cancerous breast tumor to identify the type of tumor present and help determine the patient's prognosis (projected outcome). The Scarff-Bloom-Richardson system is the most common type of cancer grade system used today. To determine a tumor's histologic grade, pathologists examine the breast cancer cells and their patterns under a microscope. A sample of breast cells may be taken from a breast biopsy, lumpectomy, or mastectomy.

Pathologists closely observe three features when determining a cancer's grade: the frequency of cell mitosis (rate of cell division), tubule formation (percentage of cancer composed of tubular structures), and nuclear pleomorphism (change in cell size and uniformity). Each of these features is assigned a score ranging from one to three (one indicating slower cell growth and three indicating faster cell growth). The scores of each of the cells' features are then added together for a final sum that will range between three and nine.

Table 7.1. Histologic Grades of Breast Cancer

Tubule Formation (% of Carcinoma Composed of Tubular Structures)	Score
> 75%	1
10–75%	2
less than 10%	3

Nuclear Pleomorphism (Change in Cells)	Score
Small, uniform cells	1
Moderate increase in size and variation	2
Marked variation	3

Mitosis Count (Cell Division)	Score
Up to 7	1
8 to 14	2
15 or more	3

Summary of Histologic Grades of Breast Cancer

A tumor with a final sum of 3, 4, or 5 is considered a Grade 1 tumor (well-differentiated). A tumor with a sum of 6 or 7 is considered a Grade 2 tumor (moderately-differentiated), and a tumor with a sum of 8 or 9 is a Grade 3 tumor (poorly-differentiated).

Pathologists also look for necrosis (areas of degenerating cancer cells) when determining a tumor's grade. Cancers with a high grade, with necrosis, close to the surrounding margin of breast tissue of a lumpectomy sample, or with large areas of DCIS are more likely to recur after breast cancer treatment than other breast cancers.[1]

Hormone Receptor Status

Physicians often examine hormone receptors in breast cancer cells at the time of biopsy or breast surgery to determine whether estrogen receptors (ER-positive) or progesterone receptors (PR-positive) are present. Patients whose cancers have ER- or PR-positive receptors tend to have a better prognosis than patients whose cancers do not have these receptors. Cancers with ER- or PR-positive receptors are also much more likely to respond to chemotherapy or hormone treatment.

Breast cancer cells that express ER-positive receptors in their nuclei also tend to respond better to hormonal manipulation. For example, the drug tamoxifen is used to block the female hormone estrogen from estrogen receptors, thus slowing the growth and reproduction of cancerous cells. Researchers know less about PR-positive receptors but have noticed that cells that contain ER-positive receptors often contain PR-positive receptors too. If a cell contains a PR-positive receptor but no ER-positive receptors, a patient's prognosis may be worsened.

HER2 (human epidermal growth factor receptor 2), a protein receptor found on the surface of cells, is a key component in regulating cell growth. When the HER2 gene (sometimes written HER2/neu) is altered, extra HER2 receptors may be produced. This overexpression of HER2 causes increased cell growth and reproduction, often resulting in more aggressive tumor cells. HER2 protein overexpression affects 25 percent to 30 percent of breast cancer patients. A new drug, Herceptin, has recently been approved by the U.S. Food and Drug Administration (FDA) to treat women with metastatic breast cancer who overexpress HER2. Metastatic breast cancer is cancer that has spread past the breast and underarm lymph nodes.

Physicians may test tumor tissue for HER2 overexpression at the time of breast biopsy or surgery. Testing may also be done on stored tumor tissue from previous biopsy. To test for HER2 overexpression, the tumor tissue will be stained by a specific solution. A pathologist

Table 7.2. Scarff-Bloom-Richardson Histologic Grade System

Grade	Description	Score	5 yr. survival	7 yr. survival
Grade 1 (lowest)	Well-differentiated breast cells; cells generally appear normal and are not growing rapidly; cancer arranged in small tubules.	3, 4, 5	95%	90%
Grade 2	Moderately-differentiated breast cells; have characteristics between Grade 1 and Grade 3 tumors.	6, 7	75%	63%
Grade 3 (highest)	Poorly differentiated breast cells; Cells do not appear normal and tend to grow and spread more aggressively.	8, 9	50%	45%

will then examine the tissue, checking for highlighted areas where high levels of overexpression are present. Depending on the level of staining, the tumor tissue sample may be classified as HER2-positive.

It is estimated that 200,000 HER2 diagnostic tests are performed each year. Women are encouraged to be tested for HER2 overexpression at the time of breast cancer diagnosis, since results of the test may help determine a course of treatment.

DNA Cytometry

Cytometry is the process of counting and measuring a patient's cells. DNA cytometry involves measuring a breast tumor's DNA to help predict the tumor's aggressiveness. Flow cytometry is one type of DNA cytometry in which lasers and computers are used to measure the amount of DNA in cancer cells suspended in liquid as they flow past a laser beam. A second type of DNA cytometry, image cytometry, involves using computers to analyze digital images of the cells from a microscope slide. Both flow cytometry and image cytometry measure the DNA ploidy (amount of DNA) of cancer cells. Ploidy is a marker that helps predict how quickly a cancer is likely to spread. Cancers with the same amount of DNA as normal cells are called diploid, and those cancers with either more or less than that amount are called aneuploid. About two-thirds of breast cancers are aneuploid.[1] Several studies have shown that aneuploid cancers tend to be more aggressive than normal cancers.

Flow cytometry can also measure a tumor's S-phase (the percentage of cells in a sample that are in the synthesis stage of cell division). Many cells in the S-phase indicate that the breast tissue is growing fast and that the cancer is likely to be more aggressive than normal cancers. Image cytometry can also estimate the growth rate of a cancer when combined with special antibody tests of the breast tissue.

References

1. The American Cancer Society provides detailed information on histologic grades at http://www3.cancer.org/cancerinfo/main_cont.asp?st=ds&ct=5.

Other Resources

O'Grady, Lois et al, *A Practical Approach to Breast Disease,* Boston: Little Brown and Company, 1995, 186–87.

To learn more about HER2 and how the drug Herceptin helps treat breast cancer patients who overexpress the HER2 gene, please visit http://www.imaginis.com/breasthealth/herceptin.asp

About Imaginis

Imaginis.com is an independent, award-winning, comprehensive resource for news and information on breast cancer prevention, screening, diagnosis, and treatment and related women's health topics such as hormone replacement therapy (HRT), multiple sclerosis, osteoporosis, and ovarian cancer. Imaginis.com also contains extensive information about medical procedures such as angiography, biopsy, CT, MR, nuclear medicine, ultrasound, x-ray imaging, and radiotherapy.

The goal of Imaginis.com is to provide women and their physicians with the most comprehensive and relevant information on breast health and related women's health issues. Imaginis content is created by an independent team of breast health specialists to ensure that it is up-to-date and accurate. Complicated medical terms are explained in everyday language to help individuals understand their options, make informed decisions, and achieve optimal health.

Chapter 8

Inflammatory Breast Cancer

What is inflammatory breast cancer?

Inflammatory breast cancer is a rare form of rapidly advancing breast cancer that usually accounts for less than 1 percent of all breast cancer diagnoses. Inflammatory breast cancer is a form of invasive breast cancer that progresses quickly and should be differentiated by physicians from other forms of advanced breast cancer with similar characteristics. Inflammatory breast cancer causes the breast to appear swollen and inflamed. This appearance is often but not always caused when cancer cells block the lymphatic vessels in the skin of the breast, preventing the normal flow of lymph fluid and leading to reddened, swollen and infected-looking breast skin—hence the designation "inflammatory" breast cancer.

With inflammatory breast cancer, the breast skin has a thick, pitted appearance that is classically described as peau d'orange (resembling an orange peel). Sometimes the skin develops ridges and small bumps that resemble hives.

How is inflammatory breast cancer diagnosed?

The symptoms associated with inflammatory breast cancer are usually the first cause of concern. These symptoms may include:

The information in this chapter is reprinted with permission from www.imaginis.com ©2004 Imaginis Corporation. All rights reserved. Complete information about Imaginis is included at the end of this chapter.

- breast redness
- swelling
- warmth
- ridges or pits in the breast skin (a condition referred to as peau d'orange; resembling an orange peel)
- a change in the size or shape of the breast
- nipple discharge or an inverted (pulled back) nipple
- swollen lymph nodes

Inflammatory breast cancer can sometimes be mistaken by patients and physicians for a breast infection because its symptoms, and the rapidity with which they appear (sometimes within weeks), resemble those associated with infections. However, while most breast infections will respond to antibiotics, inflammatory breast cancer will not. In fact, symptoms of inflammatory breast cancer do not usually get better or worse as infections do. If symptoms persist more than two or three weeks despite treatment, further testing and a breast biopsy should be performed to determine whether cancer is present.

How is inflammatory breast cancer treated?

Inflammatory breast cancer is an aggressive cancer that can grow and spread quickly. If the inflammatory cancer has not spread beyond the breast, a mastectomy (removal of the entire breast) may be performed to remove the tumor. However, because inflammatory breast cancer involves lymphatic vessels of the skin, mastectomy can increase the chances for the cancer to recur (since the skin is stitched together after mastectomy). Therefore, other treatment options (most commonly, chemotherapy) are usually considered before surgery.

Chemotherapy is treatment with anti-cancer drugs. Chemotherapy is often administered to inflammatory breast cancer patients before local treatment (such as mastectomy or radiation). One common regimen of chemotherapy used to treat inflammatory breast cancer patients is CAF (cyclophosphamide, doxorubicin, and fluorouracil). Researchers are also investigating whether high-dose chemotherapy is effective for treating inflammatory breast cancer. Because high-dose chemotherapy causes damage to bone marrow cells, a bone marrow transplant or blood stem cell transplantation may be necessary. After surgery, patients with inflammatory breast cancer are usually treated with additional chemotherapy followed by radiation therapy to the chest wall.

What is the prognosis for inflammatory breast cancer?

Because inflammatory breast cancer is an advanced cancer, it has been associated with a poor prognosis (expected outcome). Past statistics have shown the average survival rate of inflammatory breast cancer to be approximately eighteen months. However, recent studies have shown that advancements in treatment may help to extend the survival time for women with inflammatory breast cancer. Using chemotherapy, surgery (mastectomy), and radiation, the average five-year survival rate is currently 40 percent. Physicians are hopeful that advances in treatment will continue to improve the prognosis for women diagnosed with inflammatory breast cancer.

Additional Resources

Anne Preston, an inflammatory breast cancer patient, has created a website that provides information on the disease in multiple languages including English, French, German, Hungarian, Vietnamese, Spanish, Italian, and Portuguese: http://www16.brinkster.com/ibcsymptoms

The National Cancer Institute provides information on inflammatory breast cancer at http://cis.nci.nih.gov/fact/6_2.htm

The Inflammatory Breast Cancer Help Page provides information and support on inflammatory breast cancer at http://www.ibcsupport.org. Users may also subscribe to the inflammatory breast cancer support mailing list, which was created for women with inflammatory breast cancer and their loved ones.

The study, "Management of Locally Advanced Carcinoma of the Breast. II. Inflammatory carcinoma," is published in the July 1, 1994 issue of *Cancer.* An abstract of the study is available online at http://www.ncbi.nlm.nih.gov/entrez/query.fcgi?cmd=Retrieve&db=PubMed&list_uids=8004622&dopt=Abstract

About Imaginis

Imaginis.com is an independent, award-winning, comprehensive resource for news and information on breast cancer prevention, screening, diagnosis, and treatment and related women's health topics such as hormone replacement therapy (HRT), multiple sclerosis, osteoporosis, and ovarian cancer. Imaginis.com also contains extensive information about medical procedures such as angiography, biopsy, CT, MR, nuclear medicine, ultrasound, x-ray imaging, and radiotherapy.

The goal of Imaginis.com is to provide women and their physicians with the most comprehensive and relevant information on breast health and related women's health issues. Imaginis content is created by an independent team of breast health specialists to ensure that it is up-to-date and accurate. Complicated medical terms are explained in everyday language to help individuals understand their options, make informed decisions, and achieve optimal health.

Chapter 9

Paget's Disease of the Breast: Questions and Answers

What is Paget's disease of the breast?

Paget's disease of the breast is an uncommon type of cancer that occurs in 1 to 4 percent of all people with breast cancer. It is sometimes called mammary Paget's disease. Paget's disease of the breast can develop in men, but it is very rare.

This type of cancer was named after Sir James Paget, a scientist who noted an association between changes in the appearance of the nipple and underlying breast cancer. A number of other diseases have also been named after Sir James Paget, including Paget's disease of the bone, which involves genetic changes that increase the risk for osteosarcoma (cancer of the bone).

Scientists do not know exactly how Paget's disease of the breast occurs, but two major theories have been suggested. In one theory, cancer cells called Paget cells break off from a tumor (an abnormal mass of tissue) in the breast and move through the milk ducts in the breast to the surface of the nipple. In the other theory, the skin cells of the nipple spontaneously become cancerous Paget cells.

What are the symptoms of Paget's disease of the breast?

Symptoms of Paget's disease of the breast include itching, burning, redness, and scaling of the skin on the nipple and areola. The areola

Excerpted from "Paget's Disease of the Breast: Questions and Answers," National Institutes of Health, National Cancer Institute, March 2002.

is the circular area of darker-colored skin that surrounds the nipple. There may be a bloody discharge from the nipple, and the nipple may appear flattened against the breast. In up to 30 percent of cases, however, there are no visible skin changes. Almost half of all patients with Paget's disease of the breast also have a lump in the breast that can be felt at the time of diagnosis. It is important to see a health care provider about any of these symptoms, or if the symptoms do not completely disappear after treatment. They may be caused by Paget's disease of the breast, other types of breast cancer, or a less serious skin condition.

How is Paget's disease of the breast diagnosed?

If the health care provider suspects Paget's disease, a sample of any nipple discharge may be examined under a microscope for Paget cells, or a biopsy of the nipple will be done. In a biopsy, the doctor removes a small sample of nipple tissue. A pathologist examines the tissue under a microscope to see if Paget cells are present.

Most people with Paget's disease of the breast also have an underlying breast cancer. That is why the health care provider usually orders a mammogram (x-ray of the breast). However, women with symptoms of Paget's disease who do not have a lump that can be felt often have normal mammograms. These women may need to have other breast imaging techniques, such as ultrasound or MRI (magnetic resonance imaging). In an ultrasound, high-frequency sound waves that humans cannot hear are bounced off tissues and internal organs. Their echoes produce a picture called a sonogram. In an MRI, a magnet linked to a computer creates detailed pictures of areas inside the breast.

What type of breast cancer is associated with Paget's disease of the breast?

People with Paget's disease who do not have a breast lump that can be felt usually have a condition called ductal carcinoma in situ (DCIS). DCIS is also known as intraductal carcinoma. In DCIS, abnormal cells are present only in the lining of the milk ducts in the breast and have not invaded surrounding tissue or spread to the lymph nodes. People with Paget's disease of the breast who do have a lump that can be felt at the time of diagnosis usually have invasive or infiltrating ductal carcinoma. The cancer has spread to nearby tissue, lymph nodes under the arm, or other parts of the body.

How is Paget's disease of the breast treated?

Modified radical mastectomy is the usual treatment for Paget's disease when the patient has an underlying breast cancer, or when the cancer has spread beyond the central portion of the breast behind the nipple. In this operation, the surgeon removes the breast, some of the lymph nodes under the arm, and the lining over the chest muscles. The surgeon may also remove part of the chest wall muscles.

Other treatment options may be available if no underlying cancer is apparent, or when the cancer is located only in the central portion of the breast behind the nipple. Some of these patients receive radiation therapy by itself, without breast-conserving surgery, while other patients have breast-conserving surgery, which may or may not be followed by radiation therapy. Breast-conserving surgery for patients with Paget's disease of the breast involves removing all of the nipple and areola and some of the breast tissue underneath.

For patients undergoing mastectomy, the doctor will perform a biopsy of the lymph nodes. The doctor may not recommend a lymph node biopsy for patients undergoing breast-conserving surgery. Adjuvant treatment (treatment that is given in addition to surgery to prevent the cancer from coming back) may be part of the treatment plan if cancer cells have spread to the lymph nodes. Adjuvant therapy may include chemotherapy, radiation treatment, or hormonal treatment.

Are clinical trials (research studies) available for people with Paget's disease of the breast?

Yes. Clinical trials are in progress for all types of breast cancer. These studies are designed to find new treatments and better ways to use current treatments. Before any new treatment can be recommended for general use, doctors conduct clinical trials to find out whether the treatment is safe for patients and effective against the disease.

People interested in taking part in a clinical trial should talk with their health care provider.

References

Burke ET, Braeuning MP, McLelland R, Pisano ED, Cooper LL. Paget disease of the breast: A pictorial essay. *RadioGraphics* 1998; 18:1459–1464.

Jamali FR, Ricci A Jr., Deckers PJ. Paget's disease of the nipple-areola complex. *Special Problems in Breast Cancer Therapy* 1996; 76(2): 365–381.

Kaelin CM. Paget's disease. In: Harris JR, Lippman ME, Morrow M, Osborne CK, editors. *Diseases of the Breast. 2nd ed.* Philadelphia: Lippincott Williams & Wilkins, 2000.

Pierce LJ, Haffty BG, Solin LJ, et al. The conservative management of Paget's disease of the breast with radiotherapy. *Cancer* 1997; 80(6): 1065–1072.

Sakorafas GH, Blanchard K, Sarr MG, Farley DR. Paget's disease of the breast. *Cancer Treatment Reviews* 2001; 27(1):9–18.

Sheen-Chen SM, Chen HS, Chen WJ. Paget disease of the breast—an easily overlooked disease? *Journal of Surgical Oncology* 2001; 76:261–265.

Ward KA, Burton JL. Dermatologic diseases of the breast in young women. *Clinics in Dermatology* 15(1):45–52.

Part Two

Breast Cancer Statistics and Special Cases

Chapter 10

Breast Cancer Facts and Figures

Breast cancer is the most common invasive cancer in women, with more than one million cases and nearly 600,000 deaths occurring worldwide annually.[1] Incidence rates are highest in industrialized nations such as the United States, Australia, and countries in Western Europe. Breast cancer incidence increased in many countries during the twentieth century, largely reflecting global changes in reproductive patterns[2-4] and regional increases in mammography.[5,6]

Because of social and cultural considerations, breast cancer ranks highest among women's health concerns.[7] It is the most frequently diagnosed cancer in women in the United States beginning at ages thirty to thirty-nine years,[8] and the fourth most common cancer in women aged twenty to twenty-nine years after thyroid cancer, melanoma, and lymphoma. Most cases are diagnosed at local (63%) and regional (29%) stages, for which five-year relative survival rates are 97 percent and 79 percent, respectively.[9] Clinicians play a vital role in addressing concerns about breast cancer and encouraging women to follow recommended guidelines for early detection.

Approximately 211,300 new cases of invasive breast cancer will be diagnosed and 39,800 deaths will occur among women in the United

Excerpted from "Trends in Breast Cancer by Race and Ethnicity," by Asma Ghafoor, MPH, Ahmedin Jemal, DVM, Ph.D., Elizabeth Ward, Ph.D., Vilma Cokkinides, Ph.D., MSPH, Robert Smith, Ph.D., and Michael Thun, M.D., M.S., *CA Cancer J Clin* 53 (2003): 342–55. © 2003 Lippincott Williams & Wilkins. Reprinted with permission.

States in 2003. Whites account for the largest portion of estimated cases (82%) and deaths (80%). In addition to invasive breast cancers, approximately 55,700 cases of in situ cancer will be diagnosed among women in the United States in 2003.[10]

Incidence Rates

Female breast cancer incidence rates vary considerably across racial and ethnic groups. The average annual age-adjusted incidence rate from 1996 to 2000 was 140.8 cases per 100,000 among white women, 121.7 among African Americans, 97.2 among Asian Americans/Pacific Islanders, 89.8 in Hispanics, and 58 in American Indians/Alaska Natives.[9]

Female breast cancer incidence rates increased for all women combined from 1980 to 2000, although the rate of increase slowed in the 1990s. Incidence rates continue to increase in white women (0.4% per year for 1987–2000), but have stabilized in African American women since 1992. In the other racial and ethnic groups, rates increased from 1992 through 2000 in Asian Americans/Pacific Islanders (2.1% per year) and Hispanics (1.3% per year) but decreased among American Indians/Alaska Natives (3.7% per year).[9]

Mortality Rates

As with incidence rates, mortality rates vary by race and ethnicity. From 1996 to 2000, the average annual female breast cancer death rate was highest in African Americans (35.9 cases per 100,000 women), followed by whites (27.2), Hispanics (17.9), American Indians/Alaska Natives (14.9), and Asian Americans/Pacific Islanders (12.5).[9] The death rate is higher among African American than white women despite lower incidence. Similarly, the breast cancer mortality rate is higher in Hispanic and American Indians/Alaska Natives than in Asian American/Pacific Islanders despite lower incidence.

Breast cancer death rates have decreased by 2.5% per year since 1990 among white women, and by 1% per year since 1991 among African American women. From 1992 through 2000, female breast cancer death rates also decreased in Hispanics (1.4% per year), whereas rates remained unchanged among Asian Americans/Pacific Islanders and American Indians/Alaskan Natives.[9] There has been a notable divergence between long-term breast cancer mortality rate trends for white and African American women. During the early 1980s, breast cancer death rates for white and African American women were approximately equal, but by 2000, African American women had a 32% higher death rate than did white women.

Factors that may explain the difference in breast cancer death rates between African American and white women include differences in timely diagnosis through mammography and unequal access to prompt, high-quality treatment.

References

1. IARC, WHO. "Breast Cancer," in *World Cancer Report,* edited by B. Stewart and P. Kleihues, 188–19. Lyon: IARC Press, 2003.

2. B. Armstrong, "Recent Trends in Breast-Cancer Incidence and Mortality in Relation to Changes in Possible Risk Factors," *Int J Cancer* 17 (1976): 204–11.

3. S. King and D. Schottenfeld, "The 'Epidemic' of Breast Cancer in the U. S.—Determining the Factors," *Oncology* 10 (1996): 453–72.

4. K. Chu, R. Tarone, and L. Kessler, et al., "Recent Trends in U.S. Breast Cancer Incidence, Survival, and Mortality Rates," *J Natl Cancer Inst* 88 (1996): 1571–79.

5. B. Miller, E. Feuer, and B. Hankey, "Recent Incidence Trends for Breast Cancer in Women and the Relevance of Early Detection: An Update," *CA Cancer J Clin* 43 (1993): 27–41.

6. L. Garfinkel, C. C. Boring, and C. W. Heath Jr., "Changing Trends: An Overview of Breast Cancer Incidence and Mortality," *Cancer* 74 (1994): 222–27.

7. R. Smith and D. Saslow, "Breast Cancer," in *Handbook of Women's Sexual and Reproductive Health,* edited by G. M. Wingwood and R.J. DiClemente (New York: Kluwer Academics/Plenum Publishers, 2002), 345–65.

8. Surveillance, Epidemiology, and End Results (SEER) Program (www.seer.cancer.gov), SEER*Stat Database: Incidence–SEER 9 Regs Public Use, November 2002 Sub (1973–2000) < 18 Age Groups >, National Cancer Institute, DCCPS, Surveillance Research Program, Cancer Statistics Branch, released April 2003, based on the November 2002 submission.

9. L. A. G. Ries, M. P. Eisner, and C. L. Kosary, et al., *SEER Cancer Statistics Review, 1975–2000* (Bethesda, Md.: National Cancer Institute, 2003).

10. A. Jemal, T. Murray, and A. Samuels, et al., "Cancer Statistics, 2003," *CA Cancer J Clin* 53 (2003): 5–26.

Chapter 11

Lifetime Probability of Breast Cancer in American Women

A National Cancer Institute (NCI) report estimates that about one in eight women in the United States (approximately 13.3 percent) will develop breast cancer during her lifetime. This estimate is based on cancer rates from 1997 through 1999, as reported in NCI's Surveillance, Epidemiology, and End Results (SEER) Program publication *SEER Cancer Statistics Review 1973–1999*. This publication presents estimates of the risk of developing breast cancer in ten-, twenty-, and thirty-year intervals. Each age interval is assigned a weight in the calculations based on the proportion of the population living to that age.

The 1 in 8 figure means that, if current rates stay constant, a female born today has a 1 in 8 chance of being diagnosed with breast cancer sometime during her life. On the other hand, she has a 7 in 8 chance of never developing breast cancer. Because the SEER calculations are weighted, they take into account that not all women live to older ages, when breast cancer risk becomes greatest. Table 11.1 provides details about a women's chance of being diagnosed with breast cancer.

In evaluating cancer risk for a cancer-free individual at a specific point in time, age-specific (conditional) probabilities are more appropriate than lifetime probabilities. For example, at age fifty, a cancer-free black woman has about a 2.5-percent chance of developing breast cancer by age sixty, and a cancer-free white woman has about a 2.9-percent chance.

Cancer Facts, National Cancer Institute, September 2002.

Among the racial/ethnic groups studied by SEER,[1] non-Hispanic white, Hawaiian, and black women have the highest levels of breast cancer risk. Other Asian/Pacific Islander groups and Hispanic women have lower levels of risk. Some of the lowest levels of risk occur among Korean and Vietnamese women.

These probabilities are based on population averages. An individual woman's breast cancer risk may be higher or lower, depending upon a variety of factors, including family history, reproductive history, and other factors that are not yet fully understood.

The NCI is directing special attention to women with disproportionately high rates of breast cancer and poor survival rates, including members of certain minority groups and the medically underserved. Efforts targeted at these groups are under way in all components of NCI's program: basic research, early detection, clinical trials, rehabilitation, education and information dissemination, and cancer centers.

Table 11.1. A Woman's Chance of Being Diagnosed with Breast Cancer

Age	Chance of Being Diagnosed with Breast Cancer
from age 30 to age 40	1 out of 252
from age 40 to age 50	1 out of 68
from age 50 to age 60	1 out of 35
from age 60 to age 70	1 out of 27
Ever	1 out of 8

Source: National Cancer Institute Surveillance, Epidemiology, and End Results Program, 1997–99.

Reference

1. National Cancer Institute Surveillance, Epidemiology, and End Results Program, *Racial/Ethnic Patterns of Cancer in the United States 1988–1992.*

Chapter 12

Young Women and Breast Cancer

Why Do "Young" Women Get Breast Cancer?

When it comes to breast cancer, "young" usually means anyone younger than forty years old. Breast cancer is less common among women in this age group. In 2001, less than 5 percent of all breast cancer cases occurred in women under age forty.[1]

However, women who are diagnosed at a younger age are more likely to have a mutated BRCA1 or BRCA2 gene. These genes are important in the development of breast cancer, and women who carry defects on either of these genes are at greater risk of developing breast and ovarian cancer. If a woman carries a defective BRCA1 or BRCA2 gene, she may have a 50 percent to 85 percent chance of developing breast cancer in her lifetime.[2] In addition, having a mother, daughter, or sister who has or had breast cancer also increases a young woman's risk of developing breast cancer. So while the risk of breast cancer is generally much lower for younger women, there is still a high risk for some.

If you are concerned about your genetic risk, ask your doctor to refer you to a genetic counselor or a breast cancer specialist who will

discuss in detail what your own risk may be and can talk about genetic testing and prevention options.

Diagnosing breast cancer in younger women can be more difficult
because their breast tissue is often thicker than the breast tissue of
older women. By the time a lump can be felt in a younger woman, it
is often large enough and advanced enough to lower her chances of
survival. In addition, the cancer may be more aggressive and less responsive to hormone therapies. Delay of diagnosis in younger women
is a special problem because it is so rare for a younger woman to get
the disease. As a result, younger women are often told that a lump is
just a cyst and to wait and watch it. Tell your doctor if you notice a
change in either of your breasts, and think about getting a second
opinion if you are not satisfied with his or her advice.

A Helpful Tip for Younger Women

It is important for younger women to become familiar with how
their breasts look and feel through monthly breast self-exams (BSE)
beginning by age twenty. The best time to perform BSE is just as your
monthly period ends. During BSE, if you discover a lump or notice
any unusual changes in your breasts, see your health care provider
for a clinical breast exam. (For step-by-step breast self-exam instructions, go to www.komen.org/bse.)

Clinical breast exams are recommended for all women beginning
at the age of twenty, and thereafter every three years, or every year
if you are age forty or over. If you are under age forty with a family
history or other risk factors, you should talk with a your health care
provider about risk assessment, when to start getting mammograms,
and how often to have them. *If done regularly, these exams help to
detect any problems early, and increase the chances of survival.*

Hearing the Pitter-Patter of Little Feet?

In the past, doctors advised women who had had breast cancer not
to have children. Doctors thought that the added estrogen and progesterone produced by their bodies during pregnancy might promote the
growth or recurrence of breast cancer. Yet, there are no studies that
have clearly shown a link between pregnancy and recurrence of breast
cancer. Today, many doctors say it is fine for women who are free of
cancer and not undergoing treatment to become pregnant. Some suggest waiting two to five years after diagnosis—the most likely period
of recurrence—to assure that breast cancer has not returned.

Some women around age forty who are closer to menopause find that after chemotherapy, their periods do not return. For those who are in their twenties and thirties and who still have their periods after chemotherapy, the ability to have children is unaffected. If you are hoping to have children after cancer treatment, talk with your doctor about your options.

For Mothers with Breast Cancer

If you are a mother of young children and you have breast cancer, it can be hard to tell your children what you are going through. Remember that children can pick up on their parents' feelings, and may be confused if you do not talk to them about your condition. Telling your children in simple terms about your cancer and sharing some of your feelings will help them understand the changes around them. Every mother is different, and your parenting style may be different from someone else's. But in your own way, try to share with your children what you are going through. Also, trying to maintain your usual routine may help your children adjust to the changes. Talking about your breast cancer can help both you and your children be supportive and cope with the disease.

Resources

Young women with breast cancer may have special concerns that are different from those of older women. Finding the right support group can bring strength and friendship through sharing your thoughts and feelings. Many larger hospitals have or can refer you to cancer support groups in your area. Or you can contact these organizations for more information:

American Cancer Society
800-ACS-2345
www.cancer.org

The Susan G. Komen Breast Cancer Foundation
800-I'M AWARE®, www.komen.org for these booklets:

- *What's happening to me?*
- *What's happening to the woman I love?*
- *What's happening to mom?*
- *What's happening to the woman we love?*

Y-ME National Breast Cancer Organization
800-221-2141
www.y-me.org

Young Survival Coalition
212-206-6610
www.youngsurvival.org

This list of resources is made available solely as a suggested resource. Please note that it is not a complete listing of materials or information available on breast health and breast cancer. This information is not meant to be used for self-diagnosis or to replace the services of a medical professional. Further, The Susan G. Komen Breast Cancer Foundation does not endorse, recommend, or make any warranties or representations regarding the accuracy, completeness, timeliness, quality, or non-infringement of any of the materials, products, or information provided by the organizations referred to in this list.

Developed in collaboration with the Health Communication Research Laboratory at Saint Louis University.

Notes

1,2. American Cancer Society, Breast Cancer Facts and Figures 2001–2002.

Chapter 13

Breast Cancer in Women from Different Racial and Ethnic Groups

Women of different racial and ethnic backgrounds have different rates of breast cancer occurrence and survival from the disease. In general, women from lower socioeconomic groups, regardless of their race or ethnicity, have lower rates of occurrence of breast cancer but have higher death rates from breast cancer. However, there are exceptions depending on age, race or ethnicity, and place of residence. The differences in rates of breast cancer occurrence and survival appear to be the result of cultural and environmental effects rather than genetic differences between ethnic groups. Women from different ethnic groups may be given different medical treatments for breast cancer.

Are there differences in the occurrence of breast cancer among women from different racial and ethnic groups in the United States?

In the United States the risk of ever getting breast cancer differs substantially among women from different racial and ethnic groups. It is highest for white women, followed by African American or black women, Asian and Pacific Island women, Hispanic women, and finally American Indian and Alaskan native women. Occurrence or incidence of breast cancer is expressed as the number of new cases diagnosed

"Breast Cancer in Women from Different Racial/Ethnic Groups," by Barbour Warren, Ph.D., Research Associate, and Carol Devine, Ph.D., Division of Nutritional Sciences and Education Project Leader, Program on Breast Cancer and Environmental Risk Factors in New York State (BCERF), Fact Sheet #47, April 2003, © 2003 Cornell University, reprinted with permission.

per year for each 100,000 women. This rate covers a specific time period (the most recent information is for the period from 1992 to 1999) and is adjusted for the ages of the women within the group. Age-adjustment accounts for the higher occurrence of breast cancer among older women and allows comparison of groups made up of different percentages of older and younger women. The U.S. breast cancer occurrence rates (per 100,000 women) were: 139 for white women, 121 for black women, 98 for Asian and Pacific Island women, 82 for Hispanic women, and 42 for American Indian and Alaska native women.

Earlier studies (1988–1992) examined Asian and Pacific Island women in the United States in more detail. During this period the occurrence rates were highest in Hawaiian women followed by Japanese, Filipino, Chinese, Vietnamese, and Korean women. The occurrence rates discussed previously come from the SEER Cancer Registry (see "What are the cancer registries?" in the following).

Are there differences in the occurrence of breast cancer in women from different countries?

Internationally there are large differences in breast cancer occurrence. The lowest rates are found in most of Asia and Africa, where the occurrence is less than twenty-five cases a year for every 100,000 women. The highest rates are seen in North America, Western Europe, Australia, New Zealand, and the southern part of South America. In these countries the occurrence rates are more than seventy-five cases a year for every 100,000 women. The United States and the Netherlands are the countries with the highest breast cancer occurrence, with rates as much as five to eight times those reported for countries in parts of Asia and Africa. Yet, these numbers may not be directly comparable because of large differences in both the tools used for diagnosis and tumor reporting between different countries.

Why does the occurrence of breast cancer vary among women from different racial and ethnic groups?

It is not understood why breast cancer occurrence varies for women with different racial and ethnic backgrounds. Most studies of breast cancer occurrence (and survival) in racial and ethnic groups in the United States have examined differences between black and white women. Potential explanations for the racial and ethnic occurrence differences are dissimilarities in: "established" breast cancer risk factors, diet, exposure to cancer-causing agents, and socioeconomic position. Each of these topics is examined separately in the following questions.

How are women from different racial and ethnic groups affected by the "established" breast cancer risk factors?

The risk from each of the established breast cancer risk factors (such as young age of menarche, older age of menopause, and older age of first child's birth) is the same for individual women of all ethnicities; no biological difference in the size of the risk exists. For example, the risk arising from young age of menarche is the same for black women and non-black women. In other words, the potential of the risk factors to affect breast cancer occurrence is not different for black and white women.

However, the racial and ethnic groups vary in the proportion of their members who are included in either the low- or high-risk categories for some of the established risk factors. That is to say, the prevalence of some risk factors is different. For example, a large percentage of white women delay childbirth, and they are older when they have their first child, a factor for increased breast cancer risk. Accordingly, the occurrence of breast cancer in white women is affected to a greater extent by age at first birth than in other groups where earlier childbirth is more common.

The breast cancer risk factors associated with childbearing do appear to play a role in the differences in breast cancer occurrence between racial and ethnic groups. Differences between black and white women exist within four risk factors associated with breast cancer: age at menarche (first menstrual period), age at birth of first child, number of children, and age at menopause. These differences taken together are considered important and may contribute to the differences in the age at which black and white women are diagnosed with breast cancer. Yet it is important to note, especially with the preceding examples, that there is a strong connection of these risk factors (especially age of childbirth and number of children) to the socioeconomic challenges faced by the women in question. For example, poorer women, regardless of their race or ethnicity, have children early in life, and affluent women have children later or not at all.

Does diet play a role in the differences in breast cancer occurrence between racial and ethnic groups?

A number of studies have examined dietary differences between racial and ethnic groups, but very few studies have examined diet and breast cancer risk in other than white women. Levels of alcohol consumption and obesity possibly play a part in the differences in breast cancer occurrence between racial and ethnic groups.

Alcohol consumption is associated with increased breast cancer risk, and there are differences in the levels of alcohol consumption among racial and ethnic groups. White women consume alcoholic beverages more frequently than black, Hispanic, or Asian women. Nonetheless, the true effect of this racial and ethnic difference will require direct study, and this has not been done. Obesity is associated with increased breast cancer risk after menopause. Racial and ethnic differences in obesity have been reported and they may contribute to racial and ethnic difference in breast cancer occurrence. The size of the contribution will also require more study.

Racial and ethnic differences in other aspects of diet, such as consumption of fruits, vegetables, fiber, and foods containing phytoestrogens, have been described. However, the degree to which they affect breast cancer risk has not been well established and their impact on racial and ethnic differences in breast cancer occurrence is unknown.

Are there differences in exposure to cancer-causing agents between women in different racial and ethnic groups?

Numerous studies have documented that women from different racial and ethnic groups are potentially exposed to different levels of environmental health hazards. Socioeconomics play a large role as hazardous-waste facilities and treatment, storage, and disposal facilities are often located in areas with lower per capita income. While they have been inconsistently associated with breast cancer risk, studies of residues from DDT and PCBs in women of different ethnicities provide good examples for potential differences in exposure between women of different racial and ethnic groups. Generalizations could not be made from the limited number of studies that have been conducted but there was a trend in all the studies toward lower blood serum levels of DDT and PCB residues in white women and higher blood serum levels in black women. A study that also examined Asian women found they had elevated levels similar to those of black women. In another study, Hispanic women had intermediate levels for most of the residues evaluated. The results of examinations of the association of specific DDT and PCB residues and breast cancer risk within the racial and ethnic groups of women were conflicting, like examinations of risk and residue levels in women of all races and ethnicities. The extent to which exposure differences to these and potentially other cancer-causing agents contribute to the racial and ethnic differences in breast cancer occurrence is unknown.

Does socioeconomic position play a role in the differences in occurrence of breast cancer between racial and ethnic groups?

The relationship between breast cancer risk and socioeconomic position is poorly understood, but it has been found to be related to a complicated mixture of features including education, family income, related features of diet and living conditions, and access to health care. The occurrence of breast cancer is higher in women from all racial and ethnic groups who have more education or family income. Socioeconomic position as measured by either level of education or family income is considered an established risk factor for breast cancer. Since socioeconomic information for individual women is not typically collected, most studies have relied on less direct characteristics such as income within a census tract. Nonetheless, the association between education and socioeconomic position and breast cancer risk appears to be unaffected by race. Black women with higher socioeconomic position and more education have breast cancer risk similar to that of white women within the same socioeconomic position.

Is the age of occurrence of breast cancer similar for women from different racial and ethnic groups and nationalities?

The age of occurrence of breast cancer is different among racial and ethnic groups and among women from different countries. The most studied racial and ethnic groups are white and black women. Before age forty, black women have higher occurrence rate of breast cancer than white women. Yet after age forty this relationship reverses and the occurrence rate becomes higher in white women. For both groups of women the occurrence rate of breast cancer increases as women get older.

Japanese women and women from less developed countries have historically displayed a different pattern. For these women, the occurrence rate of breast cancer reaches a maximum at about the age of menopause and remains near this value or decreases among older women. However, recent examinations suggest that the pattern for women from undeveloped countries may be changing and becoming more similar to that seen in more affluent countries. Younger women in those countries are developing breast cancer, and breast cancer risk is increasing with age.

Are the differences in occurrence of breast cancer among racial and ethnic groups genetically determined?

Genetics likely plays very little role in the difference in breast cancer occurrence among different racial and ethnic groups. This is supported by several lines of evidence. First, studies of human genetics have shown that there are more genetic differences between people within the same racial and ethnic group than there are between people from different racial and ethnic groups. There are in general very few, if any, medically significant genetic differences between racial and ethnic groups of people. Second, and as discussed previously, women of different racial and ethnic groups are subject to the same level of risk from each of the established breast cancer risk factors; these risk factors affect women equally regardless of their racial and ethnic background. Third, women who are migrants to areas of higher or lower breast cancer risk adopt the level of breast cancer risk reported for women already living in the new place of residence. This suggests that, rather than genetics, there is an important role for a woman's lifestyle and environment in breast cancer risk. Finally, genetics has not been found to play a large role in breast cancer in general.

Are there differences in the risk of dying from breast cancer between racial and ethnic groups of women in the United States?

There is a considerable difference in rates of death from breast cancer between different racial and ethnic groups. Black women have the highest rate of death from breast cancer in the United States. Over the period from 1995 to 1999 the yearly rate of death from breast cancer was 37 deaths in every group of 100,000 black women. This is 32 percent higher than the rate in white women (28 deaths/100,000) and three times that of Asian and Pacific Island women (13 deaths/100,000 women), who had the lowest death rate. The rates for both American Indian/Alaska Native women (15 deaths/100,000 women) and Hispanic women (17 deaths/100,000 women) were also much lower than those of black and white women.

Survival has also been examined for different Asian and Pacific Island racial and ethnic groups over the period from 1988 to 1994. Japanese women had the best survival rate (92 percent survived five years). Chinese women and Filipino women had a survival rate about the same as white women (86 percent survived five years).

Why do death rates from breast cancer differ between different racial and ethnic groups in the United States?

The reasons for the differences in death rates from breast cancer between racial and ethnic groups are not fully understood. They are thought to involve complicated interactions between socioeconomic and medical factors such as stage or seriousness of the cancer at diagnosis, types of treatment received, tumor aggressiveness, and access to and racial discrimination within medical service systems. (These topics are examined separately in the following questions.)

Can socioeconomic factors play a role in differences in breast cancer death rates among racial and ethnic groups?

Socioeconomic factors, such as education and income, play a role in the racial and ethnic differences in breast cancer deaths but the size of this role is uncertain. Socioeconomic factors have been demonstrated to affect the stage of cancer at diagnosis, which greatly influences survival. Most studies have found that adjusting for the level of breast cancer risk associated with socioeconomic position greatly decreased, and in some cases eliminated, the differences in death rates between black and white women. Socioeconomic effects are very complicated and could affect women's survival in a number of ways, including access to medical services, treatment received, care during and after treatment, and general state of health, as well as the stage of diagnosis mentioned previously.

Does the stage or seriousness of breast cancer when it is diagnosed contribute to the differences in death rates from breast cancer of racial and ethnic groups?

The stage of breast cancer when it is detected is the main factor involved in survival. A number of studies have found that black women are more often diagnosed with late-stage breast cancer. This difference in stage of diagnosis makes a large contribution to the differences in breast cancer death rates between white and black women. Delay in seeking treatment is thought to play a major role in the differences in stage of diagnosis between black and white women. Studies examining late-stage diagnosis have shown that a number of social and cultural factors contribute, including old age, low economic status, low education, unemployment, unequal treatment due to racial and ethnic biases, marital status, beliefs about health care, and health care

71

providers and access to them. Access to health care may also be an important component in the delay in seeking treatment; examinations of white and black women in the U.S. military, where there is equal access to health care, have reported no difference in the stage of breast cancer diagnosis.

Does breast cancer treatment differ depending on a woman's racial and ethnic background?

The National Academy of Sciences recently reported that racial and ethnic minorities receive lower-quality healthcare, in general, than nonminorities. This treatment pattern also exists in the breast cancer treatment received by women of different racial and ethnic groups. A number of factors contribute to this treatment pattern, including the type of treatment examined, the age of the women examined, and the location of the study. Most studies looked at only black and white women. Breast cancer treatment was typically examined in relation to the recommended therapy at the time of the study; the results varied between the studies. The largest studies reported treatment differences between racial and ethnic groups but not for all types of treatment. For example, in some, but not all studies, breast-conserving surgery was more frequent for black than for white women. However, radiation therapy following breast-conserving surgery was consistently reported to be less frequently given to black than to white women. About half of all the studies found a difference in treatment between black and white women; in one quarter of all the studies the difference was statistically significant and unlikely to be due to chance alone.

Is breast cancer more aggressive and difficult to treat in some racial and ethnic groups of women?

It is unclear if different racial and ethnic groups have breast cancer that is more aggressive and difficult to treat. This issue has been examined in several ways and most studies have examined only black and white women.

One approach has been to examine tumor characteristics that affect treatment difficulty, such as lack of estrogen receptors. Early studies of this type suggested that black women more often have tumors that are advanced and difficult to treat. Yet, most of these studies were not designed to directly evaluate this question and in many cases did not compensate for the effect of age on their evaluations. This is an important limitation, since breast cancer in younger women is generally more difficult to treat successfully. Recent studies examining these characteristics have controlled for age and support a higher occurrence of difficult to treat breast cancer in black women. Yet, this difference is not firmly established, and further study is needed.

Other studies have approached this question in epidemiological studies that compared the survival of black and white women after attempting to eliminate the contribution of nonbiological factors, such as socioeconomic position. As mentioned previously, the effect of these nonbiological factors on breast cancer risk is complicated and is not represented by a single factor such as socioeconomic position. Accordingly, the elimination of their contribution to the observed risk is difficult. In addition, almost all of these studies have used less direct information on these factors, such as census tracts, rather than information reported by the individual women themselves. The results have been contradictory. Some studies have found no difference in breast cancer deaths between blacks and whites after adjustment for socioeconomic factors. Others have reported an excess risk for black women. Additional studies of this design have attributed differences in breast cancer death rates to other factors related to racial and ethnic biases, such as cultural attitudes leading to delays in seeking treatment.

Another approach to this question has been to compare the response of black and white women to cancer treatment in clinical trials. These studies have demonstrated that the response of black women to treatment is the same as that of white women with the same stage of breast cancer. Further support of there being no difference in black and white tumor biology is provided by examining the difference in black and white breast cancer survival over time. Only since 1982 has there been a difference in survival rates between these racial and ethnic groups; before this time the survival rates were about the same. A change, over time, in the biological behavior of the tumors of an entire racial or ethnic group is unlikely and further argues against biological differences.

What are the cancer registries?

Cancer registries play a critical role in the understanding and prevention of cancer. They are organizations that collect and organize information on the different types of cancer. This information includes patient information, tumor occurrence rate, tumor body location, severity of cancer when diagnosed, treatment received, treatment outcome, and survival time. Every state in the United States now has a

Cancer Registry. The National Cancer Institute operates an extensive cancer registry known as SEER (Surveillance, Epidemiology, and End Results Program, http://seer.cancer.gov/). This registry is composed of a number of states, cities, and counties such that it covers about one quarter of the population of the Unites States and is representative of the entire country with regard to income, education, and percentage of urban and rural areas. In addition, the SEER program includes registries to allow the collection of information on racial and ethnic minorities. Yet, at the time many of the cited studies were conducted, there were a much smaller number of registries, and the data was less representative of the country as a whole. It should also be noted that racial and ethnicity inaccuracies have been documented in the data contained within registries. These inconsistencies arise from misclassifications and are most prevalent among races and ethnicities other than white and black.

Women of different racial and ethnic backgrounds have different rates of breast cancer occurrence and survival from the disease. In general, women from lower socioeconomic groups, regardless of their race or ethnicity, have lower rates of occurrence of breast cancer but have higher death rates from breast cancer. However, there are exceptions depending on age, race and ethnicity, and place of residence. The differences in breast cancer occurrence and survival appear to be the result of cultural and environmental effects rather than genetic differences between ethnic groups. Women from different ethnic groups may be given different medical treatment for breast cancer.

—Prepared by Barbour S Warren, Ph.D.,
Cornell University Division of Nutritional Science,
and Carol Devine, Ph.D., Extension Project Leader, BCERF,
Cornell University

For More Information

Program on Breast Cancer and Environmental Risk Factors
Sprecher Institute for Comparative Cancer Research
Cornell University
Box 31
Ithaca, NY 14853
Phone: (607) 254-2893
Internet: http://envirocancer.cornell.edu
E-mail: breastcancer@cornell.edu

Chapter 14

Questions and Answers about Estimating Cancer Risk in Ashkenazi Jews

In 1995, scientists from the National Institutes of Health (NIH) discovered that a particular alteration in the breast cancer gene called BRCA1 was present in 1 percent of the general Jewish population. The researchers did a follow-up study in 1996 to estimate the cancer risk associated with this alteration as well as two other alterations subsequently reported to be present in the Ashkenazi Jewish population. This study was a cooperative effort between the Washington, D.C., Jewish community and scientists from the National Cancer Institute (NCI) and the National Human Genome Research Institute. The following questions and answers serve as background information on the follow-up study published in the May 15, 1997, issue of the *New England Journal of Medicine*.

What was the purpose of the study?

The primary purpose of the study was to estimate the risk of cancer associated with three specific alterations in the breast cancer genes BRCA1 and BRCA2. The study was conducted in the Washington, D.C., Ashkenazi Jewish population (Jews from eastern or central Europe). Two of the alterations tested were in the BRCA1 gene (185delAG and 5382insC), and one was in the BRCA2 gene (6174delT).

The researchers tested the DNA in blood provided by a finger-prick to see which of the 5,318 volunteers had an alteration. Then, using

---

Cancer Facts, National Cancer Institute, August 2000.

the family cancer histories reported by the volunteers, the scientists estimated the cancer risk by comparing the histories of cancer in the relatives of the volunteers with the alteration to the histories of cancer in the relatives of the volunteers without the alteration.

What was unique about the study?

This was the first study to test DNA from volunteers who were not selected for testing because they were part of cancer-prone families and to estimate the cancer risk associated with each alteration. (For years, researchers have studied families with breast cancer throughout several generations to help identify the altered genes passed on from one generation to the next.)

This was the first community-based study in which men and women with varying degrees of family cancer history participated. In fact, 76 percent of the volunteers had no personal or close family history of breast or ovarian cancer. About 8 percent of the women (302 of 3,742) were breast or ovarian cancer survivors.

The scientists who conducted this study had discovered in previous research that one of the alterations (185delAG) in BRCA1 was present in an unusually high proportion of anonymous stored blood samples from the general Jewish population. Even though the frequencies they found were unexpectedly high, it was impossible to estimate the cancer risk associated with the alterations because the cancer history of the blood donors was not known.

The study described here was designed both to test for the frequency of the alterations and to find out if alteration carriers from the general population were at greater risk for cancer than those without an alteration.

What is known about the BRCA1 and BRCA2 genes?

Because family history is the strongest single predictor of a woman's chance of developing breast cancer, researchers turned to cancer-prone families—those with a high incidence of cancer in several generations—to find specific inherited gene alterations that are passed on from one generation to the next. After a long search, two genes were found that are altered in many families with hereditary breast cancer. The first, BRCA1 (for BReast CAncer gene), was discovered in 1994, and the second, BRCA2, in 1995. (Alterations in other genes, including p53 and Rb, are also associated with breast cancer susceptibility. Scientists continue to search for additional genes involved in the development of breast cancer.)

Within families with cancer in multiple generations, it had been estimated previously that a woman with an alteration in the BRCA1 gene have about an 85 percent chance of developing breast cancer and a 44 percent chance of developing ovarian cancer by age seventy. Prior research in these high-risk families had reported that women with BRCA2 alterations have a lower risk of developing both breast and ovarian cancer than women with BRCA1 alterations. Previous studies had reported an increased risk of prostate cancer among alteration carriers in these same families.

Most alterations result in a shortened protein product that scientists believe prevents the protein from carrying out its normal function in the cell. The precise biological roles of BRCA1 and BRCA2 are not known.

Once the genes were isolated, it was possible to analyze the specific alterations inherited in each cancer-prone family. Today several hundred different alterations scattered throughout BRCA1 have been identified. In general, most families have a unique alteration. A similar pattern is emerging for BRCA2 alterations seen in cancer-prone families: a large number of distinct, family-specific alterations are scattered throughout the gene.

The initial impetus for this study was the observation in late 1994 that three high-risk Ashkenazi families studied at the NIH carried an identical alteration in BRCA1 (185delAG). These families were not known to be related. This observation led to the study that found that 1 percent of the Jewish population has this alteration. This was the first alteration associated with a particular ethnic group. A few other alterations that occur frequently in other ethnic groups (Icelandic, Norwegian, and Dutch) have been found since then.

Why were these particular alterations chosen to be tested?

Of the more than one hundred alterations identified in each gene (BRCA1 and BRCA2) in families with hereditary breast cancer, a few are found in subgroups of the general population. In particular, three alterations were initially identified in Ashkenazi families with hereditary breast cancer and later were found in an unusually high percentage of the general Jewish population. The estimated frequencies of the three alterations in the general Ashkenazi population, derived from previous studies, are listed in Table 14.1. In comparison, the percentage of people in the general U.S. population that have any mutation in BRCA1 has been estimated to be between 0.1 percent and 0.6 percent.

Table 14.1. Frequency of Gene Alterations in Ashkenazi Jews

Gene	Alteration	Frequency in Ashkenazi Jews
BRCA1	185delAG	1.0 percent
	5382insC	0.1 percent
BRCA2	6174delT	1.4 percent

Source: *Nature Genetics* 11(1995): 198–200; and *Nature Genetics* 14 (1996): 185–87, 188–90.

What were the findings of the 1996 study in Washington?

This study:

- Supported previous studies testing the frequency of three BRCA1 and BRCA2 alterations in the general Jewish population: The frequencies reported in this study are consistent with those previously reported for the general Jewish population. The DNA analysis in this study showed that 120 of the 5,318 volunteers had one of the three alterations, or about 1 person in 44 (2.3 percent). No individual carried more than one of the three alterations. By comparison, the frequency of all BRCA1 and BRCA2 alterations combined in the non-Jewish population is less than 1 percent.

- Estimated the average risk of breast and ovarian cancer associated with three BRCA1 and BRCA2 alterations in the general Ashkenazi population: The researchers found that women carrying one of the three alterations have, on average, a 56 percent chance (a range of 40 percent to 73 percent) of getting breast cancer by the age of seventy (compared with a 13 percent chance without the alterations) and a 16 percent chance (a range of 6 percent to 28 percent) of getting ovarian cancer by age seventy (compared with a 1.6 percent chance for noncarriers). In other words, the researchers estimate that by the age of seventy, slightly more than half of all women with an alteration will develop breast cancer, and about one out of every six carriers will develop ovarian cancer. The researchers noted that the cancer risks in this study are likely to be overestimates because people with personal or family histories of breast cancer may have been more likely than others to volunteer for the study. They estimated, for example, that the true breast cancer risk for U.S. Ashkenazi women with an alteration may be 50 percent or lower.

- Found breast and ovarian cancer risks well below previous estimates: Before this study, small studies of families with cancer in several generations had estimated that women with an alteration had a 76 percent to 87 percent chance of developing breast cancer; for ovarian cancer, the estimated risk ranged from 11 percent to 84 percent.

- Further explored the link between prostate cancer and the alterations: Previous studies had suggested a link between BRCA1 and prostate cancer. This study found an association with and showed a significant excess of prostate cancer among men with the alterations. Based on these findings, the researchers estimated that men carrying one of the three alterations have, on average, a 16 percent chance of getting prostate cancer (compared with a 3.8 percent chance for noncarriers) by the age of seventy. In other words, by age seventy the researchers estimate that about one out of every six men carrying an alteration will develop prostate cancer. However, the results of subsequent studies have been conflicting. Some studies have shown an association between BRCA1 or BRCA2 alterations and prostate cancer, while others have not.

- Found the average risks for breast, ovarian, and prostate cancers: The study estimated the average risk of cancer for alteration carriers as a group. The cancer risk for an individual man or woman who carries one of the alterations may be higher or lower than the average.

- Found no link with colon cancer: A previous report showed a link between BRCA1 alterations and colon cancer that was not confirmed in this study.

- Found that each alteration carries a similar breast cancer risk: Previous reports suggested that the risk of getting breast cancer was different for two of the alterations studied. Specifically, in studies involving Jewish early-onset breast cancer patients, data suggested that the risk associated with the 6174delT mutation (in BRCA2) was considerably lower than the risk associated with 185delAG. In this study, the risk associated with the 6174delT was slightly lower, but the risks for the three alterations were not significantly different from each other.

- Found that the three alterations account for only a small proportion of breast cancer cases in Jewish women: Of the women in this study who were breast or ovarian cancer survivors, only 9 percent had one of the alterations. In fact, only about 7 percent of breast cancer in Jewish women is due to the three alterations in BRCA1 and BRCA2.

How is inherited breast cancer different from other genetic diseases?

For many genetic diseases, such as Huntington's disease, everyone who inherits an alteration in the gene will develop the disease. This is called "complete penetrance." All cases of Huntington's disease are caused by alterations in the Huntington's disease gene. The situation with breast cancer appears to be quite different.

Breast cancer is a common disease, but only a small fraction of cases are due to the inheritance of an alteration in a single gene. In order to isolate cancer-predisposing genes such as BRCA1 and BRCA2, scientists initially studied families with many members affected by breast and ovarian cancer over several generations. Estimates of the risk of breast cancer within these families were often over 80 percent by age seventy, and 90 percent to 100 percent over a lifetime. These estimates are similar to those for other genetic diseases like Huntington's disease, with nearly complete penetrance, but whether they applied to all carriers of BRCA1 and BRCA2 alterations was unknown.

Evidence from this study suggests that they do not apply to all carriers, and that, on average, the risk of breast cancer among carriers is closer to 50 percent. This is called "incomplete penetrance" and suggests that about half of the carriers will not develop breast cancer even if they live to age seventy. Other factors, both genetic and nongenetic, are likely to affect whether someone with an alteration will develop cancer or not.

What are the chances that someone with one of these alterations in BRCA1 or BRCA2 will get breast, ovarian, or prostate cancer?

On average, by the age of seventy, women with one of the alterations tested for in this study have between a 40-percent and a 73-percent chance of being diagnosed with breast cancer and between an 8-percent and a 28-percent chance of developing ovarian cancer. Men with an alteration have about a 16-percent chance of developing prostate cancer by the age of seventy. However, for any individual with an alteration, a precise estimate of risk is not possible.

Family history helps to place an individual's cancer risk in perspective, but is also an imperfect tool. For example, family history will be most useful in determining risk if a carrier has multiple relatives affected with breast or ovarian cancer. In this case, a woman's risk of breast cancer may be higher than the average of 56 percent.

If a carrier has little or no family history of breast and ovarian cancer, his or her risk will be much more difficult to assess. This is particularly true of women in small families with very few close female relatives.

Unless someone already has a strong family history of breast or ovarian cancer, it will be very difficult to know his or her precise risk until other risk factors for cancer are identified.

What are the implications of this study for non-Jewish populations?

This is the first community-based study to estimate the cancer risk associated with alterations in BRCA1 and BRCA2 in the general population. The researchers found that the risks for breast and ovarian cancer were lower on average in this population than in hereditary breast cancer families. Even though there are no data for other ethnic groups, researchers speculate that future findings may be similar; that is, it is likely that most alterations in BRCA1 or BRCA2 that produce a shortened protein product will increase the cancer risk in the general population, but the average risk will probably not be as high as in cancer-prone families.

Do the results have implications for Jews considering whether to be tested for these alterations?

Deciding whether to be tested for a gene alteration is complex and personal. One of the factors to be considered is the cancer risk associated with having a positive or negative test result.

Based on this study, the average risk of breast, ovarian, and prostate cancer for people with BRCA1 and BRCA2 alterations is known more accurately. For example, the average risk of breast cancer is lower than previously thought, but is still significantly higher than for those who don't carry the alteration.

But gene alterations linked to cancer do not have the same effect on each person who carries them. For example, the findings from this study suggest that nearly half of the women with these alterations will not develop cancer, and since BRCA1 and BRCA2 alterations account for only a small portion of breast cancer, many women without an alteration will develop breast cancer.

Part of the complexity of the decision to be tested is that the medical consequences of an individual's test result—positive or negative— are not predictable. This is especially true of a carrier who does not have a personal or family history of cancer.

Besides the cancer risks, other considerations are important. There may be psychological and social effects of both positive and negative results for the individual tested and family members. Individuals should also consider how a positive or negative result might affect them and their relatives, especially if they have a strong history of cancer in the family.

In addition, privacy issues are important, since it is possible that having a positive or negative result may affect health insurance and employment.

Until recently, genetic testing for alterations that increase susceptibility to cancer was performed only in a research setting. However, this kind of testing is now commercially available. Still, there is no consensus about the circumstances in which genetic testing might be useful, and genetic testing is certainly not routine.

Scientists and physicians are still uncertain about how best to help alteration carriers. Even if the precise risk of cancer for an individual carrier were known, there are no proven effective risk reduction strategies. Physicians are not sure about the best ways to monitor those at high risk to assure early detection if they do develop cancer. More research is needed.

Do the results of this study have implications for the prevention or treatment of breast, ovarian, or prostate cancer?

The hope is that these gene alterations as well as any others discovered in future studies will provide novel targets for the development of anti-cancer drugs. The interaction between gene alterations and environmental factors may also present new strategies for cancer prevention.

Where can someone go to get more information about genetic testing?

Information about genetics and genetic testing may be found on NCI's CancerNet™ Web site at http://cancer.gov/cancer_information

on the internet. Several publications and other documents are available on this website, including the position papers of professional and advocacy organizations on the issue of genetic testing for susceptibility to cancer.

This website also includes a searchable directory of genetic counselors, physicians, geneticists, and nurses who have expertise in genetic testing and who will accept physicians' referrals for familial cancer risk counseling or genetic susceptibility testing. The search form for the directory is available at http://cancer.gov/search/geneticsservices on the internet. Because the issues surrounding genetic testing are highly personal and can have far-reaching consequences, a health professional trained in genetics is a good resource for exploring these issues.

Another resource is NCI's Cancer Information Service (CIS) at 1-800-4-CANCER (1-800-422-6237). The staff can send a booklet called Understanding Gene Testing and other printed information, and can answer questions about cancer and cancer genetics. The CIS can also identify facilities offering cancer risk assessment, counseling related to familial cancer and genetic susceptibility to cancer, and centers conducting research.

Chapter 15

Breast Cancer and Pregnancy

General Information about Breast Cancer and Pregnancy

Breast cancer is a disease in which malignant (cancer) cells form in the tissues of the breast. The breast is made up of lobes and ducts. Each breast has fifteen to twenty sections called lobes, which have many smaller sections called lobules. The lobes and lobules are connected by thin tubes called ducts.

Each breast also contains blood vessels and lymph vessels. The lymph vessels carry an almost colorless fluid called lymph. The lymph vessels lead to small, bean-shaped organs called lymph nodes that help the body fight infection and disease. Lymph nodes are found throughout the body. Clusters of lymph nodes are found near the breast in the axilla (under the arm), above the collarbone, and in the chest.

Breast cancer is sometimes detected in women who are pregnant or have just given birth. In women who are pregnant or who have just given birth, breast cancer occurs most often between the ages of thirty-two and thirty-eight. Breast cancer occurs about once in every three thousand pregnancies.

Diagnosing Breast Cancer in Pregnant Women

Women who are pregnant, nursing, or have just given birth usually have tender, swollen breasts. This can make small lumps difficult to

PDQ® Cancer Information Summary. National Cancer Institute, Bethesda, MD. Breast Cancer and Pregnancy (PDQ®): Treatment - Patient. Updated December 2003. Available at http://cancer.gov. Accessed December 2003.

detect and may lead to delays in diagnosing breast cancer. Because of these delays, cancers are often found at a later stage in these women.

Breast examination should be part of prenatal and postnatal care. To detect breast cancer, pregnant and nursing women should examine their breasts themselves. Women should also receive clinical breast examinations during their routine prenatal and postnatal examinations.

Tests that examine the breasts are used to find and diagnose breast cancer. If an abnormality is found, one or all of the following tests may be used:

- Ultrasound: A procedure in which high-energy sound waves (ultrasound) are bounced off internal tissues or organs and make echoes. The echoes form a picture of body tissues called a sonogram.

- Mammogram: An x-ray of the breast. A mammogram can be performed with little risk to the fetus. Mammograms in pregnant women may appear negative even though cancer is present.

- Biopsy: A procedure in which cells or tissues are removed so that they can be viewed under a microscope to check for signs of cancer.

Certain factors affect treatment options and prognosis (chance of recovery). The treatment options and prognosis depend on the stage of the cancer (whether it is in the breast only or has spread to other places in the body), the tumor size, the type of breast cancer, the age of the fetus, whether there are symptoms, and the patient's general health.

Survival rates of pregnant women with breast cancer may be lower than for women who are not pregnant. Pregnant women with breast cancer may be less likely to survive because the diagnosis of their cancer is often delayed and the cancers are more advanced when they are found. Cancers found at later stages are more difficult to treat successfully.

Stages of Breast Cancer

After breast cancer has been diagnosed, tests are done to find out if cancer cells have spread within the breast or to other parts of the body. The process used to find out if the cancer has spread within the breast or to other parts of the body is called staging. The information gathered from the staging process determines the stage of the disease. It is important to know the stage in order to plan the best treatment.

Methods used to stage breast cancer can be changed to make them safer for the fetus. Standard methods for giving imaging scans can be adjusted so that the fetus is exposed to less radiation. Tests to measure the level of hormones in the blood may also be used in the staging process.

Treatment Option Overview

Different types of treatment are available for patients with breast cancer. Some treatments are standard, and some are being tested in clinical trials. Before starting treatment, patients may want to think about taking part in a clinical trial. A treatment clinical trial is a research study meant to help improve current treatments or obtain information on new treatments for patients with cancer. When clinical trials show that a new treatment is better than the "standard" treatment, the new treatment may become the standard treatment.

Clinical trials are taking place in many parts of the country. Information about ongoing clinical trials is available from the NCI Cancer .gov website. Choosing the most appropriate cancer treatment is a decision that ideally involves the patient, family, and health care team.

Treatment options for pregnant women depend on the stage of the disease and the age of the fetus. Three types of standard treatment are used:

Surgery

Most pregnant women with breast cancer have surgery to remove the breast. Some of the lymph nodes under the arm are usually taken out and looked at under a microscope to see if they contain cancer cells.
Types of surgery to remove the breast include:

- Simple mastectomy: A surgical procedure to remove the whole breast that contains cancer. Some of the lymph nodes under the arm may also be removed for biopsy. This procedure is also called a total mastectomy.

- Modified radical mastectomy: A surgical procedure to remove the whole breast that has cancer, many of the lymph nodes under the arm, the lining over the chest muscles, and sometimes part of the chest wall muscles.

Breast-conserving surgery, an operation to remove the cancer but not the breast itself, includes the following:

- Lumpectomy: A surgical procedure to remove a tumor and a small amount of normal tissue around it. Most doctors also take out some of the lymph nodes under the arm.

- Partial mastectomy: A surgical procedure to remove the part of the breast that contains cancer and some normal tissue around it. Some of the lymph nodes under the arm may also be removed for biopsy. This procedure is also called a segmental mastectomy.

Even if the doctor removes all of the cancer that can be seen at the time of surgery, the patient may be given radiation therapy, chemotherapy, or hormone therapy after surgery to try to kill any cancer cells that may be left. Treatment given after surgery to increase the chances of a cure is called adjuvant therapy.

Radiation Therapy

Radiation therapy is a cancer treatment that uses high-energy x-rays or other types of radiation to kill cancer cells. There are two types of radiation therapy. External radiation therapy uses a machine outside the body to send radiation toward the cancer. Internal radiation therapy uses a radioactive substance sealed in needles, seeds, wires, or catheters that are placed directly into or near the cancer. The way the radiation therapy is given depends on the type and stage of the cancer being treated.

Radiation therapy should not be given to pregnant women with early stage (stage I or II) breast cancer because it can harm the fetus. For women with late stage (stage III or IV) breast cancer, it should not be given during the first three months of pregnancy.

Chemotherapy

Chemotherapy is a cancer treatment that uses drugs to stop the growth of cancer cells, either by killing the cells or by stopping the cells from dividing. When chemotherapy is taken by mouth or injected into a vein or muscle, the drugs enter the bloodstream and can reach cancer cells throughout the body (systemic chemotherapy). When chemotherapy is placed directly in the spinal column, a body cavity such as the abdomen, or an organ, the drugs mainly affect cancer cells in those areas. The way the chemotherapy is given depends on the type and stage of the cancer being treated.

Chemotherapy should not be given during the first three months of pregnancy. Chemotherapy given after this time does not usually harm the fetus but may cause early labor and low birth weight.

Hormone Therapy

Hormone therapy is not yet accepted as a standard cancer treatment, but is being tested in clinical trials. Hormone therapy is a cancer treatment that removes hormones or blocks their action and stops cancer cells from growing. Hormones are substances produced by glands in the body and circulated in the bloodstream. The presence of some hormones can cause certain cancers to grow. If tests show that the cancer cells have places where hormones can attach (receptors), drugs, surgery, or radiation therapy are used to reduce the production of hormones or block them from working.

The effectiveness of hormone therapy, alone or combined with chemotherapy, in treating breast cancer in pregnant women is not yet known.

Termination of Pregnancy

Ending the pregnancy does not seem to improve the mother's chance of survival and is not usually a treatment option. If the cancer must be treated with chemotherapy and radiation therapy, which may harm the fetus, termination of the pregnancy is sometimes considered. This decision may depend on the stage of cancer, the age of the fetus, and the mother's chance of survival.

Treatment Options by Stage

Early Stage Breast Cancer (Stage I and Stage II)

Treatment of early stage breast cancer (stage I and stage II) may be surgery followed by adjuvant therapy as follows:

- Modified radical mastectomy.

- Breast-conserving surgery: Lumpectomy, partial mastectomy, or segmental mastectomy.

- Breast-conserving surgery during pregnancy followed by radiation therapy after the baby is born.

- Surgery during pregnancy followed by chemotherapy after the first three months of pregnancy.

- Clinical trials of surgery followed by hormone therapy with or without chemotherapy.

Late Stage Breast Cancer (Stage III and Stage IV)

Treatment of late stage breast cancer (stage III and stage IV) may include the following:

- Radiation therapy

- Chemotherapy

Radiation therapy and chemotherapy should not be given during the first three months of pregnancy.

Other Considerations about Pregnancy and Breast Cancer

Breast-Feeding Concerns

Lactation (breast milk production) and breast-feeding should be stopped if surgery or chemotherapy is planned. If surgery is planned, breast-feeding should be stopped to reduce blood flow in the breasts and make them smaller. Breast-feeding should also be stopped if chemotherapy is planned. Many anticancer drugs, especially cyclophosphamide and methotrexate, may occur in high levels in breast milk and may harm the nursing baby. Women receiving chemotherapy should not breast-feed. Stopping lactation does not improve survival of the mother.

Breast Cancer and the Fetus

Breast cancer does not appear to harm the fetus. Breast cancer cells do not seem to pass from the mother to the fetus.

Pregnancy in Breast Cancer Survivors

Pregnancy does not seem to affect the survival of women who have had breast cancer in the past. Some doctors recommend that a woman wait two years after treatment for breast cancer before trying to have a baby, so that any early return of the cancer would be detected. This may affect a woman's decision to become pregnant. The fetus does not seem to be affected if the mother has previously had breast cancer.

Effects of certain cancer treatments on later pregnancies are not known. The effects of treatment with high-dose chemotherapy and a bone marrow transplant, with or without radiation therapy, on later pregnancies have not been determined.

Chapter 16

Diagnosis and Treatment of Breast Cancer in the Elderly

Introduction

Breast cancer remains the most common cancer in American women, with an estimated 211,300 new diagnoses in 2003.[1] Aging remains one of the single greatest risk factors for the development of new breast cancer, with the estimated risk of new breast cancer at 1 in 14 for women aged sixty to seventy-nine compared with 1 in 24 women aged forty to fifty-nine and 1 in 228 women aged thirty-nine and younger.[1] As a result, an estimated 35 percent of women are over the age of seventy at the time of invasive breast cancer diagnosis.[2] Almost 50 percent of women will be aged sixty-five or older at diagnosis.[3] In addition, incidence rates continue to rise for women over the age of fifty, a trend not seen in the cohort under fifty years of age.[4] Currently, the median age of breast cancer diagnosis in the United States is 62.4.

Concurrent with the increased risk of breast cancer throughout a woman's life are data outlining an increase in America's aged population. Although persons aged sixty-five and older represented 11.3 percent of the total population in 1980, this number is anticipated to rise to 20 percent by 2030.[3] In addition, age shifts within the sixty-five and older population have resulted in a greater number of persons over seventy-five years of age; by 2030, this age group is estimated to

Excerpted from "Diagnosis and Treatment of Breast Cancer in the Elderly," by Chris E. Holmes, M.D., Ph.D., and Hyman B. Muss, M.D., *CA Cancer J Clin* 53 (2003): 227–44. © 2003 Lippincott Williams and Wilkins. Reprinted with permission.

account for just under 50 percent of the total cohort over the age of sixty-five. In total, these staggering figures suggest that women over the age of sixty-five will become the most prevalent patient cohort in the breast cancer population.

A central concept in decision making in the elderly patient with breast cancer is that of life expectancy. Accurate predictions and knowledge of life expectancy are inherently important in decisions regarding screening older populations using mammography, treatment of the primary lesion, and use of systemic adjuvant therapy. Treatment options now available to the patient with breast cancer often carry short-term risks and toxicities in older women that are tempered by long-term survival gains. The estimated life expectancy for a sixty-five-year-old woman in the United States is estimated at 17.5 years. Although fifteen years older, an eighty-year-old woman is anticipated on average to live an additional 8.6 years.[5] An appreciation of this nonlinear relationship between age and life expectancy is crucial in clinical decision making, as the impact of natural disease history and risk/benefit analysis of therapeutic interventions must be made within this context.

The five-year relative (disease-specific) survival for women diagnosed with breast cancer increases with age until the age of seventy-five. Currently, the projected five-year relative survival for women younger than forty-five years of age is 83 percent, whereas women aged sixty-five to seventy-four have an expected five-year relative survival of 89 percent. Five-year relative survival rates also vary based on stage at diagnosis, with overall estimates of 96.8 percent five-year relative survival with localized disease and 78.4 percent with regional disease.[4] Disappointingly, the five-year relative survival estimate of 22.5 percent for metastatic disease has not changed appreciably over the last two decades.[4,6] Not unexpectedly, the probability of death due to causes other than breast cancer increases with increasing age.[7]

Cancer Detection and Stage at Presentation

The majority of new patients with breast cancer present with Stage I or II disease: an observation that holds true for both young and old patients.[8] In contrast, the most elderly cohort (age eighty-five) are more likely to present with metastatic disease (approximately 9 percent) or an unknown stage at the time of study analysis.[8] Based on recent data from the National Cancer Institute's Surveillance, Epidemiology and End Results Program, approximately 48 percent of women with metastatic breast cancer at presentation will be sixty-five or older.[4]

Helpful in individualized decision making are estimates for risk of women dying of breast cancer in their remaining lifetimes at a particular age. A healthy seventy-year-old has a greater chance of dying from breast cancer than the average fifty-year-old (3.3 percent versus 3.1 percent, respectively).[5] In contrast, competing comorbidities at any age over seventy result in a substantially decreased risk of breast cancer death. On a population basis, the number of patients one needs to screen with mammography to prevent one breast cancer–related death is estimated at 242 for the average seventy-year-old woman and 533 for the average eighty-year-old.

Elders and Clinical Trial Participation

As the U.S. population continues to age, the need for increased enrollment in clinical trials of elderly women with breast cancer is imperative. The discrepancy between trial eligibility and trial enrollment in patients over the age of sixty-five is substantial, with one study reporting only 35 percent of women over the age of sixty-five years offered participation, compared with 51 percent of women fewer than sixty-five years of age.[9,10] Coexisting concerns in the literature concerning the care of the elderly patient with breast cancer are an imperative to "first do no harm" and to avoid unfavorable and age-biased recommendations and treatment practices without sufficient data. This observation underscores the need to pursue rigorous clinical trials in order for the physician community to appropriately guide patients with regard to therapeutic options that contain both significant risks and benefits.

Conclusions

Pivotal concepts that guide clinical decision making and choice of treatment options in the elderly patient with breast cancer include (1) the average life expectancy of the patient at a given age, (2) comorbidities and their impact on diagnostic and therapeutic options as well as life expectancy, and (3) potential treatment benefits (including survival versus quality of life benefits) versus risks of a proposed treatment strategy. An understanding of the physiologic, physical, and psychological barriers to breast cancer diagnosis and treatment—as well as the recognition of the delicate interplay between patients' and physicians' expectations—remains pivotal in providing appropriate breast cancer care to the older patient. Despite the magnitude of the problem of breast cancer in the elderly, many issues surrounding diagnosis and treatment of the elder patient with breast cancer are complicated by inadequate representation of this group in clinical trials. As we await additional evidence to support clinical practice, physicians should encourage participation of elderly patients with breast cancer in clinical trials and emphasize shared decision making in breast cancer care.

References

1. A. Jemal, T. Murray, and A. Samuels, et al., "Cancer statistics, 2003," *CA Cancer J Clin* 53(2003): 5–26.

2. American Cancer Society, *Breast Cancer Facts & Figures 2001* (Atlanta, Ga.: American Cancer Society, 2001).

3. R. Yancik, "Cancer Burden in the Aged: An Epidemiologic and Demographic Overview," *Cancer* 80 (1997): 1273–83.

4. L. A. G. Ries, M. P. Eisner, and C. L. Kosary, *SEER Cancer Statistics Review, 1973–1999,* National Cancer Institute, Bethesda, Md. Available at: http://seer.cancer.gov/csr/ 1973_1999. Accessed August 25, 2002.

5. L. C. Walter, and K. E. Covinsky, "Cancer Screening in Elderly Patients: A Framework for Individualized Decision Making," *JAMA* 285 (2001): 2750–56.

6. R. Yancik, L. G. Ries, and J.W. Yates, "Breast Cancer in Aging Women: A Population-Based Study of Contrasts in Stage, Surgery, and Survival," *Cancer* 63 (1989): 976–81.

7. G. Swan, and C. Lin, "Survival Patterns among Younger Women with Breast Cancer: The Effects of Age, Race, Stage, and Treatment," *J Natl Cancer Inst Monogr* 16 (1994): 69–77.

8. R. Yancik, M. N. Wesley, and L.A. Ries, et al., "Effect of Age and Comorbidity in Postmenopausal Breast Cancer Patients Aged 55 Years and Older," *JAMA* 285 (2001): 885–92.

9. M. Kemeny, H. B. Muss, and A.B. Kornblith, et al., "Barriers to Participation of Older Women with Breast Cancer in Clinical Trials," *Proc Am Soc Clin Oncol* 19 (2000): 602a.

10. L. F. Hutchins, J. M. Unger, and J. J. Crowley, et al., "Underrepresentation of Patients 65 Years of Age or Older in Cancer Treatment Trials," *N Engl J Med* 341 (1999): 2061–67.

Chapter 17

Male Breast Cancer

What Is Male Breast Cancer?

All of the organs in the body are made up of cells. Cells normally divide in an orderly manner to replace old cells that have aged and died. Sometimes a cell's DNA becomes damaged, causing those normal controls to malfunction. These cells can then go on to divide uncontrollably, forming abnormal cells. These cells can grow into lumps, or tumors. The word "tumor" comes from the Latin word meaning "swelling." The tumor may be benign (not cancer) or malignant (cancer).

Breast cancer is a malignant tumor that has developed from cells of the breast. Like all cells of the body, the breast ducts in the male breast can undergo cancerous changes. Since women have many more breast cells than men and because women's breast cells are continually exposed to female hormones that promote growth, breast cancer is seen much more often in women than men. In fact, breast cancer is one hundred times more common among women.

A benign tumor won't spread to other parts of the body, but local tissue may be damaged and the growth may need to be removed.

This chapter begins with text reprinted with permission from "Male Breast Cancer" by Parma Rishel, MSN, RN, EnSURE, Inc., Department of Defense Health Services Region IV Breast Health Program, 2004. Additional information is available at http://psaweb.pcola.med.navy.mil/breasthealth. Text and graphics on self breast-examination and mammograms are reprinted with permission from the John W. Nick Foundation, an organization dedicated to educating the public about men's risk of breast cancer, http://www.johnwnick foundation.org. © 2003 John W. Nick Foundation, Inc. All rights reserved.

Malignant tumors can invade, damage, and destroy nearby tissues and spread to other parts of the body. When the cancer spreads, it is called a metastases.

Types of Breast Cancer

Noninvasive Breast Cancer: Breast cancers get their names from the part of the breast where they develop. Many breast cancers are being found in the very early stages. These breast cancers are called in situ or noninvasive cancer. In situ cancers are still inside the walls of the breast area where they developed. These very early cell changes may change over time and become invasive breast cancer.

The in situ (noninvasive) stage is not considered to be actual breast cancer, but it is a warning sign of increased risk of developing invasive cancer. For example, patients with lobular carcinoma in situ have a 25 percent chance of developing breast cancer in either breast during the next twenty-five years.

If the cancer grows through the cell walls it is called an infiltrating or invasive cancer.

All of the types of breast cancer seen in women can occur in men, but some are very rare. Many cancers are found in the lining of the milk ducts in the breast. These cancers are called ductal carcinomas (cancers) or intraductal carcinomas.

Ductal carcinoma in situ (DCIS) is an early-stage cancer. It is noninvasive, which means it has not spread out of the milk ducts to other parts of the breast, the lymph nodes under the arm, or other parts of the body. Several types of DCIS exist. Only about 5 percent of men's breast cancers are found at this early stage. Sometimes, DCIS causes a man to have a breast discharge where fluid leaks from the nipple. Comedocarcinoma is a type of DCIS in which some of the cancer cells in the duct begin to die and break down (degenerate).

These tumors need to be removed because some may change into invasive cancers. It is important to note that some of these DCIS may never progress and that there is controversy among healthcare providers about what is the best treatment. The good news is that DCIS is highly curable when treated.

Invasive Breast Cancer: In more advanced stages, breast cancer cells cross the lining of the milk duct or lobule and begin to invade, or infiltrate, the surrounding tissues. In this stage, the cancer is called "infiltrating cancer."

Invasive ductal carcinoma (also known as infiltrating ductal carcinoma) is the most common kind of invasive breast cancer in men, accounting for 80 to 90 percent of male breast cancers. This type of cancer breaks through the wall of the duct and invades (goes into) the fatty tissue of the breast. At this point, there is a significant risk that the cancer will metastasize, or spread to other parts of the body.

When the cancer begins in the lining of the milk lobule, it is called lobular carcinoma (cancer).

Lobular carcinoma in situ (LCIS) is a growth that stays in the milk lobules of the breast. According to the National Cancer Institute, however, it is a warning of increased cancer risk. Women with LCIS have about a 1 percent risk per year of developing invasive breast cancer in either breast. This type of breast cancer is very rare in men.

Invasive lobular carcinoma is found at the ends of the ducts or in the lobules and may cause widespread breast thickening rather than a specific lump. This accounts for only about 2 percent of male breast cancers.

Paget's Disease: Paget's disease is a type of cancer that starts in the breast ducts and then spreads to the skin of the nipple. The areola may also be involved. Paget's disease appears as an itchy, scaly, crusting, or ulcerating rash around the nipple and areola. The skin also looks red and there may be oozing, burning, or bleeding. This should not be mistaken for benign skin conditions such as eczema or contact dermatitis. About half of the patients with Paget's disease have a breast mass that can be felt, lymph nodes that can be felt, or both.

This accounts for about 1 percent of female breast cancer and a higher percentage in male breast cancers. However, this is still a rare condition for men and women. Since male breasts have less tissue than do female breasts, cancers start closer to the nipple and do not have as far to travel before they reach the skin and underlying tissues. This is why male breast cancers are more likely to spread to the nipple area.

Inflammatory Breast Cancer: Inflammatory breast cancer is a rare type of breast cancer that is very serious and aggressive. The breast may look red and feel warm. You may see ridges, welts, or hives on your breast; or the skin may look wrinkled. It is sometimes misdiagnosed as a simple infection. It is a separate class of breast cancer, but is treated as a stage III.

Recurrent Breast Cancer: Recurrent breast cancer means that the cancer has come back (recurred) after it has been treated. It may come back in the breast, in the soft tissues of the chest (the chest wall), or in another part of the body.

If the recurrence is local (breast or chest wall) and there is no evidence of distant metastases, the prognosis can be very good. Surgically removing the new tumor followed by radiation therapy is recommended whenever possible. If the area has already been treated with radiation therapy, this may not be an option. Recurrences that occur in other parts of the body are treated the same as metastases found at the time of diagnosis.

Incidence and Survival Rates for Men

It is estimated that 1,300 men will be diagnosed with breast cancer and 400 will die from breast cancer in 2003 (*Cancer Facts & Figures, 2003,* American Cancer Society). Male breast cancer accounts for about 0.2 percent of all cancers in men.

The overall survival rate of men five years after their breast cancer diagnosis is equal to that of women with breast cancer. It was once thought that men had a poorer survival rate than women, but studies have found this is not true. Unfortunately, breast cancer in men is often diagnosed at a more advanced stage. This can be due to a lack of awareness that men get breast cancer and the fact that there is less breast tissue in men, which makes it easier for the cancer to spread outside of the breast.

Breast cancer survival for both men and women is strongly dependent on the stage of breast cancer when it is diagnosed. The five-year survival rate based on stage at diagnosis is:

- Stages 0 and I (the earliest stages): 97%
- Stage II: 88%
- Stage III: 67%
- Stage IV (the most advanced stage): 24%.

Risk Factors

Most men who are diagnosed with breast cancer have no apparent risk factors. In fact, some men with one or more risk factors never develop breast cancer.

Known risk factors include:

- **Aging:** As men age, their risk of breast cancer increases. The average age for diagnosis of male breast cancer is sixty-five years.

- **Family history:** About 20 percent of men diagnosed with breast cancer have a close male or female family member with breast cancer. Some family members may have inherited genetic mutations that make them more likely to get breast cancer.

- **Klinefelter's syndrome:** Men with this congenital syndrome have lower levels of androgens (male hormones) and more estrogens (female hormones). Because of the increased levels of estrogen, these men often develop gynecomastia and have an increased risk for breast cancer. In fact, men with this condition are twenty times more likely to develop breast cancer, compared to an average man.

- **Radiation exposure:** Receiving radiation to the chest, usually for treatment of cancers in the chest such as Hodgkin's or non-Hodgkin's lymphoma, increases the risk of developing breast cancer.

- **Liver disease:** The liver plays an important role in the metabolism of the sex hormones. Men who have severe liver disease, such as cirrhosis, have lower levels of androgen (male hormone) activity and higher levels of estrogen (female hormone) activity. Once again, these increased levels of estrogen increase the risk of developing gynecomastia and breast cancer. Men in certain Middle Eastern and African countries have a much higher risk of breast cancer than men in the United States. This may be due to increased incidence of severe liver disease in these countries caused by certain parasites.

- **Estrogen treatment:** Men treated with hormonal therapy for conditions such as prostate cancer may have a slight increase in breast cancer risk. The risk is small compared with the benefits of this treatment in slowing the growth of prostate cancer. Men who are taking high doses of estrogen as part of a sex change procedure have a much higher chance of developing breast cancer.

- **Alcohol:** It is known that women who drink more than two drinks made with alcohol every day have more breast cancer diagnoses than women who do not drink that much alcohol. The impact on men is not known, but it is known to increase a man's risk of mouth, laryngeal, and esophageal cancer. (*American Cancer Society* 4/11/2000)

- **Smoking tobacco:** Smoking tobacco is not a known risk factor for breast cancer at this time. The BBC News reported in June 2001 that women are more likely to survive breast cancer if they do not smoke. Studies have found that women with breast cancer who smoke have two times the risk of the cancer spreading to the lungs. Once again, the exact effect on men is not known, but it is known to cause lung, mouth, and throat cancer in high numbers.

- **Obesity:** Obesity has been associated with a 12 percent increase in risk of breast cancer in women. This may be due to estrogen being stored in the fat cells—the more fat cells, the more estrogen storage capacity. This has not been studied in male breast cancer, but may contribute in a small way.

- **High-fat diet:** Eating a diet high in fat has been associated with a 26 percent increase in breast cancer risk in women. This has not been studied in male breast cancer, but may contribute in a small way.

Can Male Breast Cancer Be Prevented?

No. At this time we cannot truly prevent breast cancer. With the current knowledge, our best approach is to find breast cancers at the earliest stage before they spread outside of the breast.

What can you do to decrease your chances of getting breast cancer?

- There are many conflicting studies reporting the benefits of different dietary changes in decreasing the risk of developing breast cancer. Some research suggests that soy products may be of some benefit. In general, it is recommended that individuals maintain an ideal body weight and eat a balanced diet that is low in fat (25 percent of daily caloric intake) and high in fiber (25 grams per day).

- Some studies have suggested that about four hours of fairly strenuous activity per week may be beneficial in decreasing the incidence of breast cancer. (Source: Wynder, E., "What Can We Reasonably Recommend about Diet and Exercise to Our Patient?" *Primary Care & Cancer* March 1999, supp. 2: 11–13.)

- Do not smoke tobacco and limit the amount of alcohol you drink or stop drinking alcohol.

Awareness is probably the most important tool we have at this time to improve the outcome of a breast cancer diagnosis. By knowing the signs and symptoms of breast cancer and watching for changes in the breast we will increase the chances of finding a breast cancer early if one develops.

Signs and Symptoms of Male Breast Cancer

Signs and symptoms of breast cancer in men may include a number of changes in the breast. Men should immediately talk to their healthcare provider if they develop a lump or swelling in the breast, skin dimpling or puckering, nipple retraction (turning in), redness or scaling of the nipple or skin on the breast, pulling sensation, or a discharge (fluid) from the nipple. Breast lumps may or may not be painful.

Since most male breast cancers start under the nipple area and quickly grow into the nipple, men are more likely than women to have a nipple discharge as well as the other nipple changes described here. Many men also have axillary lymph nodes that are enlarged and can be felt when the cancer is diagnosed. This is often a sign that the cancer has spread (metastasized) out of the breast.

It is important to note that most breast lumps that are found in men are the result of gynecomastia and not breast cancer.

Early Detection

It cannot be emphasized enough that finding breast cancer at a very early stage is the key to decreasing suffering and death. While there are many ways in which breasts are the same in men and women, there are some key differences that affect early detection. The first and most obvious difference is size. Although the small amount of breast tissue in men makes it easier to feel small lumps, cancers do not need to grow far to reach the skin, nipple, and muscle underneath. Typically, the lumps start underneath the areola, where the breast tissue is the most concentrated. This is the reason that many male breast cancers quickly grow into the nipple area.

A second key difference is that female breast cancer is highly publicized and women are told from many different sources that they should do monthly breast self-examinations, get regular clinical breast examinations from their health care provider, and get regular mammograms. Because of the small numbers of male breast cancers, these recommendations are not made for men in general. Therefore, most men do not even realize that they can get breast cancer and are not concerned if they notice a lump or nipple discharge. Many men mistakenly think it is an infection or some other problem. Some men may feel embarrassed about finding a lump, since breast cancer is a "woman's disease." They may feel that this threatens their masculinity.

All of these factors can contribute to a delay in diagnosis that can be life-threatening.

Detecting Breast Cancer

The first step in evaluating (checking) a change in the breast is to take a history. The healthcare provider will ask questions about how you found the change and how long you have noticed it, and will ask you to describe the change. When describing a breast lump, it is important to know if the lump is soft or hard, painful or not, and whether it is "stuck" to the chest or if you can move it around.

The next step is to examine the breast. The healthcare provider will then discuss further testing that is needed. Tests may include a mammogram, ultrasound, or other radiologic procedure to look for abnormalities. Mammography is a test that is used as a screening tool in women to detect very early changes in the breast. Mammography, often using cone views with magnification, can also be done on men to evaluate an abnormality. This procedure uses special x-ray equipment that produces an image or film of the breast tissue. In order to get a good picture of the breast tissue, the breast is compressed between two "plates" on the special x-ray machine. This squeezing may cause temporary discomfort, but this lasts only about one minute.

If there is nipple discharge, the healthcare provider may collect some of the fluid to be looked at under the microscope for the presence of cancer cells. If there are no cancer cells seen, but the healthcare provider is concerned about a mass in the breast, a biopsy will be needed. The only way to tell if an abnormality is cancer is to do a biopsy.

Staging Breast Cancer

The process of staging breast cancers is the same for men and women. This process helps to determine how widespread the cancer is and provides important information about the best treatment plan.

Treatment of Breast Cancer

There are a number of treatment protocols that may be considered by your physician based on the stage and type of cancer you have.

Treatment options may include surgery, chemotherapy, radiation, or hormonal therapy.

Breast Conservation: Lumpectomy is an option that is often a good choice for women. However, this option is rarely used in men since there is such a small amount of breast tissue to start with and because male breast cancer frequently involves the skin and nipple area. With lumpectomy, only the lump and a small amount of tissue around the lump (called the margin) are removed. Patients who have a lumpectomy performed almost always have several weeks of radiation therapy after the surgery in an effort to kill any tiny cancer cells that may have been left behind. The lymph nodes may or may not be removed with this procedure.

Mastectomy: This is used in approximately 80 percent of surgeries performed for male breast cancer. There are a number of different types of mastectomies:

- A total (simple) mastectomy removes the entire breast, but does not remove the lymph nodes under the arm or the muscle from the chest wall.
- A modified radical mastectomy removes the entire breast and the axillary lymph nodes.
- A radical mastectomy removes the entire breast, the axillary lymph nodes, and the chest wall muscles under the breast.

Possible side effects of surgery:

- Skin in the breast area may be tight and the muscles of the arm and shoulder may feel stiff.
- Some men have some permanent loss of strength after mastectomy—for most men this is temporary.
- Nerves may be injured or cut during surgery resulting in numbness and tingling—these feelings usually go away in a few weeks or months, but can be permanent.
- Removal of lymph nodes under the arm may cause swelling from lymph buildup. This is called lymphedema.

In an effort to decrease the problems that can occur when all of the axillary lymph nodes are removed, techniques have been developed to decrease the number of lymph nodes removed. This procedure is called sentinel lymph node dissection.

Chemotherapy: There is a concern with all cancers that cancer cells may break away from the tumor and begin to spread through the bloodstream to other parts of the body. Systemic therapy reaches all parts of the body through the bloodstream. Chemotherapy is one type of systemic therapy. The goal of chemotherapy is to kill tiny hidden cancer cells.

Hormone Therapy: This is another form of systemic therapy. In women, growth of breast cancers, especially those with detectable amounts of estrogen receptor protein, is promoted by the hormone estrogen (female hormone). There are several treatment options that are aimed at blocking the effect of estrogen or lowering estrogen levels. Estrogen is the main target of hormonal therapy, and estrogen is present in both men and women. It has been found that 70 percent of male breast cancers contain progesterone receptors. Furthermore, 80 percent of male breast cancers contain estrogen receptors, and anti-estrogens are known to be effective in shrinking most of these tumors. The antiestrogen drug used most often in hormonal therapy of male and female breast cancer is tamoxifen (Nolvadex). This medication is taken as a pill every day. Other hormone therapies include LHRH analogs and anti-androgens.

Radiation Therapy: This is considered local treatment. This treatment uses high-energy rays or particles to destroy cancer cells. Sometimes this is used to shrink the size of a tumor before surgery.

Many times a combination of the above treatment options is used to gain the best control of the disease.

Clinical Trials

Another option that may be available to you is participation in a clinical trial. In cancer research, clinical trials usually evaluate new types of cancer treatment. Patients who take part in clinical trials receive the newest, most state-of-the-art treatments that have been developed before they are widely available for commercial use.

Currently, there are a number of clinical trials focusing on male breast cancer. For a list of National Cancer Institute sponsored trials, go to www.cancer.gov. Go to Clinical Trials, then Finding Trials, then PDQ Search Form, and then complete the search form to look for male breast cancer trials.

Discuss with your healthcare provider whether there are any clinical trial protocols available that might be beneficial for you.

Reconstruction

Reconstructive surgery and breast implants can help to restore the normal look of the chest after a mastectomy. This surgery can also rebuild and reform the nipple, and tattooing can recreate the areola. If you are going to have a mastectomy, it is important to talk with a plastic surgeon before your surgery to see if breast reconstruction is an option for you. This reconstruction or rebuilding of the breast can be done or started at the time of the mastectomy (called immediate reconstruction) or at a later date (called delayed reconstruction).

It is important for you to understand that reconstructive surgery does not create a "new," normally functioning breast. The goal is to create a breast form with the same general shape and texture as the other breast. The difference between the reconstructed breast and the natural breast will be able to be seen when you are undressed. However, the breasts should look like one another enough that the difference is not seen in clothing. The decision to have reconstructive surgery is very personal. The decision should be based on your feelings about your body, your sexuality, and your tolerance for more surgery. Although men rarely choose to undergo breast reconstruction, it is important that you are aware that it is an option that is not limited to women.

Some of advantages of breast reconstruction include:

- Can improve body image and self-esteem
- Fewer daily reminders of your surgery

Disadvantages of reconstruction include:

- More time required for the surgery or additional surgeries
- More pain and time needed for recovery
- May cost more
- Possible infection and surgical problems associated with more surgery

Questions to ask the plastic surgeon:

- What type of reconstruction is best for me?
- Will an implant make it harder to watch for local recurrences of breast cancer?
- May I see pictures of some of the reconstruction procedures that you have done?

- Will I have a lot of pain, and how will you treat the pain?
- How long will I be in the hospital?
- What kind of anesthesia will I need for all of the different parts of the reconstruction?
- Will I need a blood transfusion? Can I donate my own blood?
- What kind of changes to the breast can I expect over time?
- What happens if I gain or lose weight?
- How will the reconstructed breast feel to the touch? Will I have feeling in the reconstructed breast?
- Will reconstruction surgery give me more scars?
- What are the possible complications that may happen with the surgery?
- How long will it take to complete the reconstruction process?
- Am I a candidate for reconstructive surgery?

It is important to check with your insurance company to determine what is covered by your policy.

Reach to Recovery is an American Cancer Society volunteer visitation program comprised of breast cancer survivors trained to respond to the concerns of patients and their families facing the diagnosis, treatment, and effects of breast cancer. These visits are always free of charge.

To request a Reach to Recovery visit or to obtain more information, contact your nearest American Cancer Society office listed in your local telephone directory or call 1-800-ACS-2345 (1-800-227-2345).

You are the only one who can decide if breast reconstruction is the best option for you. Breast reconstruction is not an emergency. Take your time. Ask lots of questions until you feel comfortable with the information. Finally, keep in mind that the goal of breast reconstruction is improvement, not perfection.

Questions to Ask Your Physician about Male Breast Cancer

It is always important to ask your healthcare provider questions until you are comfortable with the information. Some questions that you may want to ask are:

- What type of breast cancer do I have?

- Has the cancer spread to other parts of my breast or other parts of my body?
- What stage or grade is my cancer?
- What are my treatment options? What do you recommend? Why?
- What are the risks and side effects of my treatment options?
- What can I expect during the recovery from the different treatment options?
- What do I need to do to get ready for my treatment?
- Is reconstructive surgery an option for me?
- What are the chances of the cancer recurring with the different treatment options we have discussed?
- Are there any clinical trials that I may qualify for?
- What is my expected prognosis, based on my cancer as you view it?

Emotional Considerations

A cancer diagnosis and the treatments that follow are major life changes and adjustments. This has an impact on you as well as everyone who cares for and about you. Male breast cancer survivors have a special set of challenges. Because this cancer is rare, many men feel particularly alone and helpless. This can be magnified if the physician has rarely seen or treated this disease. Second, since this is mainly a disease of women and involves hormone imbalance, many men feel a threat to their masculinity. Some of the treatments, such as hormonal therapies, result in symptoms such as hot flashes and mood swings that are traditionally "female problems." Finally, a radical mastectomy may cause the arm to be weak, which can compromise a man's work or recreation activities.

Before you get to the point where you feel overwhelmed, think about going to a meeting of a local cancer support group. If you need individualized assistance, call your healthcare provider or your local American Cancer Society for help in contacting a counselor or other services.

Self Breast Examination for Men

Feeling for changes in the shower:

1. Make yourself soapy.

2. Place your left arm above and behind your head. With your three middle fingers of your hand, press your breast against your chest wall.

3. In a circular motion feel small portions of your left breast, going around until you have covered the entire breast and underarm area. Make sure you do it slowly.

4. Repeat it again with your right arm.

Remember: look for changes, and if you find a lump or have a discharge make sure you go to a physician.

Figure 17.1. Self breast exam for men.

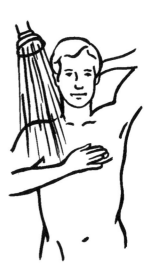

Men Have Mammograms

If a man finds a lump, a mammogram should be an automatic routine for physicians. A mammogram is essential to early detection of breast cancer, and also serves to help diagnose noncancerous breast diseases.

If a lump or abnormality is found during a self or doctor's clinical exam, an accurate mammogram reading can indicate whether there is need for further investigation.

There are no guidelines for mammography for men, and no study on male lump sizing with mammography.

When Preparing for Your Mammogram

Do not wear deodorants, creams, powders, or colognes.

Make sure your mammogram is performed and interpreted at a facility that is fully accredited (in mammography) by the American College of Radiology.

Embarrassment should never be a deterrent to getting a mammogram. Qualified and experienced healthcare technicians are trained to take the mammogram.

If your mammogram is inconclusive, your doctor will need additional tests to ensure proper treatment. An ultrasound image creates a picture of the breast with sound waves, and is a nonsurgical procedure. To further distinguish a solid lump from a fluid-filled cyst, a fine needle aspiration may be used to remove fluid or cells for microscopic study for the presence of cancer cells. Biopsy is the definitive test for breast cancer and can be performed on an outpatient basis. Needle biopsy under local anesthesia may now be performed under stereotactic x-ray or ultrasound. In some cases ultrasound is used instead of mammography. As with women, the early detection and treatment of male breast cancer vastly increases the chances of survival. Awareness can help save lives.

Part Three

Breast Cancer Risk Factors

Chapter 18

Risk Factors for Breast Cancer

Executive Summary

A wide variety of factors may influence an individual's likelihood of developing various types of cancer. These factors are usually referred to as risk factors. Different types of cancer may have different risk factors.

Some factors that influence cancer risk, such as dietary and exercise habits, are modifiable. By changing these aspects of their lifestyle, people may reduce their risk of cancer. Other factors that influence risk, such as age, gender, or family history, cannot be modified. Traditionally, it was thought that little could be done about these risk factors. However, it is now possible for individuals who are at high risk of some types of cancer because of nonmodifiable risk factors to reduce their chances of getting the disease through special measures such as chemoprevention or preventive surgery. Additionally, knowledge of risk factors can be useful when considering the benefits of early detection methods for breast cancer, including x-ray mammography, clinical breast examination, and breast self-examination.

Many possible risk factors for breast cancer have been proposed. Compelling scientific evidence supports the importance of some of these factors. These factors are referred to as "established" risk factors.

Other proposed risk factors have more limited support; the evidence for their role is inconclusive. These risk factors can be described as "speculated." Still other factors have little or no scientific support. They are primarily myths and misconceptions and are best described as "unsupported."

The established risk factors for breast cancer are female gender, age, previous breast cancer, benign breast disease, hereditary factors (family history of breast cancer), early age at menarche (first menstrual period), late age at menopause, late age at first full-term pregnancy, postmenopausal obesity, low physical activity, and high-dose exposure to ionizing radiation early in life.

Speculated risk factors for breast cancer include never having been pregnant, having only one pregnancy rather than many, not breast feeding after pregnancy, use of postmenopausal estrogen replacement therapy or postmenopausal hormone (estrogen/progestin) replacement therapy, use of oral contraceptives, prescribed diethylstilbestrol (DES), certain specific dietary practices (high intake of fat and low intake of fiber, fruits, and vegetables), alcohol consumption, tobacco smoking, abortion, breast augmentation, low intake of phytoestrogens (estrogens from plant sources), and non-use of nonsteroidal anti-inflammatory drugs (NSAIDs).

There is only limited evidence in support of the possibility that xenoestrogens (synthetic estrogens) and large breast size might increase breast cancer risk. Unsupported risk factors include premenopausal obesity, exposure to low-dose ionizing radiation in midlife, high intake of phytoestrogens, electromagnetic fields, breast trauma, and the use of antiperspirants.

For all women, American Council on Science and Health (ACSH) recommends the following.

1. Discuss your risk factors for breast cancer with your physician.

2. Stay active and watch your weight.

3. Be sure to have mammograms and breast examinations as often as your doctor recommends.

Introduction

Breast cancer is the most common type of cancer among American women. Approximately 30 percent of all cancers diagnosed in women are breast cancers.

One of the best ways to fight cancer is to prevent it from occurring, by identifying and controlling factors that increase a person's risk of developing the disease. For some types of cancer, this is a fairly straightforward process. For example, cigarette smoking greatly increases an individual's risk of developing lung cancer. In fact, at least 80 percent of all lung cancers are attributable to smoking. Therefore, not smoking cigarettes is an effective way to prevent lung cancer.

For breast cancer, however, the situation is not so simple. Many different factors may influence a woman's risk of developing this disease. The importance of some of these factors is well established; but for others, the link is a matter more of speculation than of fact. In addition, some of the factors that influence breast cancer risk cannot be modified, as they involve aspects of the woman's family and reproductive history rather than her personal habits. Thus, it is far more difficult to develop a strategy for reducing the risk of breast cancer than it is to do so for lung cancer.

This chapter reviews the scientific evidence pertaining to a variety of factors that may influence breast cancer risk and rates each of these factors as "established," "speculated," or "unsupported." (See Table 18.1.) The chapter also discusses ways in which individual women can use this information to help reduce their personal risk of breast cancer.

The Concept of Risk Factors

Unlike some other diseases, such as infections, most cancers do not have a single cause. Instead, they result from the interaction of multiple factors that range from genetic characteristics to personal lifestyle. Researchers who study the causes of cancer use the term "risk factor" to refer to anything that is associated with an increased chance of developing a particular type of cancer.

Risk factors are a matter of probability. They influence an individual's odds of developing a disease. That's not the same thing as actually causing a disease to occur. Some people with one or more risk factors for a particular type of cancer never develop it, while other people who have no known risk factors do develop that type of cancer. Most breast cancer cases fall into the second category, because they are not predicted by known risk factors. Nevertheless, identification of risk factors for cancer can be useful for risk modification or to identify individuals who may benefit more from cancer screening.

Different cancers have different risk factors. For example, smoking is the most important risk factor for lung cancer, but it is not a risk factor for skin cancer. Conversely, exposure to ultraviolet light from the sun is a risk factor for skin cancer but not lung cancer. Traditionally, scientists have divided the factors that influence an individual's odds of developing a disease into two groups: modifiable risk factors and nonmodifiable risk factors (also called predisposing factors or predispositions).

Modifiable risk factors are aspects of an individual's lifestyle that affect the risk of a disease that can be altered. Personal habits such as smoking and dietary patterns fall into this category. Individuals may be able to reduce their risk of becoming ill by changing their personal habits (for example, smokers can stop smoking). Health education efforts have usually focused on modifiable risk factors because they can be altered or eliminated.

Nonmodifiable risk factors (or predisposing factors) are inherent conditions (such as age) or aspects of an individual's genetic program

Table 18.1. Established, Speculated, and Unsupported Risk Factors for Human Breast Cancer (*continued on next page*)

Established Risk Factors

Female gender

Age

Previous breast cancer

Benign breast disease

Hereditary factors (family history of breast cancer)

Early age at menarche

Late age at menopause

Late age at first full-term pregnancy

Obesity (postmenopausal)

Low physical activity

High-dose exposure to ionizing radiation early in life

Speculated Risk Factors

Never having been pregnant[a]

Having only one pregnancy rather than many

Not breast-feeding after pregnancy

Postmenopausal estrogen replacement therapy[a]

Postmenopausal hormone (estrogen/progestin) replacement therapy

Use of oral contraceptives[a]

Prescribed diethylstilbestrol (DES)

(such as sex, ethnic background, or specific gene mutations) that increase that person's likelihood of developing a disease. Traditionally, it was assumed that little could be done about nonmodifiable risk factors. However, this is no longer true.

New techniques are being developed that can reduce the risk of cancer in high-risk individuals—even if those people are at increased risk because of inherent predispositions that cannot be changed. One such technique is chemoprevention—the use of medicines to reduce the risk of developing a disease. Another technique, which is usually used only in cases of extremely high risk, is preventive surgery. Both of these approaches have been used successfully to reduce the risk of breast cancer in high-risk women. In fact, breast cancer is the first type of cancer for which a chemoprevention drug has become available.

Table 18.1. Established, Speculated, and Unsupported Risk Factors for Human Breast Cancer (*continued*)

Speculated Risk Factors (*continued*)

Specific dietary practices (i.e., high intake of fat; low intake of fiber, fruits, and vegetables)

Alcohol consumption

Tobacco smoking

Abortion

Breast augmentation

Low intake of phytoestrogens

Non-use of nonsteroidal anti-inflammatory drugs (NSAIDs)

Unsupported Risk Factors

Obesity (premenopausal)

Exposure to low-dose ionizing radiation in midlife

High intake of phytoestrogens

Xenoestrogens[b]

Large breast size[b]

Electromagnetic fields

Breast trauma

Antiperspirants

[a] Speculated risk factors marked with an "a" are gaining scientific support.

[b] Risk factors marked with a "b" have slight scientific support but not enough to place them in the "speculated" category.

Additionally, the benefits of early detection methods for breast cancer can be maximized among women experiencing the highest risk for breast cancer, regardless of whether the risk factors are modifiable. Women at high risk for breast cancer who regularly receive mammography and clinical breast exams can benefit from early detection, even if their risk, per se, is not modified. Similar benefits may result from breast self-examination.

Women who are at increased risk of breast cancer for reasons that they cannot change should not feel that nothing can be done to help them. Thanks to early detection and chemoprevention, these women may be able to reduce their chances of developing breast cancer or the severe consequences of the disease even though they cannot change their predisposition per se.

Chemoprevention: A New Weapon against Breast Cancer

When doctors use medicines to treat cancer, they refer to it as chemotherapy. Similarly, the use of medicines to reduce the risk of cancer is called chemoprevention.

Chemoprevention is a new and promising strategy for reducing cancer risk. The first drug approved for this purpose in the United States is tamoxifen, which is used to reduce the risk of breast cancer in high-risk women. Tamoxifen is one of a group of drugs called selective estrogen receptor modulators. Drugs of this type have actions similar to those of the female hormone estrogen in some body tissues, but they block the effect of estrogen in other tissues, including breast tissue. Since estrogen promotes the development of breast cancer, drugs that block its effect may reduce breast cancer risk.

Chemoprevention is not for everyone. The women who are most likely to benefit are those who are at high risk of breast cancer. Low-risk women have less to gain because few of them will develop breast cancer anyway. Any small benefit that the medicine would give them is likely to be outweighed by the potential for side effects from the use of the drug.

Because the use of tamoxifen for breast cancer chemoprevention involves a complex mix of potential benefits and risks, decisions about its use should be made on an individual basis. Any woman who believes that she may be at high risk of breast cancer because of her age, personal medical history, family history of breast cancer, or other reasons should discuss her risk factors with her physician to find out whether she is an appropriate candidate for chemoprevention.

For more information on this subject, see Chapter 35, "Chemoprevention of Breast Cancer."

Established Risk Factors for Breast Cancer

There is clear scientific evidence linking several factors with breast cancer risk. These factors are called "established" risk factors for breast cancer. Some are inherited predispositions, while others are aspects of a woman's lifestyle or reproductive history. The established risk factors for breast cancer include female gender, age, previous breast disease, family history/genetic risk factors, early age at menarche, late age at menopause, late age at first full-term pregnancy, postmenopausal obesity, lack of physical activity, and exposure to high doses of radiation.

Gender

Simply being female is the most important risk factor for breast cancer. Although men can and do develop breast cancer, the disease is one hundred times more likely to occur in a woman than in a man. Women are at higher risk of breast cancer because they have much more breast tissue than men do. In addition, the female hormone estrogen promotes the development of breast cancer.

Age

The risk of breast cancer is higher in middle-aged and elderly women than in young women. In the United States, more than three-fourths of all breast cancers occur in women aged fifty or older.

The impact of age on breast cancer risk is sufficiently strong that many older women, especially those over the age of sixty, may be candidates for breast cancer chemoprevention with the drug tamoxifen. (See "Chemoprevention: A New Weapon against Breast Cancer.") These women should discuss the option of chemoprevention with their physicians.

Previous Breast Disease

A woman who has previously had breast cancer has a 3- to 4-fold increased risk of developing a new cancer in the other breast. Women who have had noncancerous (benign) breast problems are also at increased risk—but to a lesser extent. Benign breast disease, considered as a single condition, is associated with a 1.5- to 3-fold increase in breast cancer risk. However, the various types of benign breast disease are

119

not all associated with the same degree of risk; some types have little or no effect on risk, while others may represent early stages in the progression to breast cancer.

Women who have a history of any type of breast disease should discuss their histories with their physicians. Some women with previous breast disease (especially those who have been treated for lobular carcinoma in situ (LCIS) or ductal carcinoma in situ (DCIS)) are at sufficiently high risk of breast cancer that they may be good candidates for tamoxifen chemoprevention. (See "Chemoprevention: A New Weapon against Breast Cancer.")

Family History and Genetic Factors

The risk of breast cancer is higher among women who have a close blood relative (mother, sister, or daughter) who has had the disease. The increase in risk is especially high if the relative developed breast cancer before the age of fifty or in both breasts. According to the American Cancer Society, however, most women who get breast cancer—approximately 80 percent—have no such family history of the disease. Indeed, most women who get breast cancer would not have been considered to be in the high-risk group before their diagnosis.

The effect of family history on breast cancer risk is believed to be due primarily to genetic factors. As much as 5–10 percent of all breast cancer cases are attributable to specific inherited single-gene mutations, and many other cases have some genetic component.

Scientists compare risks of disease by using risk ratios. A risk ratio of one means that the individual's risk of developing a disease is the same as that expected among people who don't have any special risk factors. A risk ratio greater than one means that the individual has a higher risk. As Table 18.2 shows, the risk ratios for breast cancer among close relatives of breast cancer patients vary greatly, depending on the age at diagnosis and whether cancer was present in one or both breasts. A close relative of a woman who developed breast cancer in one breast after age fifty has only a slightly increased risk of developing the disease herself (risk ratio 1.2, or a 20 percent increase in risk). On the other hand, close relatives of a woman who developed cancer in both breasts before age fifty have a much larger increase in risk (risk ratio 8.8, or a nearly ninefold increase in risk). This risk ratio is similar to that seen for lung cancer among smokers, when compared to nonsmokers.

Any woman who has a family history of breast cancer should discuss that history with her physician. In some instances, the increase in risk associated with family history is substantial enough that the woman and her physician may want to consider tamoxifen chemoprevention. (See "Chemoprevention: A New Weapon against Breast Cancer.") In rare instances, if a woman's family history of breast cancer is extremely strong or if it is known that the woman carries gene mutations associated with very high breast cancer risk, the possibility of preventive surgery (mastectomy or removal of the ovaries) may also be considered.

Reproductive History

Women who reach menarche (the first menstrual period) at a relatively early age (twelve or younger) and those who reach menopause at a relatively late age (fifty-five or older) are slightly more likely than other women to develop breast cancer. These relationships are believed to be mediated through estrogen produced within the woman's body.

During the reproductive years, a woman's body produces high levels of estrogen. Women who start to menstruate at an early age or

Table 18.2. Risk Ratio for Breast Cancer in First-Degree Female Relatives of Women with Breast Cancer

Characteristics of the Breast Cancer	Risk Ratio in First-Degree Relatives
Premenopausal (before age 50)[a]	3.1
Postmenopausal (age 50 or over)	1.5
Cancer in one breast	
Premenopausal or postmenopausal	1.3
Premenopausal	1.8
Postmenopausal	1.2
Cancer in both breasts	
Premenopausal or postmenopausal	5.4
Premenopausal	8.8
Postmenopausal	4.0

Note: A woman's first-degree female relatives are her mother, sisters, and daughters.

[a] Because it is difficult to determine when individual women reach menopause, researchers generally assume that women under the age of fifty are premenopausal and that those age fifty and over are postmenopausal.

reach menopause at a late age are exposed to high levels of estrogen for more years than are women who have a late menarche or early menopause. However, the effect of age at menarche and menopause on breast cancer risk is relatively small. The increase in breast cancer risk associated with a five-year increase in age at menopause is only about 17 percent. Similarly, the decrease in breast cancer risk associated with a two-year delay in menarche is only about 10 percent.

Another aspect of reproductive history that is associated with breast cancer risk is age at first pregnancy. Women who have their first full-term pregnancy at a relatively early age have a lower risk of breast cancer than those who never have children or those who have their first child relatively late in life. The biologic basis for this relationship is not entirely clear. Scientists suspect, though, that pregnancy may lead to lasting changes in the sensitivity of breast tissue to cancer-causing agents, as well as to the maturation of breast tissue. In addition, several hormonal changes occur after a full-term pregnancy and may persist for years.

Obesity and Physical Inactivity

In scientific studies, obesity has been consistently associated with an increased risk of breast cancer among postmenopausal women. As is the case with reproductive risk factors, this relationship may be mediated by estrogen production. Fat cells produce some estrogen (though nowhere near as much as the ovaries produce during a woman's reproductive years), and obese postmenopausal women, therefore, tend to have higher blood estrogen levels than lean women do.

Obesity does not seem to be a risk factor for breast cancer in premenopausal women. In these younger women, the ovaries are the main producers of estrogen. The much smaller amount of estrogen produced by the fat cells doesn't appear to have any significant impact on breast cancer risk.

Scientific studies have consistently shown that the risk of breast cancer is lower among physically active premenopausal women than among sedentary women. Physical activity during adolescence may be especially protective, and the effect of physical activity may be strongest among women who have at least one full-term pregnancy. Scientists believe that the effect of physical activity on breast cancer risk may be due at least in part to effects of exercise on the female hormones.

Although the effects of obesity and physical inactivity on breast cancer risk are not as strong as the effects of previous breast disease or family history of breast cancer, they are important risk factors because they are modifiable. Exercise and weight control currently represent the most effective lifestyle changes that a woman can make to reduce her risk of breast cancer.

Exposure to High Doses of Radiation

Women who were exposed to high doses of radiation, especially during adolescence, have an increased risk of breast cancer. This association has been observed both among atomic bomb survivors and among women who received high-dose radiation for medical purposes. The low radiation exposures involved in modern x-rays (including chest x-rays and mammograms) have not been associated with any measurable increase in breast cancer risk.

Speculated Risk Factors for Breast Cancer

"Speculated" risk factors for breast cancer are those for which there is some scientific support but not enough to be considered conclusive. In some instances, support for these factors may increase as more research is completed. In other cases, though, future research may demonstrate that some of these factors don't relate directly to the risk of breast cancer.

Speculated risk factors include number of pregnancies, not breast-feeding, use of postmenopausal estrogen replacement therapy (ERT) or combination estrogen/progestin hormone replacement therapy (HRT), use of oral contraceptives, exposure to prescribed diethylstilbestrol (DES), specific aspects of diet, alcohol consumption, tobacco smoking, abortion, and breast augmentation. The consumption of phytoestrogens and the use of nonsteroidal anti-inflammatory drugs are speculated to be protective against breast cancer.

Number of Pregnancies

As mentioned earlier, a woman's age at the time of her first full-term pregnancy is an established risk factor for breast cancer. Whether the number of pregnancies she experiences in her lifetime is also related to breast cancer risk is less clear. There is consistent evidence that first pregnancy completed before age thirty to thirty-five lowers risk of breast cancer, and that first full-term pregnancy after age thirty to thirty-five raises risk. More limited evidence suggests that women who have many pregnancies may be less likely to develop breast cancer than those who have only one pregnancy.

Not Breast-Feeding

Some scientific studies have indicated that women who breast-feed their babies may be less likely to develop breast cancer than those who have children but do not breast-feed. Other studies, however, indicate that there may be little or no relationship between breast-feeding and breast cancer risk. If breast-feeding does protect against breast cancer, it may do so by delaying the resumption of ovulation (with its accompanying high estrogen levels) after pregnancy.

The uncertainty regarding the effect of breast-feeding on breast cancer risk should not be regarded as an argument against breast-feeding. The benefits of breast-feeding for the infant are well established, and all authorities agree that breast-feeding is the preferred method of infant feeding unless it is contraindicated for a specific medical reason.

Postmenopausal Estrogen and Hormone Replacement Therapy

As mentioned earlier, factors that influence the amount of estrogen produced by a woman's body over her lifetime (such as the ages at the onset of menstruation and at menopause) are known to influence breast cancer risk. Whether estrogen from outside sources has a similar effect on breast cancer risk is less clear.

Some scientific studies have associated long-term (more than five years) use of postmenopausal estrogen therapy (ERT) or combination estrogen/progestin hormone replacement therapy (HRT) with a small increase in breast cancer risk, but others have not found such a relationship. Women who take ERT or HRT for less than five years probably do not have an increased risk of breast cancer. The addition of progestin to estrogen does not decrease the risk of breast cancer (in the way that it does for endometrial cancer). In fact, there is some evidence—although it is not conclusive—that the increase in breast cancer risk associated with combination estrogen/progestin HRT may be greater than that associated with estrogen alone.

Possible effects on breast cancer risk are only one of the many factors that need to be considered by a woman and her physician when making decisions about ERT/HRT. Experts agree that for most women, the benefits of ERT/HRT outweigh the risks. However, decisions about ERT/HRT should be made on an individual basis, after a careful evaluation of all of the potential benefits and risks of this form of therapy.

Oral Contraceptives

Numerous scientific studies have investigated the relationship between the use of oral contraceptives (birth control pills) and the risk of breast cancer. These studies have consistently shown that oral contraceptives do not have a large effect on breast cancer risk. Whether they have a small effect on risk is less clear. A combined analysis of many studies indicates that they probably do, but that the effect decreases and eventually disappears within ten years after oral contraceptives are discontinued.

If oral contraceptives do increase breast cancer risk, it's likely that at least part of the effect is simply due to the fact that the "Pill" does its job: it prevents a woman from becoming pregnant. Pregnancy (especially a first pregnancy that occurs at an early age) is protective against breast cancer.

Diethylstilbestrol (DES)

From the late 1940s to the early 1960s, the drug diethylstilbestrol (DES) was used in the United States to reduce the risk of miscarriages, especially among women who were at high risk of miscarriage. A few scientific studies have associated the use of DES with a moderate increase in breast cancer risk later in life. Other studies, however, have not detected any association between DES and breast cancer.

Medical authorities recommend that any woman in the childbearing years avoid DES because of the risk of harm to an unborn child, even in a woman who may not be aware that she is pregnant.

Specific Dietary Factors

During the 1980s and early 1990s, there was much enthusiasm over the idea that a diet low in fat and high in fruits, vegetables, and fiber could help to prevent breast cancer. More recent research indicates, however, that these specific dietary factors may not be as important in modifying breast cancer risk as was previously supposed. Some of the effects that were once attributed to dietary fat intake were probably due to obesity (which is often linked with high fat intake) rather than to fat intake per se. And the effects of fiber, fruits, and vegetables now appear to be small, at best.

This does not mean, however, that eating plenty of fruits and vegetables and limiting fat and calorie intake is a bad idea. Diets high in fruits and vegetables and low in fat and calories are healthful for many reasons, and they may indirectly reduce the risk of breast cancer by helping to prevent obesity.

Alcohol

Women who drink moderate amounts of alcohol have been found to have a slightly higher risk of breast cancer than do those who abstain. It is uncertain, however, whether this association reflects a cause-and-effect relationship.

The mere fact that two things are associated with one another does not necessarily mean that one causes the other. The relationship could also be due to other factors that are associated with both of them. For example, if you survey a large group of people, you will probably find that arthritis is more common among those with gray hair than among those with black or brown hair. But that doesn't mean that gray hair causes arthritis (or vice versa). The relationship is due to the fact that both arthritis and gray hair are associated with a third factor—namely, age.

The weaker an association is, the more difficult it is to tell whether that association is due to a true cause-and-effect relationship or to something else. The relationship between alcohol intake and breast cancer is quite weak. It is extremely difficult for scientists to determine whether an effect of this magnitude reflects a true cause-and-effect relationship or is due to other factors—such as difficulties in measurement or differences between the lifestyles of drinkers and abstainers. The use of alcohol may vary among women who differ with regard to other factors that are known to influence breast cancer risk—such as age, obesity, and reproductive history. Failure to consider these so-called confounding factors could create the impression of a small association between alcohol intake and breast cancer even if no independent effect exists.

Tobacco

There is some evidence that cigarette smoking may be associated with a small increase in breast cancer risk. However, because the results of scientific studies have not been consistent, this relationship is currently regarded as merely speculative. Among women who have already been diagnosed with breast cancer, smoking may be associated with an increased risk that the cancer will progress more rapidly.

Abortion

Some scientific studies indicate that having an induced abortion may lead to a small increase in breast cancer risk. However, the validity of these studies has been questioned.

To investigate the relationship between abortion and breast cancer, researchers conduct surveys in which they ask women (both those with breast cancer and those who do not have the disease) whether they have ever had an abortion. Some women may not answer this extremely personal question truthfully. There's reason to suspect that women with breast cancer (who are more highly motivated to cooperate with researchers) may be more likely to admit to having had an abortion than healthy women would be. If this is the case, this bias might create the impression of a relationship between abortion and breast cancer even if none really exists.

Breast Augmentation

It has been suspected that breast augmentation surgery might increase the risk of breast cancer. However, the currently available scientific data don't support this idea.

Although breast implants probably don't cause breast cancer, it is possible that the presence of implants might delay the detection of cancer in some instances. On the other hand, women who undergo breast augmentation may have a heightened awareness of this part of their bodies, and they are likelier than other women to have regular mammograms. These factors may lead to earlier detection of tumors, perhaps offsetting any disadvantage from the implants themselves.

Phytoestrogens (as protective factors)

It has been speculated that plant substances called isoflavones most commonly found in soy products may be protective against breast cancer. These substances, sometimes referred to as phytoestrogens, appear to have effects similar to those of estrogen in some body tissues while antagonizing, or "blocking," the effects of estrogen in other tissues.

It has been suggested that the lower rate of breast cancer in Asia, as compared to North America, may be at least partly due to the higher intake of soy products in many Asian countries. Several scientific studies have demonstrated weak protective relationships between soy product intake and breast cancer. However, it is possible that constituents of soy other than phytoestrogens or aspects of diet and lifestyle other than soy product consumption might be responsible for these relationships. Thus, the evidence linking phytoestrogens with reduced breast cancer risk is regarded as inconclusive. The scientific evidence does not support the idea that high intakes of phytoestrogens could increase breast cancer risk.

Nonsteroidal Anti-Inflammatory Drugs (as protective factors)

Recent studies have suggested that aspirin and other nonsteroidal anti-inflammatory drugs (such as ibuprofen, naproxen, indomethacin, and piroxicam) may be protective against some types of cancer. Two studies in humans showed that women who regularly used aspirin or other nonsteroidal anti-inflammatory drugs had lower rates of breast cancer than those who did not. Other studies, however, have not confirmed this relationship. Since the evidence for a beneficial effect of nonsteroidal anti-inflammatory drugs is uncertain and since these drugs can have significant side effects, no recommendations have been made for the use of these drugs in breast cancer prevention.

Suggested Risk Factors That Have Little or No Scientific Support

In addition to the established and speculated risk factors listed previously, a wide variety of other factors have been suggested as possible "causes" of breast cancer. These ideas are primarily myths or misconceptions rather than true risk factors and are best described as "unsupported." Three unsupported risk factors have already been mentioned in previous sections of this chapter: premenopausal obesity, low-dose radiation, and high intake of phytoestrogens. The others are described below. Of the factors that will be discussed in this section, only two—xenoestrogens and breast size—have even slight scientific support.

Xenoestrogens

The term "xenoestrogen" refers to synthetic substances with estrogenic activity. These include certain fat-soluble organochlorine compounds, such as the insecticide DDT, its metabolite DDE, and polychlorinated biphenyls (PCBs). Some of these compounds (though not PCBs) have shown weak estrogenic effects in laboratory tests.

In several studies, the levels of certain organochlorines in breast tissue or blood samples were found to be higher in women with breast cancer than in healthy women. In other studies, however, no such relationship was found. Researchers assessing the relationship between organochlorines and breast cancer have concluded that the weak estrogenic effect of these compounds would be minimal when compared to the estrogenic activity of more significant estrogen sources, such as postmenopausal estrogen replacement therapy.

An expert panel of the National Cancer Institute of Canada recently concluded that there was no definitive evidence linking organochlorine pesticides to cancer. The panel also concluded that there is no evidence that the increased intake of pesticide residues that would result from official recommendations to increase the intake of fruits and vegetables would lead to an increase in cancer.

Breast Size

While it would seem to make sense that women with more breast tissue would be more likely to develop breast cancer, the scientific evidence on this point is actually quite unclear.

Much of the variation in breast size among women is due to differences in the amount of adipose (fat) tissue, rather than differences in the amount of glandular breast tissue (the actual tissue in which cancer develops). Most scientific studies have found no relationship between breast size and the risk of breast cancer when the degree of obesity and other related factors are taken into consideration. Nevertheless, it seems reasonable to assume that a woman who has a greater amount of glandular breast tissue might be more likely to develop breast cancer than one who has less such tissue.

Electromagnetic Fields

There is no persuasive scientific evidence to show that low-level, low-frequency electromagnetic fields can influence any of the stages in carcinogenesis. Electromagnetic fields have not been shown to be a cause of any type of cancer. The limited research that has been completed to date does not implicate electromagnetic fields as a cause of breast cancer in women.

Breast Trauma

The idea that breast trauma can cause breast cancer is widely accepted by some societal groups, including some groups of Hispanic Americans, but it is not supported by the scientific evidence. Although many women believe that childhood trauma to the breast, bruising and rough handling during breast-feeding, or fondling of the breasts during sexual relations could cause breast cancer, there is actually no cause for concern about any of these factors.

Antiperspirants

Recent rumors, spread largely through e-mail, have aroused concern over the possibility that the use of antiperspirants, especially in combination with underarm shaving, could cause breast cancer. The claims include the following.

- Underarm shaving allows cancer-causing substances in antiperspirants to be absorbed through razor nicks, and antiperspirants prevent the underarm lymph nodes from removing cancer-causing toxins from the breasts through sweating.

- Most breast cancers develop in the portion of the breast (the upper outer quadrant) that is closest to the underarm lymph nodes.

- Women are likelier than men to develop breast cancer because men do not shave their underarms; antiperspirant therefore gets caught in men's underarm hair and is not absorbed by their skin.

In actuality:

- There is no evidence that antiperspirants cause cancer.

- Antiperspirants are not absorbed through the skin, regardless of whether razor nicks are present.

- Razor nicks may increase the risk of skin infection, but they do not increase the risk of cancer.

- The lymph nodes do not remove toxins through sweating; sweat glands are located in the skin, not the lymph nodes.

- The reason that breast cancers occur most commonly in the upper outer quadrant has nothing to do with underarm lymph nodes; instead, it is due to the fact that the largest portion of breast tissue is located in this quadrant. The number of breast cancers in the upper outer quadrant is proportional to the amount of tissue located there.

- The reasons why men are less likely than women to develop breast cancer have to do with the much smaller amount of breast tissue in a man's body and with hormonal factors. The fact that men do not shave their underarm hair is not relevant.

Reducing Your Risk of Breast Cancer

When attempting to improve your health, it makes sense to focus your attention on the things that matter the most and to consider both the risks and the benefits of any action that you're planning to take.

In terms of reducing your risk of breast cancer, therefore, it's best to concentrate your efforts on the established risk factors, especially those that you can modify without risking any type of harm. For example, consider the following choices.

- Does it make sense for women to stop using antiperspirants in an effort to reduce their breast cancer risk? No. There's no scientific evidence that antiperspirants are a breast cancer risk factor, so it's not worth the trouble.

- Does it make sense for women to make a great effort to increase their intake of soy products in order to reduce their breast cancer risk? Probably not. Since the evidence linking phytoestrogens in soy products with reduced breast cancer risk is less than definitive, it's unclear whether this dietary change would really be beneficial. Of course, women who enjoy soy products can feel free to include them in their diets. But in terms of breast cancer prevention, it's better for women to focus their efforts on other factors that have been more conclusively linked to breast cancer risk.

- Does it make sense for women to exercise regularly in order to reduce their breast cancer risk? Yes, definitely. Lack of physical activity is an established risk factor for premenopausal breast cancer and represents part of a complete approach to weight management. In addition, women who stay active can also reduce their risk of other diseases, such as coronary heart disease and colon cancer, and they can increase their quality of life.

For all women, ACSH recommends three courses of action.

1. Discuss your risk factors for breast cancer with your physician. If you find out that you are at high risk, ask your physician whether chemoprevention would be appropriate for you.

2. Stay active and watch your weight. Of all the established risk factors for breast cancer, obesity and lack of physical activity stand out as the two that can be most readily and safely modified.

3. Be sure to have mammograms and breast examinations as often as recommended for women in your age group.[1] Although these screening tests do not prevent breast cancer, they do enable it to be detected early, when treatment is most likely to be effective.

Note

1. At the time that this report was written, experts agreed that all women should have screening mammograms on a regular basis starting at age fifty and continuing until about age seventy. Experts did not agree on whether screening mammograms are warranted for women in their forties and for those in their seventies or older. The U.S. government's Preventive Services Task Force has made no specific recommendation for or against screening mammography for women under age fifty or over age sixty-nine. On the other hand, the American Cancer Society has recommended annual mammograms for all women age forty and older. Recommendations about when to start and stop having mammograms may change when additional research is completed, and they may differ for low- and high-risk women. ACSH recommends that women consult their physicians for up-to-date, individualized advice on when and how often to have mammograms.

Reference

The information presented in this chapter is taken from a published scientific review that was prepared for the American Council on Science and Health. Please see:

Morgan, J., Gladson, J. E., and Rau, K. S., "Position Paper of the American Council on Science and Health on Risk Factors for Breast Cancer: Established, Speculated, and Unsupported," *Breast Journal* 4, no. 3 (1998): 177–97.

Chapter 19

Family History, Inheritance, and Breast Cancer Risk

All breast cancer results from multiple gene mutations. The initial mutation can be inherited from one's parents (familial breast cancer) or occur after conception (sporadic breast cancer). Inherited gene mutations play a role in about 27 percent of all cases of breast cancer. Mutations in two different genes, called BRCA1 and BRCA2, have been associated with early breast cancer in some families. These mutated genes can act alone, and the families that carry either of these mutations may have as many as half of their women members diagnosed with breast cancer. Yet these families are rare and are thought to account for only about 4 percent of all breast cancer cases. Most inherited breast cancer risk results from the interaction of several mutated genes. Families with this pattern of inheritance will contain only a few members with breast cancer. These mutated genes by themselves are associated with only a small increase in breast cancer risk, but when several of these genes are inherited together they can lead to a significant increase in breast cancer risk. Diet and lifestyle may modify inherited breast cancer risk but more study is needed to identify and understand how this happens.

"Family History, Inheritance, and Breast Cancer Risk," by Barbour Warren, Ph.D., Research Associate, and Carol Devine, Ph.D., Division of Nutritional Sciences and Education Project Leader, Program on Breast Cancer and Environmental Risk Factors in New York State (BCERF), Fact Sheet #48, updated March 2004, © 2004 Cornell University, reprinted with permission.

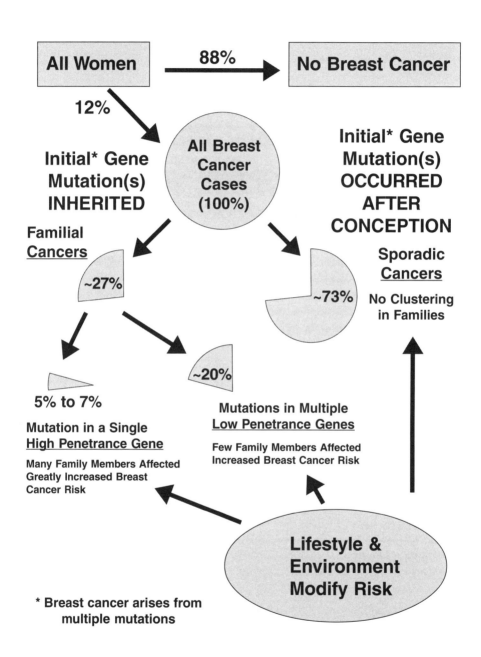

Figure 19.1. Familial and sporadic breast cancer occurrence.

How are inheritance and a family history involved in breast cancer risk?

Most women do not develop breast cancer. When it does develop it results from mutations in multiple cancer-associated genes. The first of these mutations can be either inherited from one's parents (familial cancer) or occur after conception (sporadic cancers). A few of the inherited mutations—called high-penetrance mutations—are associated with a prominent family history of breast cancer and high breast cancer risk. However, most of the inherited mutations are associated with a smaller increase in the risk of breast cancer and a less prominent family history of breast cancer (these mutations are called low-penetrance mutations). Most breast cancer cases (about two-thirds) are known as sporadic, meaning that rare mutations have occurred. In these cases the initial rare cancer gene mutations occurred after conception; these cases have no connection to family history (see Figure 19.1).

How large a role does inheritance of breast cancer risk play in a woman's chance of developing breast cancer?

Study of the differences in breast cancer risk between identical and non-identical twins has allowed a very good estimate of how much of all breast cancer risk is inherited. A recent large study using data from twin and cancer registries in Sweden, Denmark, and Finland (547 pairs of identical twins and 1,075 pairs of non-identical twins) reported that about one quarter (27 percent) of the total risk of breast cancer was due to inherited factors. While the results are most applicable to these Scandinavian countries, they would be expected to be similar in other Western countries.

How large a role does a family history of breast cancer play in a woman's chance of developing breast cancer?

Having a family history of or family member with breast cancer does not play a large role in most women's chances of developing breast cancer. Women with a family history of breast cancer make up only 5 to 7 percent of all women with breast cancer.

The mutated genes associated with a strong family history of breast cancer are known as high-penetrance genes. A breast cancer gene's penetrance is the likelihood that someone with a mutated gene will develop breast cancer during his or her lifetime. A person with a high-penetrance breast cancer gene has a high risk of breast cancer and a strong family history of breast cancer. Because high-penetrance genes are thought to largely act alone, diseases associated with them are sometimes called single-gene disorders. Yet the effects of these genes can be modified by other genes as well as by the environment inside and outside the body.

Inherited breast cancer risk seen in families with only a few cases of breast cancer results from a second type of mutated genes, low-penetrance genes. Low-penetrance genes are much more common than high-penetrance genes. The breast cancer risk of women who carry these genes depends largely on the interactions of the low-penetrance genes with other genes and with the body's internal and external environments. Since low-penetrance genes are much more common than the high-penetrance genes, low-penetrance genes account for more cases of breast cancer overall.

If inherited mutations are responsible for only about one quarter of all breast cancer risk (27 percent), what is the source of the rest of the risk?

Three-quarters of cases of breast cancer are not due to inheritance. Instead, they are the result of biological and environmental factors to which women are exposed. These factors can include: reproductive hormone levels and how long women are exposed to them (for example, age of menarche and menopause); women's child-bearing patterns (for example, at what age they bear children, how long they breast-feed, and how many children they have); medical treatments associated with breast cancer risk (for example, oral contraceptives or postmenopausal hormone treatment); women's physical characteristics (for example, body weight and where fat is carried on the body); exposure to toxic chemicals associated with breast cancer risk; exposure to radiation, especially at young ages, and parts of the diet associated with breast cancer risk (for example, alcohol use). These environmental and lifestyle factors may also act together with genetic factors.

What are breast cancer families?

Breast cancer families are families in which breast cancer is inherited and family members are at greater than average risk of breast cancer. Simply finding several cases of breast cancer within one family does not mean that a pattern of genetic inheritance exists. Determination of family inheritance requires a detailed examination of breast cancer in present and earlier generations by someone trained in genetic analysis. Breast cancer is common enough (affecting one in eight, or 12 percent, of all American women over their lifetimes) that several cases could occur within a family merely by chance alone. For example, if a woman with breast cancer has ten female relatives who have lived to eighty years old, there is a 50 percent chance that one of them will also have developed breast cancer.

Breast cancer families are frequently described as families with three or more close relatives with breast cancer. Members of these families are at high risk for developing breast cancer at a young age that may affect both breasts. The existence of breast cancer families has been noted since the mid-1800s.

Several types of family patterns exist. There are families with breast cancer alone, families with both breast and ovarian cancer, and families with several types of cancer, including breast cancer. Breast cancer families also differ in the number of family members affected with cancer. Some families have many members with breast cancer and very high risk and other families have fewer family members affected and lower, but still higher than average, breast cancer risk.

Have specific genes been linked to the high breast cancer risk seen in breast cancer families?

Mutations in two genes strongly associated with inherited breast cancer risk were identified among members of breast cancer families with the highest risk. These genes are called BRCA1 and BRCA2. Mutations in BRCA1 and BRCA2 have been linked to: the occurrence of breast cancer at a young age; the number of cases of breast cancer in a family; the occurrence of ovarian cancer as well as breast cancer in families; and breast cancer among men in the family.

BRCA1 and BRCA2 mutations are found much more often in the rare breast cancer families that have many members with breast cancer. Studies of such families have reported presence of BRCA1 or BRCA2 in as many as 87 percent of the cases. However, in breast cancer families with fewer cases of breast cancer, the presence of BRCA1 or BRCA2 mutations is much lower (15 to 20 percent of the cases). Mutations in other unidentified genes have also been implicated in these families. BRCA1 and BRCA2 mutations have rarely been found in the sporadic cancers of women with no family history of breast cancer.

How high is the risk of breast cancer for women with BRCA1 and BRCA2 mutations?

The risk of breast cancer for women who have BRCA1 and BRCA2 mutations is very high compared to that of women without these mutations, but how high is still uncertain. Early studies of the breast cancer risk associated with the mutated forms of BRCA1 and BRCA2 focused on women from the rare high-risk breast cancer families with many cases of breast cancer. Their extremely high risk made these families ideal for identifying breast cancer-associated genes. Following identification of BRCA1 and BRCA2, initial estimates indicated that all women with mutations in these genes would have breast cancer risk similar to that of women in these high breast cancer risk families. With more study, it became apparent that women in the general population with mutated versions of these genes were at higher risk of breast cancer but their risk was lower than that seen in the rare families with many cases of breast cancer.

More recent studies have evaluated the rate of occurrence of BRCA1 and BRCA2 mutations and breast cancer in women without such a strong family history of breast cancer, who were more like women in the general population. These studies have estimated that from 36 to 68 percent of the women with BRCA1 mutations in the general population would be expected to have breast cancer by age seventy. The risk associated with BRCA2 ranged between no change in risk to 37 percent of the women developing cancer by age seventy. Overall, women with a BRCA1 and BRCA2 mutations make up 15 to 20 percent of women with a family history of breast cancer. Please see "What is a woman's breast cancer risk if she has relatives who have been diagnosed with genetically undefined breast cancer?" in the following, for a discussion of breast cancer risk for women with a genetically undefined family history of breast cancer.

Are there countries or racial and ethnic groups with more women with BRCA1 and BRCA2 mutations?

Breast cancer incidence varies as much as eightfold between countries, yet in most countries 6 to 10 percent of all breast cancers are related to BRCA1 or BRCA 2 mutations. There is a considerable country-to-country difference in the proportion of cases of breast cancer in breast cancer families that are due to BRCA1 or BRCA2. Almost 80 percent of cases with a family history of breast and ovarian cancer (familial cases) in Russia have BRCA1 mutations, whereas in other European countries less than 30 percent of these familial cases are due to mutations in this gene. In the United States and Canada about 40 percent of the familial cases involve BRCA1. In the Ashkenazi Jewish population in Israel BRCA1 mutations are involved in about 50 percent of familial cases. Iceland has a high percentage (64 percent) of breast and ovarian cancer families affected by BRCA2 mutations. In the United States and Israel approximately 25 percent of breast and ovarian cancer families are due to BRCA2 mutations; in most other countries the proportion is below 20 percent.

Different racial and ethnic groups have different prevalences of BRCA1 and BRCA2 mutations. The best-studied ethnic group is the Ashkenazi Jews. More than 90 percent of the Jewish people in the United States are Ashkenazis. There are two BRCA1 mutations and one BRCA2 mutation observed frequently in Ashkenazi Jews. These mutations are also seen in the general population regardless of race or ethnicity but they are ten to fifty times more frequent in women with an Ashkenazi background. Although Ashkenazi women are more likely to be carriers of these mutations, the occurrence of these mutations is rare enough that the risk of breast or ovarian cancer for Ashkenazi women is not higher than that of non-Jewish Caucasian women.

How are mutations in BRCA1 and BRCA2 thought to increase breast cancer risk?

The majority of mutations in BRCA1 and BRCA2 have been found to result in changes in the size and function of the proteins produced by these genes. These proteins have been shown to have roles in a number of different biological processes centered around the stability of genes and the cellular response to gene damage. These are processes whose loss could be associated with increased cancer risk and may explain their linkage to high-risk breast cancer families. This is an active area of research and more definite answers should arise in the near future.

Is breast cancer seen in families with other types of inherited cancer?

Breast cancer has been associated with the following familial cancer syndromes: ataxia-telangiectasia, Muir-Torre syndrome, Cowden syndrome, Li-Fraumeni syndrome, and Peutz-Jeghers syndrome. These cancer syndromes are very rare, and their contribution to the total number of cases of breast cancer is very small.

Low-penetrance genes are thought to play a major role in breast cancer susceptibility but have any of these genes been identified?

The study of low-penetrance genes is still in its infancy. Low-penetrance genes that may be associated with breast cancer risk have been discovered, but are not yet well understood. Studies have focused on different forms (variants) of these genes, which are known as polymorphisms. Polymorphisms have been shown to have varying levels of biological activity. The different levels of biological activity of polymorphisms might link them with differing breast cancer risk. A number of classes of genes with polymorphisms have been evaluated, including genes whose products play a role in reproductive hormone action, repair gene mutations, detoxify cancer-causing chemicals, or induce or prevent cancer themselves. This area of research has the potential to identify other groups of women with increased breast cancer susceptibility.

What is a woman's breast cancer risk if she has relatives who have been diagnosed with genetically undefined breast cancer?

A woman whose close relatives have been diagnosed with breast cancer has a higher risk of breast cancer than women with no close relatives with breast cancer. The size of the breast cancer risk depends on the woman's current age, the age of relatives when they were diagnosed, and the number of relatives who were diagnosed. Table 19.1 shows how a woman's risk of breast cancer depends on her age and the number of first-degree relatives (mothers, fathers, sisters, and brothers) with breast cancer she has.

For instance, 7.8 percent of twenty-year-olds with no first-degree relative with breast cancer will develop breast cancer by the time they are eighty years old. Twenty-one percent of twenty-year-olds with two first-degree relatives will develop cancer by age eighty. Since the table looks at the percentage of women who will develop breast cancer by age eighty, the percentage decreases as the woman gets older (current age increases). Most women who develop breast cancer do so after age fifty, whether or not they have a family history.

It is important to note that most of the women in these studies who developed breast cancer did not die from it. The lifetime risk of dying from breast cancer was 2.3 percent for women with no first-degree relatives, 4.2 percent for those with one first-degree relative, and 7.6 percent for those with two first-degree relatives.

Studies have also examined how a woman's relative breast cancer risk depends on which of her family members were diagnosed with breast cancer. Women with family members with breast cancer had in general about twice the breast cancer risk of women with no family history of breast cancer. Which of a woman's relatives was diagnosed with breast cancer had a small effect on the woman's breast cancer risk.

Table 19.1. Percentage of Women Developing Breast Cancer by Age 80 as Determined by Current Age and Number of First-Degree Relatives Diagnosed with Genetically Undefined Breast Cancer

Woman's Current Age	Number of First-Degree Relatives Affected		
	None	One	Two
20 years	7.8%	13.3%	21.1%
30 years	7.7%	13.0%	20.7%
40 years	7.3%	12.0%	18.9%
50 years	6.1%	9.8%	14.7%
60 years	4.5%	7.1%	10.4%
70 years	2.5%	4.2%	5.7%

Note: First-degree relatives include mothers, sisters, and daughters.
Source: *Lancet* 358, 1389–99, 2001.

Is survival from breast cancer different for women with a family history of breast cancer?

No conclusive result can be derived from studies that have examined survival from breast cancer among women with a genetically undefined family history relative to similar-aged women with breast cancer but no family history. It is also uncertain if survival of women with BRCA1 or BRCA2 mutations is different from women diagnosed at the same age with breast cancer who do not have these mutations.

Who should be tested for BRCA1 and BRCA2 mutations?

The decision to be tested for mutations in BRCA1 or BRCA2 is best made in consultation with a genetic counselor and a medical geneticist. The National Society of Genetic Counselors maintains a website that provides the names and locations of genetic counselors, including those who specialize in cancer genetics. The address for this website is: http://www.nsgc.org/resourcelink.asp.

Are there ways that women with a family history of breast cancer can modify their breast cancer risk?

Studies of women with mutations in BRCA1 and BRCA2 argue that there are factors that modify the risk of breast cancer for women with these mutations, as well as for women with a genetically undefined family history of breast cancer. Women from the same family with the same BRCA1 or BRCA2 mutation can have different patterns of disease. Differences in whether cancer develops at all, in the age of cancer diagnosis, and in whether they develop breast or ovarian cancer can be observed. The most likely explanation for these patterns is different exposures to lifestyle and other environmental factors that modify these women's risk. However, genetic differences between these women may also contribute to differences in risk.

Many studies have evaluated whether the established risk factors for breast cancer (such as age of menarche, age of menopause, age of first child's birth) might affect women with a family history of breast cancer differently. The results of these studies have been inconsistent. However, a collaborative study pooled and reanalyzed the data from fifty-two different studies of 58,200 women with a first-degree (mother, daughter, or sister) family history of breast cancer. In this reanalysis the established breast cancer risk factors did not affect these women with a family history of breast cancer to a greater extent than women without a family history. These results support the idea that family history acts largely by itself as a risk factor.

A few studies have examined eating habits and breast cancer risk for women with a family history of breast cancer. A promising large cohort study, part of the Nurses Health Study, reported on women with a family history of breast cancer. In this study, postmenopausal women with a family history of breast cancer who ate five or more servings of fruits and vegetables a day decreased their breast cancer risk by 71 percent; no effect was reported for women without a family history. A second, more recent, study of these women reported decreased risk associated with carotene-rich foods (such as carrots, sweet potatoes, and broccoli). This study also reported a decrease in risk associated with breast-feeding and strenuous activity as a young adult. Some but not all reports associated increased risk with alcohol consumption for women with a family history of breast cancer.

Another large cohort study, based in Iowa, found a synergistic link between family history and waist-to-hip ratio, the size of the waist divided by the size of the hips. Women with a high waist-to-hip ratio (sometimes called apple shaped) and a family history of breast cancer had a 3.2-fold increase in breast cancer risk relative to women without this body characteristic or family history. In contrast, women with the same waist-to-hip ratio but without a family history of breast cancer had little or no increase in breast cancer risk.

A number of studies have specifically examined women with BRCA1 and BRCA2 mutations. Several have evaluated how these women's reproductive histories affected their breast cancer risk. The results of these studies have been inconclusive. Other studies have examined the effect of cigarette smoking and alcohol use on breast cancer risk in BRCA1 and BRCA2 mutation carriers; no conclusion could be made since the results of these studies differed. The effect of oral contraceptive use on these women's breast cancer risk is also undecided. Oral contraceptive use is an area of contention, as some reports have suggested an association of oral contraceptive use with decreased ovarian cancer in women with these mutations.

More study of how various factors might affect breast cancer risk in women with a family history of breast cancer is needed.

—Prepared by Barbour S. Warren, Ph.D., Cornell University Division of Nutritional Science, and Carol Devine, Ph.D., Extension Project Leader, BCERF, Cornell University

For More Information

Program on Breast Cancer and Environmental Risk Factors
Sprecher Institute for Comparative Cancer Research
Cornell University
Box 31
Ithaca, NY 14853
Phone: (607) 254-2893
Internet: http://envirocancer.cornell.edu
E-mail: breastcancer@cornell.edu

Chapter 20

Hormone Treatments and Breast Cancer Risk

Three recent clinical trials have changed the way postmenopausal hormone treatment is viewed. One of the trials was ended because of increases in breast cancer risk related to the treatment. Further, the decrease in the risk of heart and blood vessel disease that was expected was not found in any of these trials. Major health organizations have responded and suggested that use of this type of therapy be discontinued for health promotion and most disease prevention purposes. The decision to use birth control pills is difficult. Use of birth control pills has been associated with a small increase in breast cancer risk during the time that the pills are taken. Birth control pills also have other potential risks and benefits, beyond preventing pregnancy.

Hormone Treatment after Menopause and the Risk of Breast Cancer

What is menopause, and what physical symptoms are associated with this period of a woman's life?

Menopause is the time in a woman's life when she stops having menstrual periods completely. The average age of menopause in North

"Hormone Treatments and the Risk of Breast Cancer," by Barbour Warren, Ph.D., Research Associate, and Carol Devine, Ph.D., Division of Nutritional Sciences and Education Project Leader, Program on Breast Cancer and Environmental Risk Factors in New York State (BCERF), Fact Sheet #40, July 2002, © 2002 Cornell University, reprinted with permission.

American and European women is about fifty-one years old. Both her health and the society in which she lives affect how a woman deals with menopause. At midlife women experience a number of the physical effects of getting older, and some symptoms often associated with menopause are simply the result of aging, not of menopause itself.

Symptoms that women experience at menopause vary among cultures. North American and European women often have hot flashes, night sweats, and vaginal dryness. Hot flashes cause problems for many but not all women. The number of hot flashes increases during the time leading up to menopause. They are most frequent at about the time of menopause and then decline rapidly afterward. Symptoms that women have that may or may not be connected with menopause are incontinence (leaking urine when sneezing or laughing), forgetfulness, depression, a decrease in sexual desire, and joint pains.

How do hormone levels change during a woman's transition to menopause?

The levels of hormones that are important for childbearing change at this period of a woman's life. Hormone levels normally change during a woman's menstrual periods, but during the time before menopause the changes become more frequent. After menopause, the levels of a number of hormones change. Estrogen and progesterone levels are greatly decreased but the levels of other reproductive hormones are increased or may decrease. After menopause, women's fat tissues become the major source of estrogen and may affect estrogen levels.

Do the hormone changes at menopause carry health risks?

Lower levels of estrogen in women after menopause contribute to one type of osteoporosis (brittle bones) and may play a role in heart disease. The relationship between estrogen and osteoporosis and heart disease is discussed in the following. Changes in the levels of the other reproductive hormones have not been directly linked to adverse health effects. On the other hand, a woman's lifetime exposure to estrogen is thought to be related to her risk of breast cancer, and an earlier age at menopause and loss of estrogen are associated with lower breast cancer risk.

What is postmenopausal hormone treatment and why is it used?

Postmenopausal hormone treatment (hormone replacement therapy) is the use of estrogen alone or together with progesterone after menopause.

Postmenopausal hormone treatment has typically been prescribed to women for three purposes: (1) to limit the symptoms of menopause; (2) to reduce bone loss in women with or at risk for osteoporosis; and (3) to potentially decrease the risk of heart disease in postmenopausal women.

Estrogen may be given alone if a woman has had her uterus surgically removed (hysterectomy). Hormone treatment is also given to women whose ovaries have been removed surgically for medical reasons (ovariectomy, oophorectomy). Estrogen given alone increases the risk of uterine (endometrial) cancer. Adding progesterone to the treatment limits the negative effects of estrogen on the uterus, so women with a uterus are given progesterone with estrogen. Progesterone must be given along with estrogen treatment for at least ten days of a monthly cycle of treatment. Epidemiological studies indicate no increase in the risk of uterine cancer among women who use postmenopausal hormone treatment with estrogen and continuous progesterone but this is not yet known for certain. Hormone treatment may also be used over the short term to control some of the symptoms of menopause.

Does postmenopausal hormone treatment increase the risk of breast cancer?

Women who use postmenopausal hormone treatment have a higher risk for breast cancer compared with women who do not use hormone treatment. In the past, hormone treatment used estrogen alone, and the effects of this treatment have been studied more extensively. These early studies saw breast cancer risk increase with the length of the estrogen treatment. Breast cancer risk among women who used hormone treatment increased about 2 percent for each year of use, compared to women who did not use hormones. When hormone treatment is stopped, risk falls to previous levels over a period of five years. Today, most women who receive postmenopausal hormone treatment use estrogen combined with progesterone. A number of recent studies indicate a higher risk of breast cancer is associated with this form of hormone treatment. These studies found that estrogen with progesterone treatment increased breast cancer risk by 6 percent to 8 percent for each year of use. Confirming these results, a large clinical trial examining estrogen with progesterone treatment in healthy women, the Women's Health Initiative, was recently ended prematurely because of an association of excessive breast cancer risk with this treatment. Trials of this type are the "gold standard" for examining drug effects, and this early termination result raises strong concern about the use of estrogen with progesterone as a beneficial treatment for healthy women after menopause. [Note: Updated information regarding the Women's Health Initiative can be found online at http://www.nhlbi.nih.gov/whi or be obtained by calling the National Heart, Lung, and Blood Institute at 301-592-8573.]

Does postmenopausal hormone treatment prevent or help control heart and blood vessel disease?

It is unlikely that postmenopausal hormone treatment can prevent or help control existing heart disease. Early studies had found benefits of hormone treatment for reducing the risk of heart and blood vessel disease in women. The results of these early studies were limited because they compared women who chose to use hormone treatment to women who did not. Women in these studies who chose to use hormones may have differed from women who did not in important ways that would have affected their heart disease risk, such as diet or exercise. A more definite way to determine how hormone treatment affected heart disease is through a clinical trial. In these studies, individuals are randomly assigned to receive an active or inactive (placebo) treatment, and which treatment a person receives is unknown until the study is ended. Recent clinical trials have examined the effect of postmenopausal hormone treatment for women who already have heart disease. Two trials examined the effect of postmenopausal hormone treatment on women with existing heart and blood vessel disease. The results of both studies surprised researchers by showing no benefit of hormone treatment for women who already had heart disease These studies have questioned the idea that postmenopausal hormone treatment could help control heart disease. This question was answered by the Women's Health Initiative, the large clinical trial examining estrogen with progesterone for potential benefits including those to the heart and blood vessels. Although this study had to be terminated early, it indicated that it was unlikely that estrogen with progesterone treatment would be of benefit for heart and blood vessel disease. Both the National Heart, Lung, and Blood Institute and the American Heart Association have recommended that use of this type of therapy for women with existing disease or for prevention of heart and blood vessel disease be discontinued.

Does postmenopausal hormone treatment reduce the risk of osteoporosis?

Continuous postmenopausal hormone treatment will reduce the risk of osteoporosis and is one treatment that can be used for this disease. Osteoporosis happens when bones lose calcium and other minerals, making them more fragile and easily broken. Osteoporosis is a serious problem; broken bones can lead to pain, infection, limited ability to get around, and even death. Whether a woman develops osteoporosis as she gets older depends on how much bone she has built up by about age thirty and how quickly she loses calcium from her bones as she gets older. While some bone loss occurs in everyone with aging, some women are more likely to get osteoporosis. Risk for osteoporosis depends on a woman's family history, her estrogen levels, her diet, the amount of exercise she gets, and whether she smokes or drinks alcohol. The loss of estrogens at menopause is considered to be responsible for a short period of quick bone loss during this life period. Significant osteoporosis is seen in about a third of postmenopausal women in the United States. Prevention of osteoporosis does not necessarily require hormone treatment. Successful risk reduction has also been reported using calcium and vitamin D supplements and exercise. The best prevention is adequate calcium and vitamin D intake and physical activity in childhood and adolescence. The Women's Health Initiative (the clinical study described previously) is also studying calcium and vitamin D supplements as treatments to prevent osteoporosis in postmenopausal women.

Are there other health risks associated with postmenopausal hormone treatment?

Other studies have indicated that women who used postmenopausal hormone treatment may have higher rates of ovarian cancer, gall bladder disease, and problems associated with increased blood clotting compared to women who did not use hormone treatment. Postmenopausal hormone treatment is associated with, at most, a small increase in ovarian cancer risk. Women who used hormone therapies containing estrogen had two to four times the amount of gall bladder disease, compared to women who did not use hormone treatment.

How can women weigh the benefits and the risks of hormone treatment for themselves?

Women, with their health care providers, should decide whether to use postmenopausal hormonal treatment based on their current health, the severity of their menopausal symptoms, and their health history. Risk factors that should be considered are a family or personal history of breast cancer and other reproductive cancers, a personal history of blood clotting problems, existing heart and blood vessel disease, and a personal history of gall bladder disease. Women with a family history of heart and blood vessel disease or women at risk for osteoporosis may benefit from hormone treatment. It should also be noted that other medications and lifestyle changes could be used to control these diseases, as well as the symptoms of menopause.

Should breast cancer survivors consider hormone treatment?

Hormone treatment is not recommended for breast cancer survivors. Known or suspected breast cancer is currently considered a contraindication for hormone treatment. Investigators have suggested the need for randomized clinical trials, to assure safety, before breast cancer survivors use hormone therapy.

Use of Birth Control Pills and the Risk of Breast Cancer

What hormones are used in birth control pills and how do they work?

The birth control pills used today contain an estrogen and a progesterone. Birth control pills are thought to prevent conception by acting on the reproductive system in four complementary ways: (1) they prevent ovulation, the release of an egg; (2) they interfere with movement of the egg to the sites for fertilization and then growth; (3) they hamper preparation of the uterus (womb) to receive the fertilized egg; and (4) they change the consistency of cervical mucus, making it difficult for sperm to reach and fertilize the egg. Birth control pills are very effective. Used properly they prevent pregnancy in 97 percent to 98 percent of menstrual cycles.

Is the use of birth control pills associated with increased breast cancer risk?

Women who are currently taking birth control pills have a small increase in their risk of breast cancer relative to women who have never taken birth control. This finding is the result of the cooperative reanalysis of fifty-four studies (53,000 women with breast cancer and 100,000 women as controls) that examined the relationship between birth control pills and breast cancer risk. Ten years after women had stopped using birth control pills their risk for breast cancer was back to normal. How long birth control pills were used, the dose of hormone, or the type of the hormone used did not have an effect on breast cancer risk. However, women who began using birth control pills before age twenty may have a greater risk of premenopausal breast cancer than women who started birth control use later in life. It is currently unclear if women with a family history of breast cancer may increase their risk of breast cancer if they use birth control pills. More studies are needed examining women who began birth control pill use early in life and women with a family history of breast cancer. One of the limits to understanding how birth control pills affect breast cancer risk is that their hormone composition has changed several times since they were first released. Birth control pills in use today use lower hormone doses than those used in the past. These lower-dose pills have not been in use long enough to have been included in many of these studies. More studies are needed to determine if the lower dose of hormones in currently used birth control pills has changed their effect on breast cancer risk.

Is birth control pill use associated with other health risks?

Three other groups of health risks have been associated with birth control pill use. First, their use is linked with an increased risk of blood clots, especially in women older than thirty-five who smoke. Second, their use is potentially associated with an increase in the risk of some other cancers, such as liver and cervical cancer. Third, their use is associated with other changes in body systems and hormone levels. For example, birth control pills increase one's risk of gall bladder disease.

Are there health benefits associated with birth control pill use?

The use of birth control pills containing estrogen and progesterone has been associated with decreased risk of ovarian and uterine cancers. In general, risk of both these cancers was reduced by approximately 50 percent.

The health risks for women during pregnancy are greater than those seen among women who use birth control pills. For instance, the risk of increased blood clotting during pregnancy is higher than that seen during birth control use. Nonetheless, it should be kept in mind that a number of other safe and effective methods of birth control also exist.

Should breast cancer survivors use birth control pills?

It is not recommended that women who are survivors of breast cancer use birth control pills. As with hormone therapy, known or suspected breast cancer is a contraindication for using these drugs.

What can women do now?

- Maintain a healthy heart and bones by getting plenty of exercise.

- Maintain a healthy body weight, neither too fat nor too thin.

- Eat plenty of calcium-rich foods such as low-fat dairy products, leafy greens, and hard tofu and make sure that calcium intake is a least 1,000 mg daily before menopause and 1,200 mg daily after menopause.

- Do not smoke.

- Choose a diet low in fat, especially saturated fats from meat and dairy products.

- Choose a diet high in fiber from whole grains, vegetables, and fruits.

—Prepared by Barbour Warren, Ph.D., BCERF Research Associate, Cornell University and Carol Devine, Ph.D., BCERF Educational Project Leader, Cornell University

For More Information

Program on Breast Cancer and Environmental Risk Factors
Sprecher Institute for Comparative Cancer Research
Cornell University
Box 31
Ithaca, NY 14853
Phone: (607) 254-2893
Internet: http://envirocancer.cornell.edu
E-mail: breastcancer@cornell.edu

Chapter 21

Breast Cancer Risk and Other Known Health Effects in Women Prescribed DES while Pregnant

I was prescribed DES during my pregnancy. Am I at an increased risk for any health problems?

Women prescribed DES while pregnant are at a modestly increased risk for developing breast cancer. Studies have consistently reported an increased risk of approximately 30 percent for women prescribed DES while pregnant. The most recent study, published in the *British Journal of Cancer* (Titus-Ernstoff, 2001), included more than six thousand women and compared breast cancer rates of women exposed to DES with rates among women who were not exposed. This study followed participants over a longer period of time than did earlier research on breast cancer risks associated with DES. The researchers' findings were consistent with earlier studies, confirming an increased breast cancer risk of approximately 30 percent for women prescribed DES while pregnant. That means when considering breast cancer risks across a lifetime, one in six women prescribed DES during pregnancy will get breast cancer. In comparison, only one in eight unexposed women will get breast cancer across their lifetime.

Reprinted from "Known Health Effects for Women Prescribed DES while Pregnant," U.S. Department of Health and Human Services, Centers for Disease Control and Prevention, updated April 2004, and "DES Brand Names," U.S. Department of Health and Human Services, Centers for Disease Control and Prevention, updated April 2004.

153

Table 21.1. DES Brand Names. Following are the names under which DES has been sold in the United States:

Nonsteroidal Estrogens	**Nonsteroidal Estrogens, continued**	**Nonsteroidal Estrogens, continued**
Benzestrol	Microest	Synthosestrin
Chlorotrianisene	Methallenestrol	Tace
Comestrol	Mikarol	Vallestril
Cyren A	Mikarol forti	Willestrol
Cyren B	Milestrol	
Delvinal	Monomestrol	**Nonsteroidal Estrogen-Androgen Combination**
DES	Neo-Oestranol I	
DesPlex	Neo-Oestranol II	
Dibestil	Nulabort	
Diestryl	Oestrogenine	Amperone
Dienestrol	Oestromenin	Di-Erone
Dienoestrol	Oestromon	Estan
Diethylstilbestrol	Orestol	Metystil
dipalmitate	Pabestrol D	Teserene
Diethylstilbestrol	Palestrol	Tylandril
diphosphate	Restrol	Tylostereone
Diethylstilbestrol	Stil-Rol	
dipropionate	Stilbal	**Nonsteroidal Estrogen-Progesterone Combination**
Diethylstilbenediol	Stilbestrol	
Digestil	Stilbestronate	
Domestrol	Stilbetin	
Estilben	Stilbinol	Progravidium
Estrobene	Stilboestroform	
Estrobene DP	Stilboestrol	**Vaginal Cream Suppositories with Nonsteroidal Estrogens**
Estrosyn	Stilboestrol DP	
Fonatol	Stilestrate	
Gynben	Stilpalmitate	
Gyneben	Stilphostrol	AVC Cream with
Hexestrol	Stilronate	Dienestrol
Hexoestrol	Stilrone	Dienestrol Cream
Hi-Bestrol	Stils	
Menocrin	Synestrin	
Meprane	Synestrol	
Mestilbol		

Source: National Cancer Institute, "Exposure in utero to Diethylstilbestrol and Related Synthetic Hormones," *JAMA* 236, no. 10 (1976): 1107–9.

Table 21.2. A Woman's Chance of Being Diagnosed with Breast Cancer

from age 30 to age 40	1 out of 257 women
from age 40 to age 50	1 out of 67 women
from age 50 to age 60	1 out of 36 women
from age 60 to age 70	1 out of 28 women
from age 70 to age 80	1 out of 24 women
Ever	1 out of 8 women

Source: National Cancer Institute Surveillance, Epidemiology, and End Results Program, 1995–97.

Why haven't I heard about a connection between DES and breast cancer?

Early studies of women prescribed DES while pregnant were inconclusive. Even now, not all researchers agree that there is a link between DES exposure and breast cancer. Despite differences of opinion, the 2001 *British Journal of Cancer* study is important for two reasons. First, it is the largest study of its kind. Second, participants in the 2001 study were older than participants in previous studies; as women grow older, their chances for developing breast cancer increase, regardless of whether they were exposed to DES. Because participants were older, many more women had breast cancer in the 2001 study than in earlier studies. This provides the 2001 study with more "power" to detect meaningful differences between the rates of breast cancer among women who were and were not exposed to DES. In other words, the more women included in a study, the less likely that the results of the study can be considered chance. Now researchers can confirm with a higher degree of certainty that women prescribed DES while pregnant have a modestly increased risk of breast cancer.

How does being prescribed DES while pregnant compare with other risk factors for breast cancer?

Exposure to DES while pregnant is just one of many factors that can increase a woman's chance of developing breast cancer. Several other factors can further increase the risk for breast cancer, including personal and family history of breast cancer, genetics, diet and

155

lifestyle choices, use of hormone replacement therapy (HRT), and having children later in life. In addition, as women grow older, their chances of developing breast cancer increase, regardless of whether they were exposed to DES. Table 21.2 explains the increasing risk for breast cancer as a woman ages. This table illustrates breast cancer risk for women who were not exposed to DES while pregnant.

If I was prescribed DES while pregnant, what can I do now to increase my chances for early detection of breast cancer?

You should follow a regular schedule for the breast cancer screening recommended by your health care provider. The types and timing of the screening should be based on your risk factors for breast cancer. Talk with your health care provider about when you should start screenings for breast cancer and how often you should be checked. Your health care provider may recommend that you learn and practice breast self-examination as a way to detect any lumps in your breasts, discharge from the nipples, or skin changes (such as dimpling or puckering). Most health care providers will recommend that women forty years of age and older have a mammogram (an x-ray of the breast) every one to two years. In addition, most health care providers perform clinical breast examinations (visual and manual examination of the breast) during routine physical examinations.

For more information about breast cancer causes and prevention, visit the NCI website at www.cancer.gov or call the Cancer Information Service (CIS) toll-free 1-800-4-CANCER (1-800-422-6237).

Chapter 22

Dietary Fat and Breast Cancer

Eating large amounts of saturated fat could slightly increase the risk of breast cancer, according to a large-scale review of the evidence published in the *British Journal of Cancer*.[1]

The analysis—which included twenty-five thousand cases of breast cancer from forty-five separate studies—also found an association between high meat consumption and the risk of developing the disease.

Previous research on the effects of dietary fat has produced conflicting and confusing results. But the new Canadian report suggests the relationship between breast cancer and dietary fat may be independent of obesity or high calorie consumption, reinforcing the need for a healthy, balanced diet.

Scientists at the Ontario Cancer Institute in Canada reviewed all the published literature on dietary fat and breast cancer and combined results from 45 different studies, employing a range of methodologies. The data included 25,000 breast cancer patients and more than 580,000 healthy women worldwide.

They took into account other known and suspected risk factors for breast cancer and compared women with the highest and lowest fat intake, in order to assess whether or not dietary fat was contributing to the disease.

Women who ate high amounts of saturated fat were on average around 20 percent more likely to develop breast cancer than low consumers of fat. Eating large amounts of monounsaturated fats increased risk by about 10 percent—a nonsignificant difference—while overall fat consumption was related to a small, but statistically significant increase in risk of 13 percent.

Researchers also found a small significant increase in risk with high meat consumption. Women who ate large amounts of meat were 17 percent more likely to develop breast cancer than those who ate little or none.

Dr. Norman Boyd, lead researcher on the study, commented, "We already know that being obese can increase the risk of a range of cancers, but evidence is building that eating large amounts of fat, particularly the saturated kind, can independently increase risk. Our analysis of all the available research suggests there is indeed an association with saturated fat and breast cancer. The increase in risk seems fairly modest, even among very high consumers of fat, although the difficulties in measuring dietary intake mean we could be underestimating the true scale of the effect. In any case, the effect seems to be over and above the increase in risk from obesity and underlines the message that high consumption of fat is bad for your health."

Scientists from Cancer Research UK and the Medical Research Council recently found that one of the common methods used to measure fat in the diet may have been helping to obscure its effect on breast cancer.[2] When they asked people to remember the foods they had eaten using food frequency questionnaires, they found only a small increase in risk with dietary fat, but the effect of fat seemed to be much larger when they used food diaries to record diet on a daily basis. The new analysis combined data from both kinds of study and has strengthened the evidence that fat and meat consumption can contribute to breast cancer.

Dr. Lesley Walker, director of cancer information at Cancer Research UK, which owns the *British Journal of Cancer,* says: "It's been very difficult to separate out the effects of dietary fat and obesity, and previous studies have been inconclusive. But by combining data from a wide range of studies using different methods and including a very large number of people, this research provides the strongest indication yet that dietary fat has an independent effect on the risk of breast cancer. Tying down the various dietary contributors to cancer is important, as it will allow us to give the best possible advice about how to avoid cancer. The effect of dietary fat looks quite small, but the results add weight to the importance of a healthy, balanced diet, low in saturated fat and containing plenty of fruit and vegetables.

References

1. *British Journal of Cancer* 89(9); 2. *The Lancet* 362 (9379): 212–14.

Chapter 23

Hormones in Food and Breast Cancer Risk

This chapter addresses some of the consumer concerns that have been brought to the Program on Breast Cancer and Environmental Risk Factors in New York State (BCERF) regarding health effects of hormones used by the meat and dairy industries. Evidence available so far, though not conclusive, does not link hormone residues in meat or milk with any human health effect.

What are hormones?

Hormones are chemicals that are produced naturally in the bodies of all animals, including humans. They are chemical messages released into the blood by hormone-producing organs that travel to and affect different parts of the body. Hormones may be produced in small amounts, but they control important body functions such as growth, development, and reproduction.

Hormones can have different chemistry. They can be steroids or proteins. Steroid hormones are active in the body when eaten. For example, birth control pills are steroid hormones and can be taken orally. In contrast, protein hormones are broken down in the stomach and lose their ability to act in the body when eaten. Therefore,

"Consumer Concerns about Hormones in Food," by Renu Gandhi, Ph.D., Research Associate, and Suzanne M. Snedeker, Ph.D., Associate Director for Translational Research, Program on Breast Cancer and Environmental Risk Factors in New York State (BCERF), Fact Sheet #37, updated May 2003, © 2003 Cornell University, reprinted with permission.

ordinarily, protein hormones need to be injected into the body to have an effect. For example, insulin is a protein hormone. Diabetic patients need to be injected with insulin for treatment.

Why are hormones used in food production?

Certain hormones can make young animals gain weight faster. They help reduce the waiting time and the amount of feed eaten by an animal before slaughter in meat industries. In dairy cows, hormones can be used to increase milk production. Thus, hormones can increase the profitability of the meat and dairy industries.

Why are consumers concerned about hormones in foods?

While a variety of hormones are produced by our bodies and are essential for normal development of healthy tissues, synthetic steroid hormones used as pharmaceutical drugs have been found to affect cancer risk. For example, diethylstilbestrol (DES), a synthetic estrogen drug used in the 1960s, was withdrawn from use after it was found to increase the risk of vaginal cancer in daughters of treated women. Lifetime exposure to natural steroid hormone estrogen is also associated with an increased risk for breast cancer. Hence, consumers are concerned about whether they are being exposed to hormones used to treat animals, and whether these hormones affect human health. We try to address this complex issue based on scientific evidence that is currently available.

What is the history of hormone use in food production?

As early as the 1930s, it was realized that cows injected with material drawn from bovine (cow) pituitary glands (hormone secreting organ) produced more milk. Later, the bovine growth hormone (bGH) from the pituitary glands was found to be responsible for this effect. However, at that time, technology did not exist to harvest enough of this material for large-scale use in animals. In the 1980s, it became possible to produce large quantities of pure bGH by using recombinant DNA technology. In 1993, the Food and Drug Administration (FDA) approved the recombinant bovine growth hormone (rbGH), also known as bovine somatotropin (rbST) for use in dairy cattle. Recent estimates by the manufacturer of this hormone indicate that 30 percent of the cows in the United States may be treated with rbGH.

The female sex hormone estrogen was also shown to affect growth rates in cattle and poultry in the 1930s. Once the chemistry of estrogen was understood, it became possible to make the hormone synthetically in large amounts. Synthetic estrogens started being used to increase the size of cattle and chickens in the early 1950s. DES was one of the first synthetic estrogens made and used commercially in the United States to fatten chickens. DES was also used as a drug in human medicine. DES was found to cause cancer and its use in food production was phased out in the late 1970s.

What are the different hormones used now by the meat and dairy industries?

There are six different kinds of steroid hormones that are currently approved by the FDA for use in food production in the United States: estradiol, progesterone, testosterone, zeranol, trenbolone acetate, and melengestrol acetate. Estradiol and progesterone are natural female sex hormones; testosterone is the natural male sex hormone; zeranol, trenbolone acetate, and melengestrol acetate are synthetic growth promoters (hormone-like chemicals that can make animals grow faster). Currently, federal regulations allow these hormones to be used on growing cattle and sheep, but not on poultry (chickens, turkeys, ducks) or hogs (pigs). These hormones are not as useful in increasing weight gain of poultry or hogs. As mentioned earlier, the FDA allows the use of the protein hormone rbGH to increase milk production in dairy cattle. This protein hormone is not used on beef cattle.

How are the hormones introduced into the animals?

Steroid hormones are usually released into the animal from a pellet (ear implant) that is put under the skin of the ear. The ears of the animals are thrown away at slaughter. Improper use of pellet implants in other parts of the animal can result in higher levels of hormone residues remaining in the edible meat. Federal regulations prohibit their use in this manner. Melengestrol acetate is also available in a form that can be added to animal feed.

Dairy cattle may be injected under the skin with rbGH. This hormone is available in packages of single-dose injections to reduce chances of accidental overdose.

Do federal agencies monitor for the presence of these hormones in food?

Estradiol, progesterone, and testosterone are sex hormones that are made naturally by animals. No regulatory monitoring of these hormones is possible, since it is not possible to separate the hormones used for treatment from those made by the animal's own body. However, it is possible to detect residues of zeranol and trenbolone acetate in the animal's meat. The FDA has set the tolerance levels for these hormones. A tolerance is the maximum amount of a particular residue that may be permitted in or on food. The Food Safety Inspection Service (FSIS) of the U.S. Department of Agriculture (USDA) monitors meat from cattle for zeranol residues. The FSIS also monitors meats for DES residues from any illegal use (DES use is no longer permitted). In response to concern about cases of early puberty in Puerto Rico described in the following, a large number of meat samples were tested for hormone residues in the mid- to late 1980s. No zeranol or DES residues were found in the meat samples in this survey.

Do hormones remain in the milk or meat of treated animals?

The levels of naturally produced hormones vary from animal to animal, and a range in these levels is known to be normal. Because it is not possible to differentiate between the hormones produced naturally by the animal and those used to treat the animal, it is difficult to determine exactly how much of the hormone used for treatment remains in the meat or the milk. Studies indicate that if correct treatment and slaughter procedures are followed, the levels of these hormones may be slightly higher in the treated animal's meat or milk, but are still within the normal range of natural variation known to occur in untreated animals. Scientists are currently trying to develop better methods to measure steroid hormone residues left in edible meat from a treated animal.

Can steroid hormones in meat affect the age of puberty for girls?

Early puberty in girls has been found to be associated with a higher risk for breast cancer. Height, weight, diet, exercise, and family history have all been found to influence age of puberty. Steroid hormones in food were suspected to cause early puberty in girls in some reports. However, exposure to higher than natural levels of steroid hormones through hormone-treated meat or poultry has never been documented. Large epidemiological studies have not been done to see whether early puberty in developing girls is associated with having eaten growth-hormone-treated foods.

162

A concern about an increase in cases of girls reaching puberty or menarche early (at age eight or younger) in Puerto Rico led to an investigation in the early 1980s by the Centers for Disease Control (CDC). Samples of meat and chicken from Puerto Rico were tested for steroid hormone residues. One laboratory found a chicken sample from a local market to have a higher than normal level of estrogen. Also, residues of zeranol were reported in the blood of some of the girls who had reached puberty early. However, these results could not be verified by other laboratories. Following the CDC's investigation, the USDA tested 150 to 200 beef, poultry, and milk samples from Puerto Rico in 1985 and found no residues of DES, zeranol, or estrogen in these samples.

In another study in Italy, steroid hormone residues in beef and poultry in school meals were suspected as the cause of breast enlargement in very young girls and boys. However, the suspect beef and poultry samples were not available to test for the presence of hormones. Without proof that exposure to higher levels of steroid hormones occurred through food, it is not possible to conclude whether eating hormone-treated meat or poultry caused the breast enlargement in these cases.

Can eating meat from hormone-treated animals affect breast cancer risk?

Evidence does not exist to answer this question. The amount of steroid hormone that is eaten through meat of a treated animal is negligible compared to what the human body produces each day. The breast cancer risk of women who eat meat from hormone-treated animals has not been compared with the risk of women who eat meat from untreated animals.

Can drinking milk or eating dairy products from hormone-treated animals affect breast cancer risk?

Once again, evidence does not exist to answer this question. Use of rbGH for dairy cattle has been in practice in the United States for only six to seven years. Breast cancer can take many years to develop. It is too early to study the breast cancer risk of women who drink milk and eat milk products from hormone-treated animals.

Can hormones that remain in milk affect human health?

Scientists at the FDA's Center for Veterinary Medicine have reviewed the studies submitted by the manufacturers of rbGH. FDA scientists have concluded that eating foods with slightly higher levels of rbGH would not affect human health. This is because the amount of rbGH that is in milk or milk products as a result of treatment of the animals is insignificant compared to the amount of growth hormone that is naturally produced by our bodies. Also, rbGH is a protein hormone and is digested into smaller fragments (peptides and amino acids) when eaten. The rbGH hormone used on dairy cattle is effective in promoting growth in cows, but does not work in humans. Scientists know that rbGH is not recognized as a hormone by human cells.

There are gaps in our knowledge about whether rbGH used to treat dairy cattle can cause indirect effects. These gaps lead to uncertainties and debates, some of which are addressed in the following.

What do we know about growth factors in milk of treated animals?

The wholesomeness of milk is not affected by rbGH treatment. However, some subtle changes do take place in the treated animal. The growth hormone typically acts by triggering the cells to make other chemicals, called growth factors. These growth factors actually cause the increase in growth rate and milk production. Milk from rbGH-treated cattle has been found to have slightly higher levels of the naturally produced protein called insulin-dependent growth factor-1 (IGF-1). IGF-1 is a protein and is digested into smaller pieces in the stomach.

Scientists at the FDA have considered the evidence from studies of cancer risk in people who have naturally high body levels of IGF-1. Higher levels of IGF-1 in blood have been found in women with breast cancer compared to women without breast cancer in the Harvard-based Nurses' Health Study. Scientists are investigating if IGF-1 is just present at higher levels in breast cancer patients or if it has a role in increasing the risk for the disease. In laboratory studies, breast cancer cells growing on a plastic dish grow at a faster rate when bathed in a solution containing IGF-1. However, IGF-1 also plays an important role in helping normal cells grow. Hence, from these few studies, we cannot conclude whether IGF-1 increases breast cancer risk.

FDA scientists have concluded that IGF-1 in milk is unlikely to present any human food safety concern for the following reasons: (1) IGF-1 levels in cow's milk from untreated animals vary in nature, depending on the number of calves and the lactation stage; (2) IGF-1 is also present in human breast milk, at levels higher than in hormone-treated cow's milk; (3) IGF-1 in milk is not expected to act as a growth factor in people who drink it because it gets digested in the stomach; (4) IGF-1 needs to be injected into the blood to have a growth-promoting effect; and (5) increased IGF-1 levels in food are not expected to result in higher blood levels of IGF-1 in humans who eat the food.

What are the concerns about milk-related allergies?

A detailed discussion of this topic is beyond the scope of this chapter. A brief outline of the issue is presented here, along with references for more information. Digested or broken down fragments of proteins absorbed through the stomach can cause the immune system to produce antibodies, which sometimes can lead to milk-related allergies. There have been studies done to investigate whether the immune system can react to fragments of rbGH and IGF-1 absorbed through the stomach. Reviewers of these studies at Health Canada (the Canadian counterpart to the FDA) expressed a concern that in one study some of the laboratory rats that were fed high levels of rbGH for ninety days developed antibodies against it (http://www.hc-sc.gc.ca/english/archives/rbst). Scientists at the FDA evaluated these studies in rats and concluded that only animals that were fed a very large amount of rbGH in food produced antibodies against it. Such large amounts of rbGH are not expected to occur in the milk that humans drink ("Report on the Food and Drug Administration's Review of the Safety of Bovine Somatotropin" available at: http://www.fda.gov/cvm; a copy of this report can be requested by calling: 310-574-1755).

Studies have also looked at whether IGF-1 fed to laboratory rats and digested in the stomach can affect the immune system. No immune effects were observed in these studies, but the animals were fed IGF-1 for only two weeks. No studies have been done on the effects of feeding rats or other experimental animals with IGF-1 over longer periods of time.

Are hormone-treated animals healthy?

There is a concern that because of increased milking, hormone-treated cows may become more prone to infection of the udders, called mastitis. This could lead to more antibiotics being used to treat the cows, in turn leading to more residues of antibiotics to remain in the milk. Frequent exposure to antibiotic residues through milk or dairy products is a health concern for people over the long term. In the normal body, there are bacteria that live in the gut and mouth and help in the digestion of food in the gut. These "friendly" bacteria do not normally cause disease since the immune system keeps them in check. However, if the immune system is weak, these "friendly" bacteria can invade tissues and cause infection. Bacteria in the normal body that come across small amounts of antibiotics frequently can develop ways to survive the antibiotics and become "antibiotic resistant." In cases of infection and illness, it then becomes more difficult to control such resistant bacteria with the available antibiotics.

Some increase in incidence of antibiotic residues was observed in cow's milk following the use of rbGH. At the same time that rbGH started being used, some of the major dairy states in the United States switched over to a new and improved method to test for antibiotic residues. It is difficult to determine whether the increase in incidence of antibiotic residues in milk was due to increased use or better testing methods. New York State (NYS) was one of the states that did not change its method of testing for antibiotic residues in milk at that time. The incidence of antibiotic residues in milk from NYS was not found to be higher after the approval of rbGH use. This suggests that the increased incidence of antibiotic residues observed in some states may have been due to better testing methods rather than an increase in use of antibiotics for treatment of mastitis. An Expert Committee at the FDA's Center for Veterinary Medicine has concluded that while rbGH use may cause a slight increase in mastitis, dairy management practices that are currently in use should prevent any increase in antibiotic residues in milk.

Are growth hormones used elsewhere in the world?

The debate on whether growth hormones should or should not be used for food production has become a very political issue. In 1989, the European Community (now European Union) issued a ban on all meat from animals treated with steroid growth hormones, which is still in effect. The use of steroid hormones for beef cattle is permitted in Canada. Countries within the European Union do not allow the use of the protein hormone rbGH for dairy cattle. In 1999, the Canadian government refused approval for the sale of rbGH for dairy cattle, based on concerns about the health effects, including mastitis in treated animals.

Conclusions

Studies done so far do not provide evidence to state that hormone residues in meat or dairy products cause any human health effects. However, a conclusion on lack of human health effect can be made only after large-scale studies compare the health of people who eat meat or dairy products from hormone-treated animals to people who eat a similar diet, but from untreated animals.

Where is more research needed?

Some of the consumer concerns in this chapter cannot be answered conclusively without further studies:

- Exposure to hormones in meat was suspected as the cause for early puberty in girls in Puerto Rico and Italy, but was never verified. To conclusively answer the question, large-scale epidemiological studies would be needed to compare the age of puberty in girls who eat meat from hormone-treated animals to those who eat meat from untreated animals. Such studies would need to make sure that other known influences that affect the age of puberty in girls are not playing a role.

- Short-term studies in laboratory rats have not indicated a concern about milk-related allergies or immune effects from exposure to rbGH or IGF-1 in milk or dairy products. However, short-term studies cannot be used to rule out all possibilities of any immune or unexpected health effects after long-term exposure. Studies in laboratory animals on effects of lifelong exposure to milk from rbGH-treated cows may help answer this question.

Some healthy diet tips that also help reduce exposure to hormones used in food production.

While currently available evidence does not indicate a link between eating meat, milk, or dairy products from hormone-treated animals and any health effects, adopting some known healthy diet habits can help reduce exposure to hormones used in meat, poultry, and dairy production.

- Eat a varied diet, rich in fruits, grains, and vegetables.
- Eat meats in moderation, well cooked, but not charred.

- Eat more lean muscle meat, less liver and fat.

—Prepared by Renu Gandhi, Ph.D., Research Associate, BCERF, Cornell University and Suzanne M. Snedeker, Ph.D., Research Project Leader, BCERF, Cornell University

For More Information

Program on Breast Cancer and Environmental Risk Factors
Sprecher Institute for Comparative Cancer Research
Cornell University
Box 31
Ithaca, NY 14853
Phone: (607) 254-2893
Internet: http://envirocancer.cornell.edu
E-mail: breastcancer@cornell.edu

Chapter 24

Smoking and Breast Cancer Risk

Tobacco smoke is highly addictive and has been linked to 20 percent of all deaths in the United States. It contains many cancer-causing chemicals, and almost one-third of all cancer deaths are related to tobacco use. Tobacco smoking has generally been considered to have little or no association with breast cancer risk. Newer studies have challenged this conclusion and suggested a connection between smoking and an increased risk of breast cancer, but more investigation is needed to resolve this issue. Passive smoking has been linked with an increased risk of lung cancer and heart disease. Studies have also indicated a possible linkage between passive smoking and breast cancer risk, but settling this concern will require more study. Understanding the potential association of active and passive smoking with breast cancer risk is important, because women have some control over their exposure to tobacco smoke, unlike many other breast cancer risk factors.

Is smoking related to breast cancer risk?

The relationship between cigarette smoking and breast cancer risk is uncertain. Many studies have examined this relationship, and

"Smoking and Breast Cancer Risk," by Barbour Warren, Ph.D., Research Associate, and Carol Devine, Ph.D., R.D., Division of Nutritional Sciences and Education Project Leader, Program on Breast Cancer and Environmental Risk Factors in New York State (BCERF), Fact Sheet #46, November 2002, © 2002 Cornell University, reprinted with permission.

cigarette smoking has been considered to have little or no association with breast cancer risk. Yet recent studies of women who did not smoke but who lived or worked in environments where other people smoked (they were exposed to passive or secondhand smoke) have questioned the design and results of these earlier studies. Four studies have compared women who smoked to women who had no exposure to tobacco smoke (they had neither smoked nor had ever been passively exposed to tobacco smoke). In contrast, earlier studies had compared smokers to women who had never smoked or did not currently smoke but whose passive smoke exposure was unknown. All four of the newer studies reported increased breast cancer risk among the women who smoked cigarettes. They were all small case-control studies, and only one reported an increase in risk among women who smoked longer. Nonetheless, three of the studies reported that smokers had a statistically significantly increased breast cancer risk of two to four times that of women who neither smoked nor were ever passively exposed to tobacco smoke. This is an area of research with considerable disagreement. Recent review of this area of research by the International Agency for Research on Cancer (IARC) dismissed a linkage between smoking and breast cancer risk. A large number of women smoke or have smoked and resolution of this issue is important.

Is passive smoking related to breast cancer risk?

Although passive exposure to tobacco smoke has been linked to a number of health problems, it is unresolved whether it alters breast cancer risk. Most, but not all, studies that compared women who were passively exposed to tobacco smoke to women with no exposure to tobacco smoke reported an association of passive smoking with an increased risk of breast cancer. Only two of these studies showed a "dose-relationship," where an increase in breast cancer risk was related to more tobacco smoke exposure. Other studies, which compared the risk of breast cancer of women exposed to passive smoke to women with less clearly defined passive smoke exposure (nonsmokers or those who have never smoked), have reported conflicting associations with breast cancer risk; some studies reported increases in risk, some reported decreases in risk, and some reported no association with risk. All of these studies were also recently reviewed by the IARC. They found that it was unlikely that passive smoking increased breast cancer risk.

Several studies have found similar increases in breast cancer risk for both active and passive smoke exposures. These results have been criticized by some researchers. These researchers argue that this is an unlikely result, as smokers have much greater exposure since they are exposed to smoke both actively and passively, but further investigation will be required to resolve this issue. Possible reasons for the differences in the results of these studies are discussed in the following (see: "Why are there differences in the results of the human epidemiological studies examining breast cancer risk and passive exposure to tobacco smoke?").

Is the smoke inhaled during active smoking different from the smoke inhaled during passive smoking?

The tobacco smoke a smoker inhales is different from the smoke inhaled by those nearby. The major source of passive smoke is from the burning of the cigarette rather than what is exhaled by smokers. Both types of smoke contain thousands of chemicals. The chemicals present in both of these types of smoke are similar, but the concentrations of the chemicals are different. Many of the toxic chemicals in tobacco smoke are found in higher concentrations in the tobacco smoke as it leaves the cigarette compared to inhaled smoke; in some cases the concentrations are far higher. This smoke is largely produced from the lower-temperature burning of cigarettes between inhalations, and the chemicals are less degraded than in the smokers' inhalations. However, many factors, such room size and air flow, can affect the dilution of the smoke, and the resulting exposure can differ greatly.

How common is passive exposure to environmental tobacco smoke?

Passive exposure to tobacco smoke is very common. The most recent studies of the number of nonsmokers in the United States who are exposed to tobacco smoke were conducted in 1991. These studies used a breakdown product of nicotine, cotinine, in the blood of nonsmokers as a marker for tobacco smoke exposure. They reported that 90 percent of nonsmokers over four years old had measurable levels of cotinine. Due to changes in smoking policies since 1991, the prevalence of environmental tobacco smoke exposure may have decreased. Measurements made in 1999 of the typical levels of this marker in nonsmokers' blood were substantially lower than levels reported in

1991. Since these studies demonstrated that the typical levels of cotinine have decreased it is likely that the percentage of people who have detectable levels has also decreased.

Why are there differences in the results of the human epidemiological studies examining breast cancer risk and passive exposure to tobacco smoke?

The inconsistencies in the results of these studies arise from differences in their methodologies, the way they were carried out. The first difference is in the choice of women who served as the reference group, the women whose breast cancer risk was used as the level for risk comparison. Ideally, the women in the reference group and the women under study would differ only in their active or passive exposure to tobacco smoke. This ideal is seldom reached, and some of the differences in the results come from the extent to which these groups of women differ from this ideal.

Recent studies have used as a reference group women who had no exposure to tobacco smoke—that is, they have never actively or passively smoked. These studies in most cases have reported increases in breast cancer risk for women who smoked or were passively exposed to tobacco smoke compared to reference women who were never exposed. Critics of this approach cite studies that indicate the reference women who have never been exposed to tobacco smoke are healthier, in general. They argue that the difference in risk is due to the better health of these women used as references for risk. Older studies used as a reference group women who had never actively smoked or who were not current smokers but whose exposure to environmental smoke was unknown. These studies have largely reported no link between any exposure to tobacco smoke and breast cancer risk. Critics of this approach cite the potential for passive smoking and previous smoking to increase risk in control women and mask effects on the women under study.

A second potential source of the discrepancies may come from how the exposure or lack of exposure to environmental tobacco smoke is determined. Studies have shown that people can recall recent exposure very well but that remembering the duration and degree of distant exposure (such as whether their grandparents or baby-sitter smoked) is difficult. Yet one study examined this issue and found that women tended to underestimate their exposure, an effect that would decrease the observed risk. Thus, the information used in these studies may be inaccurate, which could influence the reported breast cancer risk association. More work is needed to resolve these issues.

How might smoking increase the risk of cancer in the breast, an organ that is not exposed to smoke?

It is biologically possible for active cigarette smoking or passive exposure to tobacco smoke to affect a woman's breast cancer risk. There is direct documentation that breasts are exposed to chemicals within tobacco smoke in active smokers. Study of the fluid in the ducts of the breast of smoking women has shown the presence of tobacco chemicals at higher concentrations than were found in blood. Women passively exposed to tobacco smoke have tobacco chemicals in their blood, too, but examinations of their breast fluid have not been carried out.

Both active and passive tobacco smoke exposure have been linked to nonrespiratory cancers. Active cigarette smoking has been associated with cancer of the bladder, cervix, stomach, pancreas, and kidney. The effects of passive exposure to tobacco smoke have been studied much less, but associations with cervical cancer in adult women, as well as leukemia and brain cancer in children, have been reported.

Does smoking at a young age or being passively exposed to tobacco smoke at a young age affect a woman 's breast cancer risk?

Exposure to tobacco smoke at a young age either by smoking or by being around people who smoke may be related to an increased breast cancer risk. Sixteen studies have examined smoking at a young age. These studies compared women who smoked at a young age to women who had never smoked or who were not currently smokers. Most studies reported a small increase in breast cancer risk associated with starting to smoke before age seventeen. Two studies used women who were never passively exposed to tobacco smoke as the comparison group and found about a doubling of breast cancer risk among young smokers; one of the studies reported this effect only for premenopausal breast cancer.

The association of exposure to passive smoke at a young age with breast cancer risk has been examined in five studies. These studies typically looked at exposure up to age nineteen. Four of these studies used women with no exposure to tobacco smoke as controls and reported approximately a doubling of breast cancer risk among women who were exposed to passive smoke. The remaining study used women who never smoked as the comparison and found no association between tobacco smoke exposure and breast cancer risk.

The breast undergoes a major period of development during adolescence, and studies in animals have demonstrated that this is a period of great susceptibility to cancer-causing agents. More study is needed in this area.

Does the number of years a woman has been smoking or the amount she smokes affect her breast cancer risk?

Increases in breast cancer risk, relative to how long a woman has smoked or the number of cigarettes she smoked a day, have been found in several studies. However, the relationship between breast cancer and the level of smoking exposure is not as clear as it is for lung cancer. For example, people who smoke the least (or for the shortest time) have the lowest risk of lung cancer, while people who smoke the most (or for the longest time) have the highest risk. People who smoke amounts between these two extremes have risks that fall between the two extremes. This is called a "dose-relationship" between lung cancer risk and smoking; the risk of lung cancer increases with the dose or amount a person smokes. Most breast cancer studies have not seen a dose-relationship between smoking and breast cancer risk. A possible explanation would be that there is an exposure level that must be exceeded for risk to increase; such a level is called a threshold. A threshold effect is possible but has not been described for other smoking-related diseases.

Why did some earlier studies report an association of active smoking and decreased breast cancer risk?

Most of the epidemiological studies that compared breast cancer risk of active smokers to women who were not smokers (regardless of their passive smoke exposure) found no association between smoking and breast cancer risk. Yet several studies found that women who smoked had a decreased breast cancer risk. It is not uncommon for epidemiological studies to come to different assessments of health risk, especially when, as in these studies, the associated risk is not large. Epidemiological studies differ in many ways, such as the groups of women being studied, how information is obtained, and what other exposures and risk factors are taken into consideration. These differences can affect the study's outcome. For this reason, many epidemiological studies must be conducted and evaluated before there is an agreement on the relationship between a potential risk factor and a disease.

The clarity of these studies' results is also affected by the very complicated relationship between tobacco smoke exposure and breast cancer risk—which could support associations with either increased or decreased risk. Smoking has effects that can both increase and decrease breast cancer risk. On the one hand, tobacco smoke contains chemicals that can cause breast cancer in animals and could thus be associated with an increase in breast cancer risk. On the other hand, smoking has been shown to have many effects that suggest an opposition of the effects of estrogen and could decrease breast cancer risk. The interplay between the effects of the cancer-causing chemicals and the apparent opposition of estrogen is critical to breast cancer risk. The nature of this interplay is poorly understood.

Does quitting smoking affect breast cancer risk?

Quitting smoking may lead to a temporary increase in breast cancer risk. Most of the studies that have examined the breast cancer risk of women who have quit smoking have reported an increase in breast cancer risk. In many of these studies, breast cancer risk was highest shortly after the women stopped smoking and gradually decreased over five years to twenty years, depending on the study.

It is possible that the interplay between the effects of toxic tobacco chemicals and the effects that may oppose estrogen matter here. Opposition of estrogen's effects is lost in women who quit smoking, and this may allow the expression of the accumulated toxic effects of cigarette smoke.

The increase in breast cancer risk associated with quitting smoking should be considered in the context of overall health. After quitting smoking, a woman's risk of breast cancer temporarily increases between 25 and 450 percent (depending on the study examined). This is in sharp contrast to the high risks for other health problems associated with continued smoking. For example, there is a well-established 1,000 to 2,000 percent increase in lung cancer risk associated with smoking. Without question, the effects of quitting smoking on overall health are beneficial.

Does smoking marijuana affect breast cancer risk?

The relationship between smoking marijuana and breast cancer risk has not been studied. Marijuana smoke has been shown to contain many of the toxic substances found in tobacco smoke. Unfortunately, there has not been enough study to evaluate a possible link of marijuana smoking with breast or even lung cancer.

Are some women more susceptible to tobacco smoke?

Studies have shown that people differ in how their bodies process different chemicals, including the toxic chemicals in tobacco. Examinations of the connection between breast cancer risk and differences in the processing of these toxic tobacco chemicals have produced conflicting results. This is an active area of research that may allow the identification of women who are more susceptible to the cancer-causing chemicals in tobacco smoke.

Does smoking affect the survival of women with breast cancer?

The effect of smoking on the survival of women with breast cancer is unclear. Some studies have reported an association between smoking and an increase in the risk of death, while others have found no association with the risk of death from breast cancer. Smokers may be at increased risk for metastasis (the spread of cancer). Two studies have reported an increase in the spread of tumors from the breast to the lungs in women who smoked. The survival of women with breast cancer who stopped smoking has been examined in one study. Their survival rate was found to be similar to that of women with breast cancer who never smoked.

What can women do now?

Quitting smoking and avoiding passive exposure to tobacco smoke makes good sense. Although it is unclear if smoking and passive exposure to tobacco smoke are associated with breast cancer risk, women can control their exposure to these potential risk factors. There are also many other health benefits to be gained by decreasing or eliminating either of these exposures.

Quitting smoking is difficult, but a number of drug and behavioral programs have been shown to increase the likelihood of success. Quitting smoking will not only make one ultimately feel better, but will decrease the risk of many diseases, including heart disease, stroke, many respiratory diseases, cancer of the lung, mouth, larynx, kidney, pancreas, stomach, and some types of leukemia. The effects of passive exposure to tobacco smoke are just beginning to be understood. Until more is known, decreasing exposure is desirable. Minimizing tobacco smoke exposure is particularly important for children, who appear to be more sensitive to its toxic effects.

—Prepared by Barbour Warren, Ph.D., Research Associate, BCERF, Cornell University and Carol Devine, Ph.D., R.D., Division of Nutritional Sciences and Education Project Leader, BCERF, Cornell University

For More Information

Program on Breast Cancer and Environmental Risk Factors
Sprecher Institute for Comparative Cancer Research
Cornell University
Box 31
Ithaca, NY 14853
Phone: (607) 254-2893
Internet: http://envirocancer.cornell.edu
E-mail: breastcancer@cornell.edu

Chapter 25

Environmental Chemicals and Breast Cancer Risk

There has been growing interest in whether environmental factors, including exposures to certain chemicals or changes in lifestyle, may increase the risk of breast cancer. This chapter will discuss research linking environmental chemicals and the risk of breast cancer. This will include exposures of concern in the home and workplace and chemicals known to cause mammary (breast) tumors in laboratory animals. The chapter will also discuss new emerging data on how exposures to certain chemicals early in life may affect breast development and breast cancer risk, as well as new work identifying important gene-environmental interactions. Current challenges and new avenues of research also will be discussed.

What are the established risk factors for breast cancer?

Risk factors consistently associated with a higher breast cancer risk are called "established" risk factors. Established risk factors include getting older, having regular menstrual periods earlier, going through menopause later in life, having a first child late in life, not having any children, having a mother or sister with breast cancer, past exposure of breasts to ionizing radiation, or having certain types of

"Environmental Chemicals and Breast Cancer Risk: Why Is There Concern?" by Suzanne Snedeker, Ph.D., Associate Director for Translational Research, Program on Breast Cancer and Environmental Risk Factors in New York State (BCERF), Fact Sheet #45, May 2002, © 2002 Cornell University, reprinted with permission.

benign breast disease. Yet these factors explain only about 25 to 50 percent of breast cancer cases (Madigan et al., *JNCI* vol. 87, pp. 1681–85, 1987; Rockhill et al., *Am. J. Epidemiol.* vol. 147, pp. 826–33, 1998).

Are there environmental links to breast cancer risk?

Breast cancer rates vary widely in different parts of the world. Rates are the highest in North America, Northern Europe, and Australia. Breast cancer rates are much lower in Japan, China, Africa, and India (IARC [International Agency for Research on Cancer], GLOBOCAN, 2000). It is not clear why there are geographical differences in breast cancer rates. Differences in age of childbearing, diet, lifestyle, and exposure to environmental chemicals have been offered as possible explanations. Studies of breast cancer rates of Japanese women who migrate to the United States suggest an environmental influence on the risk of breast cancer. Within one or two generations the breast cancer rates of descendants of Japanese women migrating to the United States increase and become similar to the higher breast cancer rates of Western women (Shimizu et al., *Br. J. Cancer* vol. 63, pp. 963–66, 1991). Results of studies on twins in Scandinavia also suggest that a woman's environment plays a significant role in determining her breast cancer risk. In this study inherited factors accounted for about 27 percent of breast cancer risk, suggesting that environmental factors play a major role in determining the risk of breast cancer (Lichtenstein, *N. Engl. J. Med.* vol. 343, pp. 78–85, 2000).

How can you be exposed to environmental chemicals?

We are exposed to thousands of naturally occurring and synthetic chemicals over a lifetime. Many chemicals are essential for life and are beneficial, while exposures to other chemicals can be harmful and affect our health. There are many ways our bodies can be exposed to chemicals. This includes exposure in the air we breathe, in the food and beverages we eat, and by contact with our skin. Fetuses can be exposed to chemicals that cross the placenta during pregnancy. Some environmental contaminants can pass from a mother's body to an infant through breast milk. Certain chemicals can be stored in the fat of fish or animals, becoming more concentrated as they pass up the food chain. These chemicals can be stored in the body for a long time. Other chemicals may be broken down and are quickly eliminated from the body. Some chemicals first need to be "activated" by enzymes in the body to become cancer-causing chemicals (carcinogens). Other chemicals pose no cancer risk, while still others may act as beneficial "anti-cancer" agents. It is impossible to make generalizations about environmental chemicals. Each chemical has a unique pattern in the way it is handled by the body, and has a different potential for whether it can contribute to breast cancer risk.

Are there concerns about chemicals in the home and workplace?

We can be exposed to a variety of synthetic chemicals in many different settings, including in our homes and workplaces. Some chemical exposures in the workplace have been associated with a higher risk of breast cancer (see Table 25.1). More research is needed to help identify the chemicals of concern for different workplace situations. There are relatively few studies of women in the workplace (most occupational studies of cancer risk have been done on men). There is a need for better-quality studies to give us better answers. Many of the studies done so far had very limited data on exposure to specific chemicals, and usually only small groups of women were followed for a limited time period.

Several groups that need further evaluation because of potential exposures to known or potential carcinogens include those employed in the chemical and pharmaceutical industries; laboratory and biomedical workers; cosmetologists and hairdressers; workers in semiconductor, printing, and textile-dyeing industries; airline personnel; health care workers; and metal plate workers (Aaronson and Howe, *JOEM* vol. 36, pp. 1174–79, 1994; Cantor et al., *JOEM* vol. 37, pp. 336–48, 1995; Habel et al.,

Table 25.1. Examples of Chemical Exposures in the Workplace Associated with Some Evidence of a Higher Breast Cancer Risk

Acid mists	Lead oxide
Benzene	Methylene chloride
Carbon tetrachloride	Styrene
Formaldehyde	

References:
Blair and Kazerouni, *Cancer Causes & Control* vol. 8, pp. 473–90, 1997.
Cantor et al., *JOEM* vol. 37, pp. 336–48, 1995.
Goldberg and Lebreche, *Occup. Environ. Med.* vol. 53, pp. 145–56, 1996.
Hansen, A. J. *Int. J. Epidemiol.* vol. 36, pp. 43–47, 1999.
Norman et al., *Int. J. Epidemiol.* vol. 24, pp. 276–84, 1995.
Spiritas et al., *Br. J. Ind. Med.* vol. 48, pp. 515–30, 1991.

Table 25.2. National Toxicology Program's Cancer Bioassays Examples of Chemicals that Cause Breast Tumors in Laboratory Animals (continued on next page).

Chemical solvents

Benzene

1,1-Dichloroethane

1,2-Dichloropropane

Methylene chloride

Nitromethane (also used in rocket and engine fuels)

1,2,3-Trichloropropane

Chemicals used or formed in the manufacturing of dyes

C.I. acid red 114

C.I. basic red 9

2,4-Diaminotoluene

3,3'-Dimethlybenzidine dihydrochloride

3,3'-Dimethoxybenzidine dihydrochloride

2,4-Dinitrotoluene

Hydrazobenzene

o-Nitrotoluene

o-Toluidine hydrochloride

Chemicals used in the manufacturing of rubber, vinyl, polyurethane foams, or neoprene

Benzene (rubber manufacturing)

1,3-Butadiene (rubber manufacturing)

Chloroprene (neoprene manufacturing)

2,4-Diaminotoluene (polyethylene manufacturing)

1,2-Dichloroethane (vinyl chloride manufacturing)

Chemicals used in the manufacturing of rubber, vinyl, polyurethane foams, or neoprene, continued

Glycidol (vinyl manufacturing)

o-Nitrotoluene (rubber manufacturing)

2,4-2,6-Toluene diisocyanate (polyethylene foam manufacturing)

Chemical intermediates

Ethylene oxide (anti-freeze products)

Isoprene (formed during ethylene production)

Flame retardants

2,2-Bis(bromomethyl)-1,3-propanediol

2,3-Dibromo-1-propanol

Food additive

Methyleugenol (flavoring)

Fumigants and pesticides

Clonitralid (molluscicide)

1,2-Dibromoethane (also called ethylene dibromide)

1,2-Dibromo-3-chloropropane (soil fumigant)

1,2-Dichloroethane (soil/grain fumigant)

1,2-Dichloropropane (soil/grain fumigant)

Dichlorvos (insecticide)

Sulfallate (herbicide)

Table 25.2. National Toxicology Program's Cancer Bioassays Examples of Chemicals that Cause Breast Tumors in Laboratory Animals (continued from previous page).

Gasoline additives

Benzene 1,2-Dibromoethane (lead scavenger)

1,2-Dichloroethane (lead scavenger)

Microelectronics

Indium phosphide (used in semi-conductors)

Mycotoxin

Ochratoxin A (toxin produced by molds)

Pharmaceutical drugs

Acronycine (anti-cancer drug)

Cytembena (cytostatic drug)

Furosemide (diuretic)

Hydrazobenzene (used in making phenylbutazone, an antiarthritic drug)

Isophosphamide (anti-cancer drug)

Nitrofurazone (anti-bacterial agent)

Phenesterin (anti-cancer drug)

Procarbazine hydrochloride (anti-cancer drug)

Reserpine (anti-hypertension drug)

Sterilizing agent for medical instruments

Ethylene oxide

Research chemical

5-Nitroacenaphthenol

Riot control/Tear gas

2-Chloroacetophenone

References:

Dunnick et al., *Carcinogenesis* vol. 16, pp. 173–79, 1995.

Bennett and Davis, *Environ. Mol. Mutagen.* vol. 39, pp. 150–57, 2002.

NTP, 9th Report on Carcinogens, 2000.

NTP, Chemicals associated with site-specific tumor induction in the mammary gland, http://ntp-server.niehs.nih.gov/htdocs/Sites/MAMM.HTML, cited June 2002.

JOEM vol. 37, pp. 349–56, 1995; LaBreche, vol. 2., sect. 4, http://www.breast.cancer.ca, posted 2001).

Of recent interest is whether breast cancer risk may be indirectly affected in night-shift workers exposed to "light at night," which may affect melatonin synthesis (Steven and Rea, *Cancer Causes Control*, vol. 12, 279–87, 2001). Scientists are exploring whether changes in melatonin levels may affect levels of estrogen and breast cancer risk (Davis et al., *JNCI* vol. 93, pp. 1557–62, 2001; Hansen et al., *Epidemiology* vol. 12, pp. 74–77, 2001; Schernhammer et al., *JNCI* vol. 93, pp. 1563–68, 2001).

Researchers are also interested in measuring chemicals women may be exposed to every day at home. Researchers on Long Island, New York, and on Cape Cod, Massachusetts, are measuring levels of environmental chemicals in the homes of women with and without breast cancer (see Long Island Breast Cancer Study Project's website http://epi.grants.cancer.gov/LIBCSP/; Cape Cod Breast Cancer Study; Rudel et al., *J. Air Waste Manage. Assoc.* vol. 51, pp. 499–513, 2001). Such studies may help identify the types of chemicals in the home that may be linked to a higher risk of breast cancer. It is important to characterize the types of chemicals found in the home environment. These studies help to identify sources and patterns of exposure, and prioritize chemicals that need further study.

Why is there concern that pesticides may affect breast cancer risk?

There has been concern about exposure to pesticides because of their widespread use in agriculture for crop and livestock protection; for public health in controlling disease-bearing insects; and for pest control in homes, schools, workplaces, gardens, and recreational areas such as parks and athletic fields. Currently, there are about 865 pesticide active ingredients registered with the Environmental Protection Agency (EPA), and thousands of products containing these chemicals singly or in combination.

Much of the concern about whether pesticides affect breast cancer risk stems from observations of higher rates of cancer in male workers with high exposures to pesticides. There are higher rates of some cancers in male farmworkers, including lip and skin cancer, non-Hodgkin's lymphoma, and cancer of the stomach, brain and prostate (Blair and Zahm, *Environ. Health Perspect.* vol. 103 [Suppl. 8], pp. 205–8, 1995). Some of these cancers are due to excessive exposure to ultraviolet radiation from the sun (lip and skin cancer). There are many types of exposures on the farm that may affect cancer risk, including exposures to pesticides, solvents, fuel exhaust, and toxins (called mycotoxins) from molds that form in stored crops. While some scientists have found higher cancer rates in farmers exposed to certain pesticides, other studies have not supported an association. An ongoing, large-scale study that will help provide better answers to whether specific chemicals used in agriculture affect cancer risk is the "Agricultural Health Study" (for more information go to http://www.aghealth.org/index.html).

Are breast cancer rates higher in women living or working on a farm?

There are very few studies that have evaluated whether farm women have a higher risk of breast cancer (Blair and Zahm, *Environ. Health Perspect.* vol. 103 [Suppl. 8], pp. 205–8, 1995). In a study of North Carolina farm women, overall breast cancer rates were lower in women who lived or worked on a farm compared to women who did not work or live on a farm. It has been suggested that these farm women may have lifestyles or risk factors that could have reduced their risk of breast cancer (later age at menarche, earlier age at first birth, higher number of pregnancies, less likely to smoke or drink alcohol, higher level of exercise). However, in this study, one group of farm women who did not wear protective clothing or gloves when applying pesticides had a twofold higher risk of breast cancer compared to women who did take proper precautions. The results of this small study suggest that breast cancer risk may be increased in some farm women with high exposures to pesticides. This study illustrates the importance of reducing exposures to pesticides in workplace situations (Duell et al., *Epidemiology* vol. 11, pp. 523–31, 2000).

Do organochlorine pesticides affect breast cancer risk in women?

Organochlorine pesticides were used extensively during and after WWII because of their long-lasting effects in controlling insects. Most were banned during the 1970s and 1980s in the United States, Canada, and Europe because of human health and ecological concerns. Some examples of organochlorine pesticides include: dichlorodiphenyltrichloroethane (DDT; used in mosquito control and agriculture), dieldrin (used to control termites and other soil insects), chlordane and heptachlor (used to control termites and fire ants), lindane (currently used in agriculture and in anti-lice shampoos), beta-hexachlorocyclohexane (by-product of lindane manufacture), and hexachlorobenzene (fungicide used to prevent mold on crops). These long-lasting chemicals concentrate as they pass up the food chain and are stored in the body fat of animals, fish, and humans. Some are endocrine disruptors that affect reproduction in wildlife, especially birds and reptiles. While there are links to some types of cancers (for instance, several organochlorines induce liver or thyroid tumors in laboratory animals), effects on breast cancer risk in humans have been studied only recently.

The organochlorine pesticide that has been studied the most extensively is the insecticide DDT. Over time, DDT breaks down in the environment to a very long-lasting chemical called dichlorodiphenyl-dichloroethylene, or DDE. Early reports suggested that women with high levels of DDE in their blood or fat had a higher risk of breast cancer. However, the majority of the more recent, well-controlled studies have not been able to confirm these findings. Most of these studies have looked at breast cancer risk in white women living in North America and Europe. These studies of Western women have not shown a higher risk of breast cancer in those with higher levels of DDT or DDE. Other populations, including different ethnic groups, have not been studied as well. The results from several studies suggest that breast cancer risk may be higher in African American women who have higher body levels of DDE. We don't have clear answers to whether breast cancer risk is higher for women who live in less industrialized tropical countries that still use DDT against mosquitoes for malaria control. More studies are needed to explore these areas.

For many of the other organochlorines, we have very limited data from human studies. Breast cancer risk was higher in Danish women with high blood levels of dieldrin, but the few studies done on American women have not confirmed this finding. For dieldrin, and other organochlorine pesticides, there are too few studies in women to make a conclusion of whether or not body levels are associated with breast cancer risk (Snedeker, *Environ. Health Perspect.* vol. 109 [Suppl. 1], pp. 35–47, 2001).

What can we learn from animal studies?

While human studies are given the greatest weight when deciding whether or not a chemical causes cancer, there is little or no information on the cancer-causing potential of most chemicals in people. Much of the information on chemicals and cancer risk comes from carefully controlled laboratory animal studies called "cancer bioassays." Animal studies are used by federal agencies to identify the hazard and to estimate the cancer risk to humans. These studies are important to help predict cancer risk when human studies are unavailable. In a cancer bioassay, male and female animals from two species (usually mice and rats) are exposed for most of their lives to a range of levels (doses) of the chemical. This approach is intended to maximize the likelihood of detecting cancer-causing chemicals. Before the EPA allows a pesticide to be registered for use, the primary manufacturer (registrant) must submit the results of cancer bioassays conducted in laboratory animals. The EPA can ask for additional studies to be conducted when a pesticide is reviewed for re-registration (for more information on how EPA assesses the health risks of pesticides see http://www.epa.gov/pesticides/citizens/riskassess.htm).

Animal studies are also conducted by the National Toxicology Program, a federal agency that screens a variety of chemicals for their cancer-causing potential (see http://ntp-server.niehs.nih.gov). Of the 509 chemicals tested by this agency, 42 chemicals were found to cause breast tumors (called mammary gland tumors) in laboratory animals. There is a wide range of different types of chemicals that cause breast tumors in laboratory animals. Some examples include several pharmaceutical drugs, chemical solvents, and flame retardants; a variety of chemicals used in the manufacturing of dyes, rubber, vinyl, and polyurethane foams; a sterilizing agent for medical instruments; a food additive; several fumigants and pesticides; a metal used in microelectronics; a mycotoxin produced by molds; and a gasoline additive (see Table 25.2). Some of these chemicals are still used and produced (for instance, methylene chloride). Others are no longer manufactured or limits have been placed on the maximum exposure allowed in workplaces. This includes the herbicide sulfallate (registration canceled by EPA), the soil fumigant 1,2-dibromo-3-chloropropane (banned by EPA), 1,2-dibromoethane used as a soil fumigant and as an anti-knock compound in gasoline (uses have been limited and maximum exposure standards have been set in the workplace), and ethylene oxide (limits have been placed on workplace exposures).

There is concern because some of these chemicals are environmentally persistent pollutants. One example is the soil fumigant 1,2-dibromo-3-chloropropane. Low levels of this persistent pesticide are still detected in well water in California and other states, even though all uses were banned by the EPA between 1979 and 1985 (CA EPA, EH95-06, 1995). Researchers from Finland reported that a chemical found in chlorinated drinking water called "MX" can cause a variety of cancers in laboratory animals, including mammary tumors in rats

(Komulainen et al., *JNCI* vol. 89, pp. 848–56, 1997). Researchers are monitoring levels and trying to find ways to reduce the level of this disinfection by-product in drinking water supplies (Wright et al., *Environ. Health Perspect.* vol. 110, pp. 157–64, 2002).

There are few studies available on the human breast cancer risk of the chemicals that are known to cause mammary tumors in laboratory animals. Ethylene oxide is an example of one of the few chemicals where we have evidence of a moderately higher breast cancer risk in women exposed to this chemical and evidence of mammary tumors in laboratory animals (Norman et al., *Int. J. Epidemiol.* vol. 24, pp. 276–84, 1995). Ethylene oxide is used to sterilize medical instruments. For other chemicals, species differences may influence the interpretation of results. Reserpine is an anti-hypertension drug known to increase levels of prolactin (Lee et al., *JAMA* vol. 235, pp. 2316–17, 1976), a hormone that plays a strong role in inducing breast tumors in rodents, but plays less of a role in human breast cancer. This species difference may explain why reserpine has been shown to be a mammary carcinogen in rodent bioassays but there is not strong evidence that it affects breast cancer risk in women taking this drug (Curb et al., *Hypertension* vol. 4, pp. 307–11, 1982; Horwitz and Feinstein, *Arch. Intern. Med.* vol. 145, pp. 1873–75, 1985; Laska et al., *Lancet* vol. 2, pp. 296–300, 1975; Mack et al., *N. Engl. J. Med.* vol. 292, pp. 1366–71, 1975).

Several polycyclic aromatic hydrocarbons (PAHs) have been identified as potent mammary carcinogens in animal studies. In the environment, PAHs are formed during the burning of fossil fuels (gasoline, coal, wood, oil), when tobacco is burned or when meats or fatty fish are char-broiled. While workplace exposures to mixtures of PAHs increases the risk of lung cancer, most studies have not shown a higher risk of breast cancer. One limitation of some of the workplace studies has been the small size of the studies. One larger study is evaluating whether exposures to PAHs affect breast cancer risk in women from Long Island, New York.

Do endocrine-disrupting chemicals affect breast cancer risk?

Hormones and growth factors act as chemical messengers in the body. Certain hormones and growth factors are important in normal growth and functioning of the breast, but they also can have a role in the cancer process. Examples of these hormones include estrogen, progestins, prolactin, and growth hormone (Nandi et al., *Proc. Natl. Acad. Sci. USA* vol. 92, pp. 3650–57, 1995; Russo and Russo, *JNCI*

Monograph vol. 27, pp. 17–37, 2000). Examples of growth factors include insulin-like growth factors (Kleinberg et al., *Br. J. Cancer Res. Treat.* vol. 47, pp. 201–8, 1998), and members of the epidermal growth factor family. In many cases these chemical messengers affect the rate of cell division in the breast, or they may work with hormones to help support the growth of breast tumor cells.

Breast cancer takes many years to develop—often up to thirty or more years—because of the many changes that must occur before a normal cell becomes a cancerous cell that divides out of control. Scientists are concerned that some environmental chemicals can either mimic the effects of hormones or growth factors or affect how fast the body makes or breaks down these hormones. Through these actions an environmental chemical could affect the delicate balance that controls cell division. More than half of all breast tumors depend on estrogen for growth. Chemicals that mimic the effect of estrogen may play a role in supporting the growth of estrogen-dependent breast tumors. For example, preliminary research suggests that occupational exposure to the environmental estrogen 4-octylphenol is associated with a higher risk of breast cancer (Aschengrau, et al., *Am. J. Ind. Med.* vol. 34, pp. 6–14, 1998).

In addition to concerns about how environmental estrogens may affect breast cancer risk, there also is evidence that these "xenoestrogens" can affect reproduction in wildlife and possibly in humans (Crisp et al., *Environ. Health. Perspect.* vol. 106 [Suppl. 1], pp. 11–56, 1998; McLachlan, *Endocrine Rev.* vol. 22, pp. 319–41, 2001). Because of these concerns, the U.S. Congress passed the Food Quality Protection Act in 1996. This legislation mandates that all pesticide active ingredients be tested for their estrogen-mimicking and other hormone-disrupting effects. The EPA is currently validating the screening tests that will be used. After these screening tests are validated, the EPA expects to test more than 865 pesticide active ingredients and about 150 high-volume industrial chemicals for endocrine-disrupting effects (for more information go to http://www.epa.gov/scipoly/oscpendo).

Do chemical exposures early in life affect breast cancer risk?

Childhood and adolescence are critical periods of breast development. Exposures to cancer-causing chemicals when the breast is developing may affect breast cancer risk later in life. Studies have shown that the developing mammary glands (breast tissue) of young rats and mice have budlike structures composed of rapidly dividing cells. These dividing immature breast cells are more susceptible to the damaging effects of cancer-causing chemicals. During pregnancy breast cells undergo changes making them more mature. Mature breast cells appear to be more resistant to the effects of carcinogens, and can more easily repair damage caused by cancer-causing chemicals.

In utero exposures to estrogenic chemicals may increase breast cancer risk. A drug that acts like estrogen, called diethylstilbestrol (DES), was prescribed to pregnant women from the mid-1940s to the 1970s, to prevent spontaneous abortions. Women who were treated with DES during pregnancy have a moderately higher breast cancer risk (Calle et al., *Am J. Epidemiol.* vol. 144, pp. 645–52, 1996; Colton, et al., *JAMA* vol. 269, pp. 2096–2100, 1993; Greenberg et al., *N. Engl. J. Med.* vol. 311, 1393–98, 1984). DES can also cause mammary (breast) tumors in mice (IARC, Suppl. 7, 1987). This is one of the reasons researchers are interested in whether early exposures to chemicals in the womb affect breast cancer risk later in life.

Results from animal studies have shown that early exposures to some chemicals can have permanent effects on the way the breast develops and its susceptibility to carcinogens. Early exposure to certain environmental chemicals may keep the mammary gland in an immature state for longer periods of time, increasing its susceptibility to carcinogens (Fenton et al., *Toxicol. Sci.* vol. 67, pp. 63–74, 2002). So, many chemicals may not cause a tumor to develop directly, but they may work in subtle ways to increase breast cancer risk. For instance, in one study female rats were exposed prenatally to an environmental contaminant, a dioxin called TCDD. When these dioxin-exposed rats were older, they were also exposed to a known breast carcinogen called dimethylbenz[a]anthracene (DMBA). The female rats pretreated with dioxin developed more breast tumors than the rats not pretreated with dioxin. The researchers suggested that the dioxin treatment prenatally changed how the breast tissue developed, keeping the breast in an immature state with a greater number of dividing bud structures for a longer time (Brown et al., *Carcinogenesis* vol. 19, pp. 1623–29, 1998). Similarly, results of preliminary studies conducted by EPA researchers have suggested that prenatal treatments with the herbicide atrazine can also help keep rat breast tissue in an immature state for prolonged periods of time (Fenton and Davis, *Toxicol. Sci.* vol. 66, pp. 185, 2002). While the implications for human cancer risk are not yet known, it is important that researchers fully explore the many ways chemicals may affect breast cancer risk.

How can genes influence responses to environmental chemicals?

Many chemicals have to become "activated" in the body to become carcinogens. Some people have differences (also called variations or polymorphisms) in certain genes that control these activation pathways. If a person has a variation in such genes, this may result in more activation and a higher level of the active form of the carcinogen. This may put the person at greater risk for developing certain cancers, including breast cancer. For example, women with high body levels of environmental chemicals called polychlorinated biphenyls (PCBs) usually do not have a higher risk of breast cancer. However, in one study breast cancer risk was higher in a group of women who had both a high level of PCBs and a variation in an activation gene called CYP1A1 (Moysich et al., *Cancer Epidemiol. Biomark. Prev.* vol. 8, pp. 41–44, 1999). This is an example of a "gene-environment interaction." More research is being done to identify important gene-environment interactions. This will help identify groups of women who may have a higher breast cancer risk if they are exposed to certain chemicals.

What are the challenges and new avenues for research?

There are many challenges that face scientists as they evaluate how breast cancer risk may be affected by exposure to environmental chemicals. Some of the greatest challenges are the complexity of the disease and that it takes many years for most breast cancers to develop. It is very difficult to characterize chemical exposures that occurred ten, twenty, or even thirty years before a breast tumor is detected. It is also hard to determine how individual chemicals may affect breast cancer risk when we are exposed to low levels of thousands of chemicals over a lifetime.

What are potential avenues of future research? More studies are needed to explore the wide variety of chemicals that may affect breast cancer risk. For instance, there is interest in whether certain antihistamines and antidepressants affect breast cancer risk. There also is interest in whether environmental chemicals, such as certain phthalates used in plastics, play a role in premature breast development and later risk of breast cancer. We need better tools to identify potential cancer-causing chemicals and better ways to measure exposures to chemicals. New powerful molecular techniques are being developed that may help to identify "molecular" footprints, including identifying chemicals that activate specific cancer genes or that turn off genes that can suppress cancer. While studies are ongoing to screen for and identify breast carcinogens in animal cancer bioassays, new screening techniques are being developed that will allow for more rapid screening of a larger number of chemicals.

More research is needed to identify gene-environmental interactions that may help identify groups of women who may be at higher risk when exposed to certain chemicals, and identify endocrine-disrupting chemicals that can support the growth of breast tumors. More research is needed not only to define the types of exposures encountered in the workplace and the home, but also to evaluate how exposure during critical periods of breast development may affect cancer risk later in life. A combination of human, animal, and molecular-based studies is needed to address how environmental chemicals may affect the risk of breast and other cancers.

—Prepared by Suzanne Snedeker, Ph.D., Associate Director for Translational Research, BCERF, Cornell University

For More Information

Program on Breast Cancer and Environmental Risk Factors
Sprecher Institute for Comparative Cancer Research
Cornell University
Box 31
Ithaca, NY 14853
Phone: (607) 254-2893
Internet: http://envirocancer.cornell.edu
E-mail: breastcancer@cornell.edu

Chapter 26

Study Shows Link between Antibiotic Use and Increased Risk of Breast Cancer

A study published in the *Journal of the American Medical Association* (*JAMA*) provides evidence that use of antibiotics is associated with an increased risk of breast cancer. The authors—from Group Health Cooperative (GHC) in Seattle; the National Cancer Institute (NCI), a part of the National Institutes of Health in Bethesda, Maryland; the University of Washington, Seattle; and the Fred Hutchinson Cancer Center, also in Seattle—concluded that the more antibiotics the women in the study used, the higher their risk of breast cancer.

The results of this study do not mean that antibiotics cause breast cancer. "These results only show that there is an association between the two," explained co-author Stephen H. Taplin, M.D., of NCI's Division of Cancer Control and Population Sciences and formerly of the GHC. "More studies must be conducted to determine whether there is indeed a direct cause-and-effect relationship."

"This trial suggests another piece in the puzzle of factors that may potentially be involved in the development of breast cancer," said NCI director Andrew C. von Eschenbach, M.D. "The NCI will continue to support research into underlying mechanisms of cancer risk."

The authors of this *JAMA* study found that women who took antibiotics for more than five hundred days—or had more than twenty-five prescriptions—over an average period of seventeen years had more than twice the risk of breast cancer as women who had not taken

Reprinted from "Study Shows Link between Antibiotic Use and Increased Risk of Breast Cancer," National Cancer Institute, February 16, 2004.

any antibiotics. The risk was smaller for women who took antibiotics for fewer days. However, even women who had between one and twenty-five prescriptions over an average period of seventeen years had an increased risk; they were about 1.5 times more likely to be diagnosed with breast cancer than women who didn't take any antibiotics. The authors found an increased risk in all classes of antibiotics that they studied.

"Breast cancer is the second leading cause of cancer deaths among women in the United States—with an estimated forty thousand deaths this year—and is the most common cancer in women worldwide," said first author Christine Velicer, Ph.D., of GHC's Center for Health Studies. "Antibiotics are used extensively in this country and in many parts of the world. The possible association between breast cancer and antibiotic use was important to examine."

To gather the necessary data, the researchers used computerized pharmacy and breast cancer screening databases at GHC, a large, nonprofit health plan in Washington state. They compared the antibiotic use of 2,266 women with breast cancer to similar information from 7,953 women without breast cancer. All the women in the study were age twenty and older, and the researchers examined a wide variety of the most frequently prescribed antibiotic medications.

The authors offer a few possible explanations for the observed association between antibiotic use and increased breast cancer risk. Antibiotics can affect bacteria in the intestine, which may impact how certain foods that might prevent cancer are broken down in the body. Another hypothesis focuses on antibiotics' effects on the body's immune response and response to inflammation, which could also be related to the development of cancer. It is also possible that the underlying conditions that led to the antibiotics prescriptions caused the increased risk, or that a weakened immune system—either alone, or in combination with the use of antibiotics—is the cause of this association.

The results of the study are consistent with an earlier Finnish study of almost ten thousand women. "Further studies must be conducted, though, for us to know why we see this increased risk and the full implications of these findings," said Velicer. Studies are also necessary to clarify whether specific indications for antibiotic use, such as respiratory infection or urinary tract infection, or times of use, such as adolescence, pregnancy, or menopause, are associated with increased breast cancer risk. Additionally, breast cancer risks could differ between women who take low-dose antibiotics for a long period of time and women who take high-dose antibiotics only once in a while.

Antibiotics are regularly prescribed for conditions such as respiratory infections, acne, and urinary tract infections, in addition to a wide range of other conditions or illnesses. In this *JAMA* study, for example, more than 70 percent of women had used between one and twenty-five prescriptions for antibiotics to treat various conditions over an average seventeen-year period, and only 18 percent of women in the study had not filled any antibiotic prescriptions during their enrollment in the health plan.

Over the past decade, overuse of antibiotics has become a serious problem. According to the Centers for Disease Control and Prevention (CDC), tens of millions of antibiotics are prescribed for viral infections that are not treatable with antibiotics, contributing to the troubling growth of antibiotic resistance. Efforts are underway such as the "Get Smart: Know When Antibiotics Work" campaign—unveiled last year by the Department of Health and Human Services' CDC and the Food and Drug Administration (FDA) and other partners—to lower the rate of antibiotic overuse.

"These study results do not mean that women should stop using antibiotics to treat bacterial infections," stressed Taplin. "Until we understand more about the association between antibiotics and cancer, people should take into account the substantial benefits that antibiotics can have, but should continue to use these medicines wisely."

Chapter 27

Alcohol and Breast Cancer in Women

Background

Many studies have shown an increased risk of breast cancer with alcohol consumption. The mechanism is not completely understood, but some studies have shown an increased estrogen level in women who have a moderate to high alcohol daily intake. Most are small studies or meta-analysis, which have their inherent biases. The Pooling Project of Prospective Studies of Diet and Cancer was established to evaluate associations between lifestyle factors and breast cancer.

Methods

Seven prospective studies of lifestyle and cancer risks were deemed eligible for evaluation:

1. Canadian National Breast Screening Study
2. Iowa Women's Health Study
3. Netherlands Cohort Study
4. New York State Cohort
5. Nurses' Health Study '80–'86
6. Nurses' Health Study '87–'91
7. Sweden Mammography Cohort

197

All studies had food frequency questionnaires that included detailed inquiries about alcohol consumption. Calculations were made such that a standardized amount was agreed upon. Grams of alcohol consumption were the basis for comparison. Ten grams of alcohol are equal to one drink. Over four thousand cases were assessed. The studies had a range of 23 percent to 55 percent nondrinkers, to which the other cases were compared.

Results

The mean alcohol consumption ranged from 3.22 grams/day for the Swedish group to 12.58 grams/day for the Canadians. The relative risk for breast cancer seemed to be little affected by average consumption in the range of less than 15 grams/day. The relative risk increased to 16 percent above nondrinkers when consumption was 15 to less than 30 grams/day. When the alcohol intake is 30 to less than 60 grams/day (two to five drinks), the relative risks were 41 percent greater than for nondrinkers. Beyond that, the risk plateaus without incremental increase.

Type of alcohol was not a significant factor in predicting risk. Associated factors of menopausal status, family history of breast cancer, hormone replacement therapy, and obesity were evaluated and not found to be of significance in relative risk.

Discussion

The investigators conclude that breast cancer risk is positively correlated with alcohol consumption rate. Their results seem to confirm the 1994 meta-analysis (Longnecker, M.P. *Cancer Causes Control* 5 (1994): 73–82) that quoted a 9 percent increase in relative risk of breast cancer for every 10 grams/day of alcohol consumption.

There were inherent limitations of this study, some of which were detailed by the authors. Only the initial baseline alcohol consumption was known. Over time, the drinking habits of most individuals change. Taking, essentially, what seems to be a snapshot of a person's life to determine overall lifetime risk cannot be fully valid. As with all survey or questionnaire types of studies, the validity of the data relies on the recall ability and also somewhat on the interpretive abilities of those surveyed. This leads to many opportunities for misrepresentation.

While there are many health-related reasons to avoid alcohol consumption, breast cancer risk cannot be fully validated as being increased. There have been as many studies disproving the theory as supporting it. As with everything, moderation is the important step.

Chapter 28

No Link Found between Abortion, Miscarriage, and Breast Cancer Risk

Introduction

A woman's hormone levels normally change throughout her life for a variety of reasons, and these hormonal changes can lead to changes in her breasts. Many such hormonal changes occur during pregnancy, changes that may influence a woman's chances of developing breast cancer later in life. As a result, over several decades a considerable amount of research has been and continues to be conducted to determine whether having an induced abortion or a miscarriage (also known as spontaneous abortion) influences a woman's chances of developing breast cancer later in life.

Current Knowledge

In February 2003, the National Cancer Institute (NCI) convened a workshop of over one hundred of the world's leading experts on pregnancy and breast cancer risk. Workshop participants reviewed existing population-based, clinical, and animal studies on the relationship between pregnancy and breast cancer risk, including studies of induced and spontaneous abortions. They concluded that having an abortion or miscarriage does not increase a woman's subsequent risk of developing breast cancer. A summary of their findings, titled Summary Report: Early Reproductive Events and Breast Cancer Workshop, can be found at http://cancer.gov/cancerinfo/ere-workshop-report.

Cancer Facts, National Cancer Institute, May 30, 2003.

199

Background

The relationship between induced and spontaneous abortion and breast cancer risk has been the subject of extensive research since the late 1950s. Until the mid-1990s, the evidence was inconsistent. Findings from some studies suggested there was no increase in risk of breast cancer among women who had had an abortion, while findings from other studies suggested there was an increased risk. Most of these studies, however, were flawed in a number of ways that can lead to unreliable results. Only a small number of women were included in many of these studies, and for most, the data were collected only after breast cancer had been diagnosed, and women's histories of miscarriage and abortion were based on their "self-report" rather than on their medical records. Since then, better-designed studies have been conducted. These newer studies examined large numbers of women, collected data before breast cancer was found, and gathered medical history information from medical records rather than simply from self-reports, thereby generating more reliable findings. The newer studies consistently showed no association between induced and spontaneous abortions and breast cancer risk.

Chapter 29

Antiperspirant and Deodorant Use Not Found to Be Linked to Breast Cancer

Articles in the press and on the Internet have warned that underarm antiperspirants or deodorants cause breast cancer. The reports have suggested that these products contain harmful substances, which can be absorbed through the skin or enter the body through nicks caused by shaving.

Scientists at the National Cancer Institute (NCI) are not aware of any research to support a link between the use of underarm antiperspirants or deodorants and the subsequent development of breast cancer. The U.S. Food and Drug Administration, which regulates food, cosmetics, medicines, and medical devices, also does not have any evidence or research data to support the theory that ingredients in underarm antiperspirants or deodorants cause cancer.

The results of a study looking for a relationship between breast cancer and underarm antiperspirants or deodorants were reported in the *Journal of the National Cancer Institute* in October 2002. The findings did not show any increased risk for breast cancer in women who reported using an underarm antiperspirant or deodorant. The results also showed no increased breast cancer risk for women who reported using a blade (non-electric) razor and an underarm antiperspirant or deodorant, or for women who reported using an underarm antiperspirant or deodorant within one hour of shaving with a blade razor. These conclusions were based on interviews with 813 women with breast cancer and 793 women with no history of breast cancer.

Cancer Facts, National Cancer Institute, February 4, 2003.

People who are concerned about their cancer risk are encouraged to talk with their doctor. More information about cancer is available on the NCI's website (http://cancer.gov). Also, U.S. residents may wish to contact the NCI's Cancer Information Service (CIS) with any remaining questions or concerns about breast cancer.

Cancer Information Service
Toll-free: 1-800-4-CANCER (1-800-422-6237)
TTY (for deaf and hard of hearing callers): 1-800-332-8615

Inquirers who live outside the United States may wish to contact the International Union Against Cancer (UICC) for information about a resource in their country. The UICC website is located at http://www.uicc.org on the internet.

Chapter 30

Study Finds No Link between Silicone Breast Implants and Breast Cancer Risk

In one of the largest studies on the long-term health effects of silicone breast implants, researchers from the National Cancer Institute (NCI) in Bethesda, Maryland, found no association between breast implants and the subsequent risk of breast cancer. The study is published in the November issue of Cancer Causes and Control. The study is titled, "Breast Cancer Following Augmentation Mammoplasty (United States)." The authors are Louise A. Brinton, Jay H. Lubin, Mary Cay Burich, Theodore Colton, S. Lori Brown, and Robert N. Hoover. It is published in the November 2000 issue of *Cancer Causes and Control,* vol. 11(9):819–27.

Breast Implant Study

Breast implants first appeared on the market in 1962. Manufacturers initially assumed that the implants were biologically inactive and, therefore, would have no harmful effects. However, over the past two decades there have been a number of reports of connective tissue disorders and cancers among implant patients.

In 1992, because of the lack of sufficient evidence on the long-term safety of implants, the Food and Drug Administration (FDA) restricted the use of silicone breast implants to women seeking breast reconstruction in controlled clinical trials, and Congress directed the National

"Silicone Breast Implants Are Not Linked to Breast Cancer Risk," National Institutes of Health, Office of Cancer Communications, Building 31, Room 10A19, Bethesda, MD 20892; Press Release dated October 2, 2000.

Institutes of Health to undertake a large follow-up study to evaluate the long-term health effects of the implants.

"This is the first part of our analysis of the health risks from the study," said Louise A. Brinton, Ph.D., principal investigator from NCI's Division of Cancer Epidemiology and Genetics (DCEG) in Bethesda, Maryland. "For women followed for more than ten years, there was no change in breast cancer risk. Our results do not confirm the findings from several other studies that exposure to implants reduces a woman's risk for breast cancer. This may relate to the longer follow-up in this study as compared with most others."

The average length of follow-up was 12.9 years among the implant patients and 11.6 years among the comparison patients. In previous studies, women with implants were generally followed for less than 10 years.

The participants included 13,500 women who had implant surgery for cosmetic reasons in both breasts sometime between 1962 and 1989 and, for comparison, about 4,000 women similar in age who had some other type of plastic surgery, such as removal of fat from the stomach, or wrinkles from the face and neck. Both groups of women were selected from eighteen plastic surgery practices in which the surgeons had performed large numbers of cosmetic breast implant surgeries prior to 1989 and were willing to give the investigators access to their records. The practices were located in six geographic areas: Atlanta, Georgia; Birmingham, Alabama; Charlotte, North Carolina; Miami and Orlando, Florida; and Washington, D.C.

In order to carry out the study, researchers reviewed the medical records from the plastic surgery practices and collected data about the surgical procedures, types of implants, and complications, if any, as well as factors affecting health status, such as weight and medical history. Patients who were located were asked to complete a mailed questionnaire in order to collect information about their health status, factors that might affect their health, and short- and long-term complications that might be associated with the implants. No clinical exams were done on the patients, but attempts were made to verify patient reports of cancer and connective tissue disease from the medical records of the physicians who diagnosed or treated the diseases. For patients who had died, death certificates were collected to verify the causes of death.

Study Groups

Besides the size of the study and the length of follow-up, another unique feature of the NCI study is that the researchers compared the breast implant patients to both the general population and to women who had received other types of plastic surgery. In previous reports, the general population was used as the control group. However, NCI investigators found in an earlier study that women with implants tend to share more breast cancer risk factors with women who had received other types of plastic surgery than with the general population. (The study is titled: "Characteristics of a Population of Women with Breast Implants Compared with Women Seeking Other Types of Plastic Surgery." The authors are Louise A. Brinton, S. Lori Brown, Theodore Colton, Mary Cay Burich, and Jay H. Lubin. *Plastic and Reconstructive Surgery* 105, no. 3 (2000): 919–27.) These risk factors include histories of previous gynecologic operations and operations for benign breast disease. Therefore, they believe that women who received other types of plastic surgery may be a more appropriate comparison group than the general population. However, when compared to either the general population or women with other types of plastic surgery, there was no evidence of a change in breast cancer risk in the implant group.

Typically, implants are soft silicone sacs, inflated with either saline solution (salt water) or a synthetic silicone gel. Both have been marketed since 1962. Before the 1992 FDA ban, 90 percent to 95 percent of the implants contained silicone gel because they had a more pleasing look and feel than the saline-filled implants. Since 1992, 90 percent to 95 percent of the implants have been saline-filled. It is not known how many women currently have silicone vs. saline implants.

Of the implant patients in the study, 49.7 percent received silicone gel implants, 34.1 percent double lumen implants, 12.2 percent saline-filled implants, 0.1 percent other types of implants, and 3.8 percent unspecified types of implants. (Double lumen implants have two shells; the inner sac is filled with silicone gel and the outer with saline.) The participants had cosmetic surgery during a time (between 1962 and 1988) when a great number of changes were taking place in the manufacturing of breast implants such as the shell thickness, the type of shell coating, and the gel composition. However, the researchers found there was no altered breast cancer risk associated with any of the types of implants.

Implants and Cancer Diagnosis

One of the controversial issues is whether women with breast implants have more advanced breast cancer at diagnosis than women without implants. In the current study, NCI researchers found a somewhat later stage at detection of breast cancer among the implant patients compared to the controls and a smaller percentage of *in situ* (early-stage) cancers among the implant patients. However, the differences were not statistically significant and there was no significant difference in breast cancer mortality between the implant and comparison group.

"This is an issue that needs further study," said Brinton. "This would include continuing to follow participants in this study to see if their breast cancer death rate changes with time."

About 80 percent of breast implants in the United States are for cosmetic reasons and 20 percent for breast reconstruction. This study does not include women undergoing breast reconstruction after breast cancer surgery, so it is not possible to predict whether similar results would be found for this population. The majority of the previous studies have also focused on women who received implants for cosmetic reasons.

It is estimated that between 1.5 million and 2 million U.S. women have had breast implants since they first appeared on the market in 1962.

Future analyses of the data will evaluate the risk of other cancers, connective tissue disorders, and causes of death.

Part Four

Prevention of Breast Cancer

Chapter 31

Genetic Testing for BRCA1 and BRCA2: It's Your Choice

What are BRCA1 and BRCA2?

Each year, more than 192,000 American women learn they have breast cancer. Approximately 5 to 10 percent of these women have a hereditary form of the disease. Changes, called alterations or mutations, in certain genes make some women more susceptible to developing breast and other types of cancer. Inherited alterations in the genes called BRCA1 and BRCA2 (short for breast cancer 1 and breast cancer 2) are involved in many cases of hereditary breast and ovarian cancer. Researchers are searching for other genes that may also increase a woman's cancer risk.

The likelihood that breast or ovarian cancer is associated with BRCA1 or BRCA2 is highest in families with a history of multiple cases of breast cancer, cases of both breast and ovarian cancer, one or more family members with two primary cancers (original tumors at different sites), or an Ashkenazi (Eastern European) Jewish background. However, not every woman in such families carries an alteration in BRCA1 or BRCA2, and not every cancer in such families is linked to alterations in these genes.

How do alterations in BRCA1 and BRCA2 affect a person's risk of cancer?

A woman's lifetime chance of developing breast or ovarian cancer is greatly increased if she inherits an altered BRCA1 or BRCA2 gene.

Cancer Facts, National Cancer Institute, February 6, 2002.

209

Women with an inherited alteration in one of these genes have an increased risk of developing these cancers at a young age (before menopause), and often have multiple close family members with the disease. These women may also have an increased chance of developing colon cancer.

Men with an altered BRCA1 or BRCA2 gene also have an increased risk of breast cancer (primarily if the alteration is in BRCA2), and possibly prostate cancer. Alterations in the BRCA2 gene have also been associated with an increased risk of lymphoma, melanoma, and cancers of the pancreas, gallbladder, bile duct, and stomach in some men and women.

According to estimates of lifetime risk, about 13.2 percent (132 out of 1,000 individuals) of women in the general population will develop breast cancer, compared with estimates of 36 to 85 percent (360–850 out of 1,000) of women with an altered BRCA1 or BRCA2 gene. In other words, women with an altered BRCA1 or BRCA2 gene are three to seven times more likely to develop breast cancer than women without alterations in those genes. Lifetime risk estimates of ovarian cancer for women in the general population indicate that 1.7 percent (17 out of 1,000) will get ovarian cancer, compared with 16 to 60 percent (160–600 out of 1,000) of women with altered BRCA1 or BRCA2 genes. No data are available from long-term studies of the general population comparing the cancer risk in women who have a BRCA1 or BRCA2 alteration with women who do not have an alteration in these genes. Therefore, these figures are estimated ranges that may change as more research data are added.

Some evidence suggests that there are slight differences in patterns of cancer between people with BRCA1 alterations and people with BRCA2 alterations, and even between people with different alterations in the same gene. For example, one study found that alterations in a certain part of the BRCA2 gene were associated with a higher risk for ovarian cancer in women, and a lower risk for prostate cancer in men, than alterations in other areas of BRCA2.

Most research related to BRCA1 and BRCA2 has been done on large families with many affected individuals. Estimates of breast and ovarian cancer risk associated with BRCA1 and BRCA2 alterations have been calculated from studies of these families. Because family members share a proportion of their genes and, often, their environment, it is possible that the large number of cancer cases seen in these families may be partly due to other genetic or environmental factors. Therefore, risk estimates that are based on families with many affected members may not accurately reflect the levels of risk in the general population.

Are specific alterations in BRCA1 and BRCA2 more common in certain populations?

Specific gene alterations have been identified in different ethnic groups. For example, among individuals of Ashkenazi Jewish descent, researchers have found that about 2.3 percent (23 out of 1,000 persons) have an altered BRCA1 or BRCA2 gene. This frequency is about five times higher than that of the general population. Among people with alterations in BRCA1 or BRCA2, three particular alterations have been found to be most common in the Ashkenazi Jewish population—two in the BRCA1 gene and one in the BRCA2 gene. It is not known whether the increased frequency of these alterations is responsible for the increased risk of breast cancer in Jewish populations compared with non-Jewish populations. Other ethnic and geographic populations, such as the Norwegian, Dutch, and Icelandic people, also have a higher rate of certain genetic alterations in BRCA1 and BRCA2. This information about genetic differences between ethnic groups may help health care providers determine the most appropriate genetic test to select.

What does a positive BRCA1 or BRCA2 test result mean?

In a family with a history of breast or ovarian cancer, it may be most informative to first test a family member who has the disease. If that person is found to have an altered BRCA1 or BRCA2 gene, the specific change is referred to as a "known mutation." Other family members can then be tested to see if they also carry that specific alteration. In this scenario, a positive test result indicates that a person has inherited a known mutation in BRCA1 or BRCA2 and has an increased risk of developing certain cancers, as described previously. However, a positive result provides information only about a person's risk of developing cancer. It cannot tell whether cancer will actually develop—or when. It is also impossible to predict the effectiveness of special screening or preventive medical procedures for people with alterations in BRCA1 or BRCA2. Not all women who inherit an altered gene will develop breast or ovarian cancer.

A positive test result may have important health and social implications for family members, including future generations. Unlike most other medical tests, genetic tests can reveal information not only about the person being tested, but also about that person's relatives. Both men and women who inherit an altered BRCA1 or BRCA2 gene, whether or not they get cancer themselves, may pass the alteration

211

on to their sons and daughters. However, not all children of people who have an altered gene will inherit the alteration.

What does a negative BRCA1 or BRCA2 test result mean?

A negative test result will be interpreted differently, depending upon whether there is a known mutation in the family. If someone in a family has a known mutation in BRCA1 or BRCA2, testing other family members for that specific gene alteration can provide information about their cancer risk. In this case, if a family member tests negative for the known mutation in that family, it is highly unlikely that he or she has an inherited susceptibility to cancer. This test result is called a "true negative." Having a true negative test result does not mean that a person will not get cancer; it means that the person's risk of cancer is the same as that of the general population.

In cases where no known mutation in BRCA1 or BRCA2 has previously been identified in a family with a history of breast or ovarian cancer, a negative test is not informative. It is not possible to tell whether a person has an alteration in BRCA1 or BRCA2 that was not identified by the test (a false negative), or whether the result is a true negative. In addition, it is possible for people to have an alteration in a gene other than BRCA1 or BRCA2 that increases their cancer risk but is not detectable by this test.

What does an ambiguous BRCA1 or BRCA2 test result mean?

If the test shows a change in BRCA1 or BRCA2 that has not been associated with cancer in other people, that person's test result may be interpreted as ambiguous or uncertain. One study found that 10 percent of women who underwent BRCA1 and BRCA2 testing had this type of ambiguous genetic change. Because everyone has genetic alterations that do not increase the risk of disease, it is sometimes not known whether a specific change affects a person's risk of developing cancer. As more research is conducted and more people are tested for BRCA1 or BRCA2 alterations, scientists will learn more about these genetic alterations and cancer risk.

What are the options for a person who tests positive?

Several approaches are available for managing cancer risk in individuals with alterations in their BRCA1 or BRCA2 genes. However, limited data exist on the effectiveness of these approaches.

Surveillance: If cancer develops, it is important to detect it as soon as possible. Careful monitoring for symptoms of cancer may allow a person to catch the disease at an earlier stage. Surveillance methods for breast cancer may include mammography and a clinical breast exam. Some health professionals also recommend breast self-exams, but this surveillance method should not be used in place of clinical exams. Studies are currently being conducted to test the effectiveness of other breast cancer screening methods in women with an altered BRCA1 or BRCA2 gene. With careful surveillance, many cancers will be diagnosed early enough to be successfully treated.

For ovarian cancer, surveillance methods may include transvaginal ultrasound, CA-125 blood testing, and clinical exams. Surveillance can sometimes find cancer at an early stage, but it is uncertain whether these methods can reduce a person's chance of dying from ovarian cancer.

Prophylactic Surgery: This type of surgery involves removing as much of the at-risk tissue as possible in order to reduce the chance of developing cancer. Preventive mastectomy (removal of healthy breasts) and preventive salpingo-oophorectomy (removal of healthy fallopian tubes and ovaries) do not, however, offer a guarantee against developing these cancers. Because not all at-risk tissue can be removed by these procedures, some women have developed breast cancer, ovarian cancer, or primary peritoneal carcinomatosis (a type of cancer similar to ovarian cancer) even after prophylactic surgery.

Risk Avoidance: Behaviors that may decrease breast cancer risk include exercising regularly and limiting alcohol consumption. Research results on the benefits of these behaviors are based on studies in the general population; the effects of these actions in people with BRCA1 or BRCA2 alterations are not yet known.

Chemoprevention: This approach involves the use of natural or synthetic substances to reduce the risk of developing cancer, or to reduce the chance that cancer will come back. For example, the NCI-supported Breast Cancer Prevention Trial found that the drug tamoxifen reduced the risk of invasive breast cancer by 49 percent in women at increased risk for developing the disease. Few studies have been performed to test the effectiveness of tamoxifen in women with a BRCA1 or BRCA2 alteration. One study found that tamoxifen reduced the incidence of breast cancer by 62 percent in women with alterations in BRCA2. However, the results showed no reduction in breast cancer incidence with tamoxifen use among women with BRCA1 alterations. Additional chemoprevention studies with tamoxifen and other substances in women with an altered BRCA1 or BRCA2 gene are anticipated.

Gene Therapy: At present, altered BRCA1 and BRCA2 genes cannot be repaired. Some day it may be possible to fix or manipulate the genes or sets of genes that increase one's risk of cancer.

What are some of the benefits of genetic testing for breast and ovarian cancer risk?

There can be benefits to genetic testing, whether a person receives a positive or a negative result. The potential benefits of a negative result include a sense of relief and elimination of the need for special preventive checkups, tests, or surgeries. A positive test result can bring relief from uncertainty and allow people to make informed decisions about their future, including taking steps to reduce cancer risk. In addition, many people are able to participate in medical research that may, in the long run, decrease the risk of death from breast cancer.

What are some of the risks of genetic testing for breast and ovarian cancer risk?

The direct medical risks of genetic testing are very small, but test results may have an impact on a person's emotions, social relationships, finances, and medical choices. People who receive a positive test result may feel anxious, depressed, or angry. They may choose to undergo preventive measures that have serious long-term implications and whose effectiveness is uncertain. People who receive a negative test result may experience "survivor guilt" caused by avoiding a disease that affects a loved one. They may also be falsely reassured that they have no chance of developing cancer, even though people with a negative test result have the same cancer risk as the general population. Because genetic testing can reveal information about more than one family member, the emotions caused by test results can create tension within families. Test results can also affect personal choices, such as marriage and childbearing. Issues surrounding the privacy and confidentiality of genetic test results are additional potential risks.

What can happen when genetic test results are placed in medical records?

Clinical test results are normally included in a person's medical records, and the inclusion of genetic test results in a patient's records may have serious implications. For example, when applying for medical, life, or disability insurance, people may be asked to sign forms that give the insurance company permission to access their medical records. The insurance company may take genetic test results into account when making decisions about coverage. An employer may also have the right to look at an employee's medical records. Individuals considering genetic testing must understand that when test results are placed in their medical records, the results might not be kept private.

Some physicians keep test results out of medical records. However, even if genetic test results are not included in a person's medical records, there may still be some risk of discrimination. Information about a person's genetic profile can sometimes be gathered from that person's family medical history.

What is genetic discrimination, and what laws protect people from this type of discrimination?

Genetic discrimination occurs when people are treated differently by their insurance company or employer because they have a gene alteration that increases their risk of a disease, such as cancer. People who undergo genetic testing to find out whether they have an alteration in their BRCA1 or BRCA2 gene may be at risk for genetic discrimination.

A positive genetic test result may affect a person's insurance coverage, particularly their health insurance. A person with a positive result may be denied coverage for medical expenses related to their genetic condition, dropped from their current health plan, or unable to qualify for new insurance. Some insurers view the affected individual as a potential cancer patient whose medical treatment would be costly to the insurance company.

The Health Insurance Portability and Accountability Act (HIPAA) of 1996 provides some protection for people who have employer-based health insurance. The act prohibits group health plans from using genetic information as a basis for denying coverage if a person does not currently have a disease. However, the act does not prohibit employers from refusing to offer health coverage as part of their benefits, or prevent insurance companies from requesting genetic information.

In 2000, the Department of Health and Human Services released the HIPAA National Standards to Protect Patients' Personal Medical Records. This regulation covers medical records maintained by health care providers, health plans, and health care clearinghouses. Although the standards are not specific to genetic information, they provide the first comprehensive federal protection for the privacy of health information.

A person who tests positive for a BRCA1 or BRCA2 alteration may also experience genetic discrimination in the workplace if an employer learns about the test result. Although there are currently no federal laws specific to genetic nondiscrimination, some protection from discrimination by employers is offered through the Americans with Disabilities Act of 1990 (ADA). In 1995, the Equal Employment Opportunity Commission (EEOC) expanded the definition of "disabled" to include individuals who carry genes that put them at higher risk for genetic disorders. The extent of this protection, however, has not yet been tested in the courts.

Several states also have laws that address genetic discrimination by employers and health insurance companies. The degree of discrimination protection varies from state to state. Therefore, the decisions that people make about genetic testing while living in one state may have repercussions in the future if they move to another area.

How are the tests for BRCA1 or BRCA2 performed?

Testing for alterations in a person's BRCA1 or BRCA2 gene is done on a blood sample. The person's blood is drawn in a laboratory, doctor's office, hospital, or clinic, and the blood sample is sent to a laboratory to check for alterations in the BRCA1 and BRCA2 genes.

How much does testing cost and how long does it take to get the results?

The cost for genetic testing can range from several hundred to several thousand dollars. Insurance policies vary with regard to whether the cost of genetic testing is covered.

As addressed previously, because the results of genetic tests can affect a person's health insurance coverage, some individuals may not want to use their insurance to pay for testing. Some people may choose to pay out-of-pocket for the test, even when their insurer would be willing to cover the cost. To protect their privacy, some may not even want their insurer to know they are thinking about genetic testing. Others may decide to ask their insurance company to cover these costs. People who are considering genetic testing may want to find out more about their particular insurance company's policies and the privacy protection laws in their state before submitting the charge for the test.

From the date that blood is drawn, it can take several weeks or months for test results to become available. The length of time depends on the tests performed and other factors. Individuals who decide to get tested should check with their doctor or genetic counselor to find out when test results might be available.

What factors increase the chance of developing breast or ovarian cancer?

The following factors have been associated with increased breast or ovarian cancer risk. It is not yet known exactly how these factors influence risk in people with BRCA1 or BRCA2 alterations.

Age: The risk of breast and ovarian cancers increases with age. Most breast and ovarian cancers occur in women over the age of fifty. Women with an altered BRCA1 or BRCA2 gene often develop breast or ovarian cancer before age fifty.

Family History: Women who have a first-degree relative (mother, sister, or daughter) or other close relative with breast or ovarian cancer may be at increased risk for developing these cancers. In addition, women with relatives who have had colon cancer are at increased risk of developing ovarian cancer.

Medical History: Women who have already had breast cancer are at increased risk of developing breast cancer again, or of developing ovarian cancer. Women who have had colon cancer also have an increased risk of developing ovarian cancer.

Hormonal Influences: Estrogen is naturally produced by the body and stimulates the normal growth of breast tissue. It is suspected that excess estrogen may contribute to breast cancer risk because of its natural role in stimulating breast cell growth. Women who had their first menstrual period before the age of twelve or experienced menopause after age fifty-five have a slightly increased risk of breast cancer, as do women who had their first child after age thirty. Each of these factors increases the amount of time a woman's body is exposed to estrogen. Removal of a woman's ovaries, which produce estrogen, reduces the risk of breast cancer.

Birth Control Pills (Oral Contraceptives): Most studies show a slight increase or no change in breast cancer risk in women taking birth control pills. Some studies suggest that a woman who has taken birth control pills for a long period of time, and began taking them at an early age or before her first pregnancy, has a small increase in her risk for developing breast cancer. In contrast, taking birth control pills may decrease a woman's risk of ovarian cancer.

Hormone Replacement Therapy: A woman's risk for developing breast cancer may be increased by hormone replacement therapy (HRT), especially when it is used for a long period of time. Doctors may prescribe HRT to reduce the discomfort from symptoms of menopause, such as hot flashes. Some evidence suggests that women who use HRT after menopause may also have a slightly increased risk of developing ovarian cancer. HRT may have positive health effects as well, such as lowering a woman's risk of heart disease and osteoporosis. These protective effects diminish after a woman discontinues therapy. The risks and benefits of HRT should be carefully considered by a woman and her health care provider.

Dietary Fat: Although early studies suggested a possible association between a high-fat diet and increased breast cancer risk, more recent studies have been inconclusive. It is not yet known whether a diet low in fat will lower breast cancer risk.

Physical Activity: Studies of the relationship between physical activity and breast cancer have had mixed results. However, some studies suggest that regular exercise, particularly in women age forty and younger, may decrease breast cancer risk.

Alcohol: Alcohol use may increase breast cancer risk, but no biological mechanism for the relationship between alcohol and breast cancer risk has been established.

Environmental Factors: Exposure of the breast to ionizing radiation, such as radiation therapy for Hodgkin's disease or other disorders, is associated with an increased risk of breast cancer, especially when the exposure occurred at a young age. Evidence for the effect of occupational, environmental, or chemical exposures on breast cancer risk is limited. For example, there is some evidence to suggest that organochlorine residues in the environment, such as those from insecticides, might be associated with an increase in breast cancer risk. However, the significance of this evidence has been debated. Scientific research is currently in progress to study the effects of various environmental factors on breast cancer risk.

Where can people get more information about genetic testing for cancer risk?

A person who is considering genetic testing should speak with a professional trained in genetics before deciding whether to be tested. These professionals may include doctors, genetic counselors, and other health care workers trained in genetics (such as nurses, psychologists, or social workers). For more information on genetic testing or for help finding a health care professional trained in genetics, contact the National Cancer Institute's Cancer Information Service (CIS) at 1-800-4-CANCER (1-800-422-6237). The CIS can also provide information about clinical trials (research studies with people) and answer questions about cancer.

References

Aziz S, G. Kuperstein, and B. Rosen, et al. "A Genetic Epidemiological Study of Carcinoma of the Fallopian Tube." *Gynecologic Oncology* 80, no. 3 (2001): 341–45.

Breast Cancer Linkage Consortium. "Cancer Risks in BRCA2 Mutation Carriers." *Journal of the National Cancer Institute* 91, no. 15 (1999): 1310–16.

Brekelmans, C. T. M., C. Seynaeve, and C. C. M. Bartels, et al. "Effectiveness of Breast Cancer Surveillance in BRCA1/2 Gene Mutation Carriers and Women with High Familial Risk." *Journal of Clinical Oncology* 19, no. 4 (2001): 924–30.

Fisher, B., J. P. Constantino, and D. L. Wickerham, et al. "Tamoxifen for Prevention of Breast Cancer: Report of the National Surgical Adjuvant Breast and Bowel Project P-1 Study." *Journal of the National Cancer Institute* 90, no. 18 (1998): 1371–88.

Garber, J. "A 40-Year-Old Woman with a Strong Family History of Breast Cancer." *Journal of the American Medical Association* 282, no. 20 (1999): 1953–60.

Hartge, P., J. P. Struewing, S. Wacholder, L. C. Brody, and M. A. Tucker. "The Prevalence of Common BRCA1 and BRCA2 Mutations among Ashkenazi Jews." *American Journal of Human Genetics* 64 (1999): 963–70.

King, M., S. Wieand, and K. Hale, et al. "Tamoxifen and Breast Cancer Incidence among Women with Inherited Mutations in BRCA1 and

BRCA2." *Journal of the American Medical Association* 286, no. 18 (2001): 2251–56.

Kodish, E., G. L. Wiesner, M. Mehlman, and T. Murray. "Genetic Testing for Cancer Risk: How to Reconcile the Conflicts." *Journal of the American Medical Association* 279, no. 3 (1998): 179–81.

Malone, K. E., J. R. Daling, J. D. Thompson, C. A. O'Brien, L. V. Francisco, and E. A. Ostrander. "BRCA1 Mutations and Breast Cancer in the General Population: Analyses in Women before Age 35 Years and in Women before Age 45 Years with First-Degree Family History." *Journal of the American Medical Association* 279, no. 12 (1998): 922–29.

Martin, A. M., and B. L. Weber. "Genetic and Hormonal Risk Factors in Breast Cancer." *Journal of the National Cancer Institute* 92, no. 14 (2000): 1126–35.

Newman, B, H. Mu, L. M. Butler, R. C. Millikan, P. G. Moorman, and M. C. King. "Frequency of Breast Cancer Attributable to BRCA1 in a Population-Based Series of American Women." *Journal of the American Medical Association* 279, no. 12 (1998): 915–21.

Peshkin, B. N., T. A. DeMarco, B. M. Brogan, C. Lerman, and C. Isaacs. "BRCA1/2 Testing: Complex Themes in Result Interpretation." *Journal of Clinical Oncology* 19, no. 9 (2001): 2555–65.

Rebbeck, T. R. "Prophylactic Oophorectomy in BRCA1 and BRCA2 Mutation Carriers." *Journal of Clinical Oncology* 18, no. 21s (2000): 100s–103s.

Thompson, D., and E. Easton, on behalf of the Breast Cancer Linkage Consortium. "Variation in Cancer Risks, by Mutation Position, in BRCA2 Mutation Carriers. *American Journal of Human Genetics* 68, no. 2 (2001): 410–19.

Warner, E., W. Foulkes, and P. Goodwin, et al. "Prevalence and Penetrance of BRCA1 and BRCA2 Gene Mutations in Unselected Ashkenazi Jewish Women with Breast Cancer." *Journal of the National Cancer Institute* 91, no. 14 (1999): 1241–47.

Welch, H. G., and W. Burke. "Uncertainties in Genetic Testing for Chronic Disease." *Journal of the American Medical Association* 280, no. 17 (1998): 1525–27.

Chapter 32

Breast Feeding May Reduce Breast Cancer Risk

Breast feeding may offer some modest protection against the development of breast cancer, particularly in young women. Considering the other health benefits of breast feeding for both mothers and their babies, this information should encourage new mothers to try to arrange their schedules to accommodate breast feeding.

Does breast feeding influence the risk of breast cancer?

Breast feeding may modestly reduce the risk of developing breast cancer. Out of thirty-one studies, more than half reported that women who breast fed had a decreased risk of developing breast cancer (ranging from 10 percent to 64 percent) compared to women who never breast fed. The rest of the studies reported that breast feeding had no influence on the risk of developing breast cancer.

The results of these studies may vary because of differences in the pattern of breast feeding among women in different cultures, such as when solid foods are added, how often a child is fed, and the reasons for stopping breast feeding. Another reason may be that some studies used information on the average length of time of breast feeding per child, while others asked for the total length of time of breast

"Breast Feeding and Breast Cancer Risk," by Julie A. Napieralski, Ph.D., Research Associate, and Carol Devine, Ph.D., R.D., Division of Nutritional Sciences and Education Project Leader, Program on Breast Cancer and Environmental Risk Factors in New York State (BCERF), Fact Sheet #29, updated May 2003, © 2003 Cornell University, reprinted with permission.

feeding all children combined. In addition, other reproductive factors, such as number of children and a woman's age at first birth, are very closely related to breast feeding and may also influence breast cancer risk. Other issues being studied include whether the age at which a woman first breast feeds is important, and the effects of breast feeding in women with a family history of breast cancer. Finally, it is also possible that breast feeding has different effects on the risk of developing premenopausal breast cancer compared to postmenopausal breast cancer.

Does breast feeding influence the risk of premenopausal and postmenopausal breast cancer differently?

Breast feeding may be more protective against the development of premenopausal compared to postmenopausal breast cancer. In some studies where there was no overall reduction in breast cancer risk associated with breast feeding, an analysis of the data by menopausal status revealed a slight protective effect of breast feeding in younger premenopausal women. Many other studies that focused specifically on young women reported that the incidence of premenopausal breast cancer was lower among women who breast fed. Many researchers think that premenopausal breast cancer and postmenopausal breast cancer are different diseases. However, it is not clear why breast feeding may be more protective against premenopausal breast cancer than postmenopausal breast cancer.

How long should women breast feed?

Although there are a few studies that report a decrease in the risk of breast cancer after only three or more months of breast feeding, the evidence for risk reduction becomes more consistent the longer women breast feed. The most consistent evidence of a relationship between breast feeding and the risk of breast cancer has been reported in studies of Chinese women who breast fed for long periods of time. In these studies, women who breast fed for a total of six years or more (all children combined) over the course of their lives had as much as a 63 percent decrease in breast cancer incidence compared to women who never breast fed.

The American Academy of Pediatrics recommends that women begin breast feeding within the first hour after birth if possible. For most women, exclusive breast feeding is recommended for about the first six months, and breast feeding should continue for at least twelve months thereafter. In the report Healthy People 2000, the U.S. Department of Health and Human Services set goals to: (1) increase to at least 75 percent the proportion of mothers who breast feed their babies in the early postpartum period, and (2) increase to at least 50 percent the proportion who continue breast feeding until their babies are five to six months old.

Is there any evidence that drugs used to suppress lactation influence breast cancer risk?

Studies that examined the use of drugs to suppress lactation reported that these drugs do not have any influence on the risk of developing breast cancer.

Should breast cancer survivors breast feed?

Since there are relatively few cases of breast cancer in premenopausal women, there are also very few studies that have looked at the effects of treatment for breast cancer on breast feeding. The ability to breast feed after treatment for breast cancer depends on the individual and on the treatment she received. Surgery and radiation may impair a woman's ability to breast feed on the affected side. Radiation may cause skin damage during treatment similar to sunburn or chapped skin and, in order to avoid infection so treatment can continue, it is usually recommended that breast feeding from the breast being treated be stopped. In some cases, women reported that there seemed to be less milk produced in the irradiated breast. However, they were able to breast feed from the untreated breast. Other women have reported that they were able to breast feed from both the treated and the untreated breast after radiation treatment.

Lumps are common in the breasts of women who are breast feeding. Not all are cancer, but all should be evaluated seriously by a health care provider. Women should feel comfortable getting a second opinion about a persistent lump. Although physical changes in the breasts of women who are pregnant or breast feeding may hide a lump, women who are breast feeding should examine their breasts for changes or abnormalities. The best time to examine the breasts is immediately after a feeding. Women should talk to their health care providers about any unusual physical changes in their breasts while they are breast feeding.

Women needing to undergo any kind of treatment for breast cancer, including surgery, chemotherapy, or radiation should talk with their health care providers if breast feeding is a concern. It may be possible to breast feed before and after surgery and through radiation, though probably not on the side being irradiated. Since many drugs may be passed to an infant through breast milk, breast feeding women should always talk with their health care providers about any medications they are taking.

How might breast feeding influence the risk of breast cancer?

There are several ways that breast feeding may influence the risk of developing breast cancer. Breast feeding may

- Cause hormonal changes, such as a decrease in the level of estrogen.

- Lower levels of estrogen, which may decrease a woman's risk of developing breast cancer.

- Suppress ovulation. According to some studies, women who have fewer ovulatory cycles over the course of their reproductive lives may have a decreased risk of developing breast cancer.

- Remove possible carcinogens that are stored in the adipose tissue of the breast (see following for more information).

- Cause physical changes in the cells that line the mammary ducts. These changes may make the cells more resistant to mutations that can lead to cancer.

Does breast feeding influence the risk of breast cancer for the baby?

There is some preliminary evidence that there may be a slight decrease in the risk of developing breast cancer among women who were breast fed as infants. This protection may be due to the hormones and immune factors present in breast milk. It may also be due to the fact that babies who are breast fed take in fewer calories and gain weight more slowly than babies who are bottle-fed. There are some studies that report that earlier maturation in childhood may increase the risk of developing breast cancer later in life.

In other preliminary studies, no association was found between being breast fed as an infant and the development of breast cancer later in life. In addition, one study reported that there was no difference in the risk of breast cancer among women who had been breast fed by a mother who eventually developed the disease.

Are there any health concerns associated with breast feeding?

Breast milk is considered to be the ideal nutrient source for infants. However, because certain chemicals persist in the environment, are stored in fat, and are secreted in breast milk, they have been studied by researchers at the National Institute of Environmental Health Sciences (NIEHS). These researchers concluded that in the vast majority of women the benefits of breast feeding appear to outweigh possible risks.

In only a few cases, women should consult with their health care providers before breast feeding. These cases include women with certain infectious diseases, women who have been taking prescription or street drugs, or women who may be exposed to high levels of certain environmental contaminants. There are only a few circumstances that may lead to some women having high levels of chemicals in their breast milk. These circumstances are (1) having a history of workplace exposure to environmental chemicals, (2) having a large accidental exposure, and (3) regularly consuming fish that are caught in contaminated waters (this does not include fish bought in supermarkets).

Women can obtain information on the safety of consuming fish caught in bodies of water throughout the United States by calling the Environmental Protection Agency at: 513-489-8190. Also, researchers at the Bureau of Toxic Substance Assessment in the New York State Department of Health (DOH) are continuing to assess the effects of various environmental chemicals on human health.

For more information, women can obtain a helpful review from the U.S. Department of Health and Human Services by calling 703-356-1964 and requesting a copy of the "Maternal and Child Health Technical Information Bulletin: A Review of the Medical Benefits and Contraindications to Breastfeeding in the United States" by Dr. Ruth Lawrence.

What are the other health benefits of breast feeding?

There are many important health benefits associated with breast feeding for both the mother and the baby. Babies who are breast fed have a lower incidence or severity of several childhood illnesses, including diarrhea, lower respiratory infections, ear infections, and bacterial meningitis. Other possible protective effects have been reported against sudden death infant syndrome, allergic diseases, and chronic digestive diseases.

Women who breast feed their infants have less postpartum bleeding and may have an earlier return to pre-pregnant weight. There is also some evidence that they have improved bone remineralization after they stop breast feeding, which may lead to a reduction in hip fractures during the postmenopausal years.

An extensive bibliography on breast feeding and the risk of breast cancer is available on the BCERF web site: http://envirocancer .cornell.edu.

—Prepared by Julie A. Napieralski, Ph.D., Research Associate, BCERF, Cornell University and Carol Devine, Ph.D., R.D., Education Project Leader, BCERF, Cornell University

For More Information

Program on Breast Cancer and Environmental Risk Factors
Sprecher Institute for Comparative Cancer Research
Cornell University
Box 31
Ithaca, NY 14853
Phone: (607) 254-2893
Internet: http://envirocancer.cornell.edu
E-mail: breastcancer@cornell.edu

Chapter 33

Physical Activity Can Cut Breast Cancer Risk

Women who take part in strenuous leisure-time activities vigorous enough to work up a sweat appear to cut their risk of developing breast cancer, University at Buffalo (UB) researchers have shown.

The study asked women between the ages of forty and eighty-five how much physical activity they took part in at two, ten, and twenty years prior to the interview and at age sixteen.

Findings showed the strongest protective effect from strenuous exercise at a point twenty years in the past. All women who reported an average of 3.5 hours per week of sweat-producing physical activity at that point in their lives cut their risk of developing breast cancer later in life in half.

Being active in their teens also appeared to be protective. Strenuous activity at age sixteen produced a 35 to 45 percent reduction in risk, findings showed.

The study appears in the February issue of *Medicine and Science in Sports and Exercise.*

"This is one more small piece of a really large puzzle concerning what protects against breast cancer," said lead author Joan Dorn, assistant professor of social and preventive medicine in the School of Public Health and Health Professions. "To date, few factors related to breast cancer have emerged as being strongly protective, particularly factors that women can modify, so even a modest effect is important."

Reprinted with permission from "Strenuous Physical Activity throughout Life Can Cut Breast Cancer Risk," by Lois Baker, *University at Buffalo Reporter,* Vol. 34, No. 15, February 27, 2003.

The Study

Physical activity has received much attention recently as a lifestyle component that could offer some potential protection against breast cancer, but study results remain mixed and some research indicated different effects for pre- and postmenopausal women, Dorn said. In addition, researchers have been interested in determining if physical activity at any particular point in a woman's life was particularly protective, she noted.

To attempt to answer these questions, Dorn and colleagues turned to UB's Western New York Diet Study, a population-based, case-control study of newly diagnosed breast cancer patients and randomly selected healthy women in Western New York conducted from 1986–91. One of the study's aims was to examine the association between lifetime physical activity and breast cancer risk.

The study group consisted of 301 menopausal women and 439 postmenopausal women with breast cancer, and 316 premenopausal and 494 postmenopausal controls. During the initial interview, women were asked to report on time spent per week in physical activity strenuous enough to make them sweat at four points (two, ten, and twenty years in the past and at age sixteen) in their lives. From this information, Dorn and colleagues calculated an average hours-per-week of exercise for each participant at those four points in her life.

The Results

Looking at each time period separately, results showed generally a modest protective effect of exercise for both pre- and postmenopausal women who were active at any one time period, Dorn said. Postmenopausal women who were active at all four time periods had a 50 percent decrease in risk, but this protective effect didn't show up for the younger women in the study for reasons that weren't immediately clear, she noted.

However, being active at age sixteen and at a point twenty years in the past appeared to be particularly significant. Dorn speculated that these time points may have coincided with significant physiological events in the women's lives.

"The age of menarche and age at first birth have been identified as potentially important periods in the life history of breast cancer," she said. "For the premenopausal women whose mean age was forty-six at the time of the interview, twenty years prior may have placed them, on average, around the time of first pregnancy. It's possible that our observation of a protective effect coincides with this important time period.

"Twenty years post-interview for the postmenopausal women would put them around their mid-forties, when many would be approaching menopause," Dorn noted. "It's possible that strenuous exercise during this period of a woman's life has an impact on breast cancer by favorably affecting a hormonal milieu in the process of change.

"These results, combined with what we know about the benefits of physical activity in protecting against other chronic diseases, are enough to tell women to get out there and get some exercise," she said.

Additional authors on the study, all from the Department of Social and Preventive Medicine in the School of Health and Health Professions, were John Vena, John Brasure, Jo Freudenheim, and Saxon Graham.

Chapter 34

Phytoestrogens and Breast Cancer

Phytoestrogens are estrogen-like chemicals found in plant foods such as beans, seeds, and grains. Foods made from soybeans have some of the highest levels of phytoestrogens and have been studied the most. In spite of initial optimism, it is not clear whether eating foods rich in phytoestrogens decreases breast cancer risk. This is an active area of research, with much work needed to resolve this issue. This chapter presents the most current information and indicates where more research would be helpful.

What are phytoestrogens?

Phytoestrogens are a group of chemicals found in plants that can act like the hormone estrogen. Estrogen is a hormone necessary for childbearing and is involved with bone and heart health in women. However, higher exposure to estrogens over a lifetime is linked with increased breast cancer risk.

What foods contain phytoestrogens?

More than three hundred foods have been shown to contain phytoestrogens. Most food phytoestrogens are from one of three chemical

"Phytoestrogens and Breast Cancer," by Barbour Warren, Ph.D., Research Associate, and Carol Devine, Ph.D., R.D., Division of Nutritional Sciences and Education Project Leader, Program on Breast Cancer and Environmental Risk Factors in New York State (BCERF), Fact Sheet #01, updated July 2002, © 2002 Cornell University, reprinted with permission.

classes, the isoflavonoids, the lignans, or the coumestans. Isoflavonoid phytoestrogens are found in beans from the legume family; soybeans and soy products are the major dietary source of this type of phytoestrogens. Lignan phytoestrogens are found in high-fiber foods such as cereal brans and beans; flaxseeds contain large amounts of lignans. The coumestan phytoestrogens are found in various beans such as split peas, pinto beans, and lima beans; alfalfa and clover sprouts are the foods with the highest amounts of coumestans.

Can phytoestrogens from soy foods affect breast cancer risk?

It is currently unclear whether phytoestrogens from soy foods affect breast cancer risk. Studies looking directly at breast cancer risk and soy in the diet are not in agreement. Almost half of the studies have reported no effect of soy on breast cancer risk. In addition, animal and cellular studies of soy phytoestrogens have generated both enthusiasm and concern. Animal studies have shown that soy phytoestrogens can decrease breast cancer formation in rats. However, animal and human studies suggest that soy phytoestrogens can behave like estrogen and potentially increase breast cancer risk. Some scientists have suggested that women should be cautious about eating large amounts of the soy products or soy supplements, because of the possible harmful effects of soy phytoestrogens. These concerns and areas of research are discussed in the following in more detail.

How do phytoestrogens act in the body?

There are many different ways that phytoestrogens may work in the body. The chemical structure of phytoestrogens is similar to estrogen, and they may act as mimics (copies) of estrogen. On the other hand, phytoestrogens also have effects that are different from those of estrogen.

Working as estrogen mimics, phytoestrogens may either have the same effects as estrogen or block estrogen's effects. Which effect the phytoestrogen produces can depend on the dose of the phytoestrogen. The phytoestrogen can act like estrogen at low doses but block estrogen at high doses. Estrogen activates a family of proteins called estrogen receptors. Recent studies have shown that phytoestrogens interact more with some members of the estrogen receptor family, but more information is needed about how these receptors work, especially in breast cancer. Finally, phytoestrogens acting as estrogen mimics may affect the production or the breakdown of estrogen by the body, as well as the levels of estrogen carried in the bloodstream.

Phytoestrogens—acting differently from estrogen—may affect communication pathways between cells, prevent the formation of blood vessels to tumors, or alter processes involved in the processing of DNA for cell multiplication. Which of these effects occur is unknown. It is very possible that more than one of them may be working. Also, the effects in various parts of the body may be different.

What have human studies on soy in the diet and breast cancer risk found?

The results of the case-control human studies of the connection between eating soy products and breast cancer risk are conflicting. Some studies have reported no link and others have reported a decrease in the risk of breast cancer among women eating soy compared to women who did not eat soy; no studies have reliably demonstrated an increase in the risk of breast cancer among women eating soy. In addition to the conflicting results, there are four problems with these studies. First, the number of studies is small; only ten studies have examined soy in the diet and breast cancer risk. Second, most of the studies examined small numbers of women; only four of the studies included more than two hundred patients. Third, all but two of the studies were limited to women from Asia. The effect of soy in Asian women may not best reflect its effect on much of the population of Western countries like the United States. Women in Asia differ in important ways. Many of them have eaten soy products all their lives, and their usual diets contain large amounts of soy products. Also, Asian women have low rates of breast cancer compared to Western women, which may be related to other factors besides soy in their diet. Fourth, most of these studies are limited by their focus on the general diet of women rather than soy products in detail. More carefully controlled studies are needed that examine the effect of soy products on breast cancer risk in women from cultures outside of Asia, and more in-depth studies are needed of Asian women.

What is the effect of eating soy on women's hormone levels and growth within the breast?

Soy phytoestrogens could change breast cancer risk by changing the production or breakdown of reproductive hormones such as estrogen. The results of studies examining hormone changes among

233

women eating soy have not been consistent, but recent studies suggest there may be a small decrease in the levels of estrogens in the body. Some studies have also shown that eating soy phytoestrogens is associated with a decrease in the formation of forms of estrogens that may directly lead to cancer-causing mutations.

One of the ways higher estrogen exposure may be linked to breast cancer risk is through its ability to increase growth of milk ducts in the breast. Most breast cancer arises from these ducts. Several but not all studies examining the effect of soy phytoestrogens on breast growth in women have suggested that phytoestrogens have a weak estrogen-like effect. The longest examination followed twenty-eight women for a year. These women received a soy supplement for six months. While they were taking this supplement the women were found to have more growth of the milk ducts in their breasts. These studies are not conclusive, but such growth could increase breast cancer risk. More study is needed to evaluate the possible effects of soy phytoestrogens on growth within the breast and hormone levels in the body.

What are the results of the animal and cellular studies examining soy phytoestrogens and breast cancer?

Animals that were given soy phytoestrogens developed fewer mammary (breast) tumors in many, but not all, studies. The decrease in tumor formation was dependent on the age at which the animals were given the soy. Animals given a soy phytoestrogen before sexual maturity had about half as many tumors as animals given a soy phytoestrogen as adults. A similar effect of the age of treatment was also seen when animals were given a synthetic estrogen or estrogen together with progesterone. More studies are needed to understand this effect of phytoestrogens and of estrogen itself.

Studies of breast cells in tissue culture have shown that soy phytoestrogens can either encourage or discourage growth within the breast. This effect depends on the amount of the soy phytoestrogen the cells are exposed to (See "How do phytoestrogens act in the body?" in the preceding). It is unclear if these effects on cells in the laboratory are the same or different from those on breast cells in the body.

Have other classes of phytoestrogens been examined for their effect on breast cancer risk?

Both lignan (from brans, beans, and seeds) and coumestans phytoestrogens (from beans and sprouts) have been studied for a possible effect on breast cancer risk. Two studies have found higher levels of lignan phytoestrogens in the urine of women who may be at lower risk for breast cancer, such as Japanese women and women eating a macrobiotic diet. Other studies compared women without cancer to women with breast cancer; the women with breast cancer had significantly lower levels of lignan phytoestrogens in their urine. Phytoestrogen levels in urine are an accurate measure of phytoestrogens in the body, but it is uncertain how levels in the women with cancer compare to levels in these women during the decades when cancer was developing.

A lignan phytoestrogen found in flaxseed, secoisolariciresinol diglycoside (SDG) has been shown to interfere with mammary (breast) tumor formation in rats. SDG has similar effects on the development of the mammary gland to the soy phytoestrogen genistein. (But see the discussion of potential SDG/flaxseed toxicity in the question on pregnancy and nursing in the following.)

Coumestans are the least studied phytoestrogens. Treatment of rats with a coumestan phytoestrogen had no effect on mammary (breast) tumor formation but this phytoestrogen has been examined in only one study of this type. Some coumestans have strong interactions with estrogen receptors. This makes them like the strongest estrogens made by the body and suggests that they may also have estrogen-like actions.

Is there any harm in taking phytoestrogen supplements or eating large amounts of foods with phytoestrogens?

Care should be taken in the use of phytoestrogen supplements that may contain phytoestrogens at levels far higher than in food. Since phytoestrogens can have estrogen-like effects in humans, use of these supplements for a long time could increase breast cancer risk.

Moderate consumption of foods high in phytoestrogens is unlikely to have any adverse effects, and these foods are generally healthful.

Is there a certain time during a woman's life when eating phytoestrogens can be of the greatest benefit?

One recent study of Chinese women suggests that eating large amounts of soy during adolescence may reduce the risk of breast cancer. Studies in animals have demonstrated that the period of breast development is critical for mammary tumor inhibition by phytoestrogens. It is currently unclear if the results in Chinese women reflect a similar critical period or a lifetime of eating soy products.

Human epidemiological studies suggest that if breast cancer risk reduction is linked to eating soy phytoestrogens, the effect may be greater on premenopausal breast cancer. More studies are needed to determine if soy phytoestrogen and other phytoestrogens act largely on premenopausal breast cancer and whether the effectiveness of phytoestrogens is related to the period of life when they are eaten.

Should breast cancer survivors eat more phytoestrogens?

No studies have examined the health effects of eating phytoestrogens among breast cancer survivors. Drugs or chemicals that cause growth of breast tissue are generally not recommended for breast cancer survivors. Phytoestrogen supplements have been shown to cause growth of breast tissue in animals and healthy women.

No human studies have assessed the effects of combining tamoxifen (an anti-estrogenic drug prescribed for many breast cancer survivors and some women at high risk for breast cancer) and phytoestrogens in breast cancer survivors. Women taking tamoxifen are usually not included in studies where concentrated supplements of phytoestrogens are given. Studies examining the actions of tamoxifen and genistein in the laboratory using isolated breast cancer cells have produced conflicting results. In some studies the two chemicals acted together, and in others their effects were opposing. More studies are needed to understand potential favorable or conflicting actions between these two chemicals.

Should I eat more phytoestrogens if I am taking estrogen for treatments such as birth control or postmenopausal hormone therapy?

The effects of phytoestrogens on women taking birth control pills or being treated with postmenopausal hormonal therapy have not been examined. Both of these treatments use estrogen, and since phytoestrogens can act like the hormone estrogen, phytoestrogens might disrupt or amplify the effect of the estrogen in individuals with a diet very high in phytoestrogens. However, such effects have not been reported in groups of women who have diets high in phytoestrogens.

Should infants and young children eat phytoestrogens?

The regulatory bodies of several countries, including Great Britain, Switzerland, Australia, and New Zealand, have suggested that soy infant formulas be used only in children who are not breast-fed and are definitely intolerant to cow's milk. Soy formulas contain much higher amounts of phytoestrogens than is seen in human breast milk. In addition, infants fed soy formula have blood levels of phytoestrogens that are far greater than normal levels of estrogen in infants. No studies have examined the health effects of children eating phytoestrogen-rich foods. Long-term studies that look at the health benefits and risks of soy-based infant formulas and eating phytoestrogen-rich foods as a child are needed.

Should I eat phytoestrogens if I am pregnant or breast-feeding?

Pregnant or breast-feeding women should not use phytoestrogen supplements or consume substantial amounts of flaxseeds on a regular basis. In animal studies, the phytoestrogens found in high amounts in flaxseeds have been shown to cause developmental abnormalities, and some studies of soy phytoestrogens have shown a possible increase in susceptibility to cancer in offspring. Eating moderate amounts of soy or flax products should present no problem. Women in China and Japan regularly eat foods containing soy phytoestrogens during pregnancy and while breast-feeding and no adverse health affects have been reported in these countries.

Do phytoestrogens have other health benefits?

Phytoestrogens are actively being researched for beneficial effects on cardiovascular and bone health. Studies are also examining various phytoestrogens for relieving some of the symptoms associated with menopause.

What can women do now?

It is unclear what role foods containing phytoestrogens play in decreasing breast cancer risk. Women can help themselves stay healthy by eating plenty of fruits, vegetables, whole grains, and beans and by getting plenty of exercise and maintaining a healthy weight.

What scientific studies need to be done?

The following aspects of phytoestrogens especially need further study:

- Effects of phytoestrogens, especially from soy, on breast cancer risk in humans

- Actions of soy phytoestrogens on breast development in humans

- Health effects of soy phytoestrogens on individuals who used soy formula as an infant

- Consequences of phytoestrogens on breast cancer survival

—Prepared by Barbour S. Warren, Research Associate, BCERF, Cornell University and Carol Devine, Ph.D., R.D., Educational Project Leader, BCERF, Cornell University

For More Information

Program on Breast Cancer and Environmental Risk Factors
Sprecher Institute for Comparative Cancer Research
Cornell University
Box 31
Ithaca, NY 14853
Phone: (607) 254-2893
Internet: http://envirocancer.cornell.edu
E-mail: breastcancer@cornell.edu

Chapter 35

Chemoprevention of Breast Cancer

Executive Summary

1. The U.S. Food and Drug Administration has approved the drug tamoxifen for breast cancer risk reduction in high-risk women. This is the first time that any drug has been approved for cancer chemoprevention.

2. Several studies in high-risk women have shown that the use of tamoxifen may reduce a woman's risk of breast cancer by 40–50 percent.

3. There is suggestive evidence that the drug raloxifene, which is used in the prevention and treatment of osteoporosis, may also reduce breast cancer risk. However, the evidence for a chemopreventive effect of this drug is less compelling than the evidence for tamoxifen. The FDA has not approved raloxifene for breast cancer chemoprevention. Therefore, unless ongoing research on raloxifene in the STAR (Study of Tamoxifen and Raloxifene) trial indicates otherwise, tamoxifen remains the only agent with FDA approval for reducing the risk of breast cancer.

4. Physicians should discuss breast cancer chemoprevention with all high-risk women unless there is a medical contraindication

"Chemoprevention of Breast Cancer" by Kathleen Meister is reprinted with permission of the American Council on Science and Health (ACSH). ©2000 American Council on Science and Health, Inc. For additional information about ACSH, visit their website at www.acsh.org.

to its use. The decision to start chemoprevention should rest on two major factors: a woman's actual risks and what those risks mean to her. Women who are considering chemoprevention need to be aware of all of the potential benefits and risks, and to weigh these factors carefully, before making a final decision. Women have the right to know all the information necessary to make educated choices in this important area of their personal health.

Introduction

Each year, approximately 175,000 women in the United States are diagnosed with breast cancer and about 43,000 die of it. Among American women, breast cancer is the most common cancer and the second-most common cause of death from cancer (after lung cancer).

In recent years, researchers have developed better ways to treat breast cancer, and they have devised screening methods that enable the detection of many breast cancers early, when the likelihood of a cure is greatest. Until very recently, however, scientists did not make much progress in developing ways to prevent breast cancer.

People can help protect themselves against some types of cancer (such as lung cancer and skin cancer) by making changes in their lifestyles (such as choosing not to smoke and limiting exposure to the sun). However, lifestyle changes can't do much to protect one against breast cancer. The most important factors associated with breast cancer risk—age, family history of the disease, and reproductive factors such as age at menopause—are difficult or impossible to modify. Therefore, other approaches to prevention are needed.

Very recently, scientists have developed a new method—called "chemoprevention"—to reduce the risk of breast cancer in women who are at high risk of this disease. This chapter summarizes the current scientific evidence on chemoprevention of breast cancer and describes the issues that an individual woman and her physician need to consider when deciding whether chemoprevention is appropriate for her. This chapter includes a discussion of the comparative risks and benefits of tamoxifen, the only drug recommended for reducing breast cancer risk, and raloxifene, a promising drug that currently is undergoing rigorous testing in this setting.

Risk Factors for Breast Cancer

Unlike some other diseases, such as infections, most cancers do not have a single cause. Instead, they result from the interaction of multiple factors. Researchers who study the causes of cancer use the term "risk factor" to refer to anything that is associated with an increased chance of developing a particular type of cancer.

Different cancers have different risk factors. For example, smoking is the most important risk factor for lung cancer, but it is not a risk factor for skin cancer. Conversely, exposure to ultraviolet light from the sun is a risk factor for skin cancer but not for lung cancer.

The principal risk factors for breast cancer are described below.

Gender

Breast cancer is primarily a woman's disease. Although it can occur in men, it is about one hundred times more common in women.

Age

As is true for many forms of cancer, the risk of breast cancer increases with age. More than 75 percent of all cases of breast cancer occur in women over the age of fifty.

Family History and Genetic Risk Factors

The risk of breast cancer is higher among women whose close blood relatives have had the disease. Having one first-degree relative (mother, sister, or daughter) with breast cancer doubles a woman's breast cancer risk; having two first-degree relatives with breast cancer increases risk fivefold (500 percent). The increase in risk is especially high if the relative or relatives developed the disease before age fifty or in both breasts. In one study, women who had a first-degree relative who developed cancer in both breasts before the age of fifty had an eightfold (800 percent) increase in the risk of breast cancer, while those whose relative developed cancer in one breast after the age of fifty showed only a slight (20 percent) increase in risk.

Genetic factors may contribute to the increased risk associated with a family history of breast cancer. About 10 percent of all cases of breast cancer are hereditary, resulting from mutations in specific genes, such as the BRCA1, BRCA2, or p53 genes. The other cases may also have a genetic component.

Personal Medical History

A woman who has previously had breast cancer has a three- to four-fold increased risk of developing a new cancer in the other breast.

241

Women who have had certain other breast conditions—such as lobular carcinoma in situ (LCIS) or ductal carcinoma in situ (DCIS)—are also at increased risk. Another breast condition, called "atypical ductal hyperplasia" (ADH), is also associated with an increase in risk. A history of benign breast disease, such as fibroadenoma, may also increase risk.

Reproductive History

Certain aspects of a woman's reproductive history are associated with increases or decreases in breast cancer risk. At least some of these factors are believed to exert their effects by modifying a woman's lifetime exposure to the female hormone estrogen, which may promote breast cancer.

Reproductive factors associated with increased risk include the following:

- Early age at menarche (first menstrual period)
- Late age at menopause
- Never having a full-term pregnancy
- Giving birth for the first time at a relatively late age, i.e., after age thirty-five

Lifestyle Factors

Several aspects of a woman's lifestyle have been associated with relatively small increases or decreases in breast cancer risk. Obesity is associated with an increased risk of breast cancer after menopause but not before. Physical activity helps to protect one against breast cancer. There may be a small increase in breast cancer risk associated with long-term postmenopausal estrogen replacement therapy; the evidence for increased risk with oral contraceptive use and alcohol consumption is not conclusive.

What Is Chemoprevention?

When doctors use medicines to treat cancer, they refer to it as chemotherapy. The use of medicines to prevent or reduce the risk of cancer is called "chemoprevention."

The word "chemoprevention" is easy to remember, but it can be misleading. When people hear that an agent "prevents" a disease, they may expect that it will provide nearly 100 percent protection, which many vaccines do. Cancer chemoprevention, however, is not so effective. A chemopreventive agent can reduce an individual's risk of cancer, but it does not eliminate that risk completely.

Cancer chemoprevention is much like the use of cholesterol-lowering drugs to help prevent heart disease. These drugs do not eliminate the risk of a heart attack, but they do decrease that risk substantially. Similarly, chemoprevention substantially decreases a woman's risk of breast cancer, but it doesn't guarantee that she will not develop this disease.

Another important point to remember about chemoprevention is that it has risks as well as benefits. Any agent that is strong enough to reduce the risk of cancer is also likely to have other effects on the body, some of which may be undesirable. Thus, decisions about the use of chemoprevention should be based on a thorough understanding of both its risks and its benefits.

The idea of giving healthy people strong medicine for a prolonged period of time in an effort to prevent cancer is a new one, and it makes some people (including some physicians) uncomfortable. However, chemoprevention is not very different from other, well-accepted types of risk reduction—such as the use of hormone replacement therapy to reduce the risk of osteoporosis, the use of blood pressure–lowering medications to reduce the risk of stroke, or the use of aspirin or cholesterol-lowering drugs to reduce the risk of a heart attack. In all of these instances, people who are essentially healthy—except for their increased risk of a particular disease—are given medicines to reduce their risk of developing that disease. And in all of these instances, the medicines can, at least occasionally, have significant harmful effects.

The people who are most likely to benefit from the use of a risk-reducing agent are those who are at high risk of the disease that the agent protects against. Low-risk individuals have less to gain because few of them will develop the disease anyway. Any small benefit that the medicine would offer them is likely to be outweighed by the potential for side effects.

For example, doctors often recommend that their sixty-year-old patients take a small dose of aspirin every day to reduce their risk of a heart attack, but they almost never recommend this to their twenty-year-old patients. The reason is simple: heart attacks are common in sixty-year-olds, but rare in twenty-year-olds. However, both younger and older people are at risk of developing side effects—such as stomach bleeding—from aspirin therapy. The benefits of aspirin outweigh the risks for the sixty-year-old, but they do not outweigh the risks for the younger person. Similar considerations apply to cancer chemoprevention.

The Use of Tamoxifen for Breast Cancer Chemoprevention

The drug tamoxifen (brand name Nolvadex) has been used for more than twenty years to treat breast cancer. Tamoxifen is one of a group of drugs called "selective estrogen-receptor modulators." Drugs of this type have actions similar to those of the female hormone estrogen in some body tissues, but they block the effect of estrogen in other tissues, including breast tissue.

In 1998 the U.S. Food and Drug Administration (FDA) approved the use of tamoxifen for the reduction of risk of breast cancer in healthy high-risk women. This was the first time the FDA had ever approved an agent for the prevention of cancer in healthy people.

FDA approval of tamoxifen was based on several studies that evaluated the effect of this drug on the risk of breast cancer in high-risk women. The most important of these studies was the Breast Cancer Prevention Trial (BCPT), in which more than thirteen thousand women were randomly assigned to receive either tamoxifen or an inactive placebo for five years. The women chosen for this study were at higher-than-average risk of breast cancer because they either (1) were age sixty or over, (2) had a history of LCIS, or (3) were thirty-five to fifty-nine years old with other risk factors (such as family history of breast cancer) that increased their risk to the level usually seen in older women. At the end of the study, the researchers found that women taking tamoxifen had developed only half as many breast cancers as had those taking placebo. In other studies, tamoxifen produced a similar (40–50%) reduction in breast cancer risk in women who were at increased risk because of a history of previous breast cancer or DCIS.

In these studies, the overall benefits of tamoxifen outweighed the overall risks. Nevertheless, the risks were significant. Women taking the drug had increased risks of endometrial cancer (cancer of the lining of the uterus), problems related to blood clots, and cataracts. Most of the women taking tamoxifen also experienced hot flashes as a result of taking the drug; although this side effect is not medically serious, it can be severe enough to reduce the quality of life for some individuals. In specific cases—depending on age, baseline risk levels, and other factors—the risk of taking tamoxifen may outweigh the benefits to a person. There is a comprehensive risk assessment (by Gail and colleagues) available through doctors' offices and university and college medical centers that can help a woman determine whether her potential risks would outweigh her potential benefits from tamoxifen.

Some people may wonder why anyone would even consider trying to prevent one type of cancer—breast cancer—with a drug that increases the risk of another type of cancer—endometrial cancer. This is not, however, as strange as it may seem, for two reasons. First, breast cancer is more common than endometrial cancer (especially in women with increased breast cancer risk factors); in the BCPT, five women developed breast cancer for every one who developed endometrial cancer. Second, in women who get regular gynecological care and who promptly report unusual symptoms, such as vaginal bleeding, endometrial cancer can usually be found at an early stage, when treatment is very effective. This may not be true for breast cancer, which is a more common and generally a more serious cancer.

Although the FDA and the American Society of Clinical Oncology have recommended tamoxifen for breast cancer chemoprevention in high-risk women, the use of tamoxifen for this purpose has not gained wide acceptance in the community. The underutilization of tamoxifen may be based partly on an understandable reluctance to administer a drug with well-known adverse effects to healthy women.

Is Raloxifene Useful for Breast Cancer Chemoprevention?

Like tamoxifen, raloxifene (brand name Evista) is a selective estrogen-receptor modulator. Raloxifene has been approved by the FDA for both the treatment and prevention of osteoporosis (loss of bone density) in postmenopausal women. Like tamoxifen, raloxifene can increase the risk of blood clots. However, unlike tamoxifen, raloxifene does not appear to increase the risk of endometrial hypertrophy (growth) or cancer.

In 1999, scientists who were conducting a large controlled study of raloxifene for fracture prevention in women with osteoporosis reported that women in their study who were taking the active drug had a lower rate of breast cancer than those who were taking the placebo. The extent of the reduction in breast cancer risk was even greater than that seen with tamoxifen.

After these findings were made public, physicians and patients responded enthusiastically to the idea that raloxifene might be useful for breast cancer chemoprevention. This reaction was probably related to the belief that raloxifene could be as effective as tamoxifen in reducing breast cancer risk, but with less risk of endometrial cancer and valuable protection against bone fractures. However, as of now, the use of raloxifene for breast cancer chemoprevention does not have as firm a scientific basis as does the use of tamoxifen.

245

The evidence that tamoxifen is beneficial in breast cancer chemoprevention comes from several studies that were specifically designed to address this relationship, using groups of women who were chosen for study because of their increased risk of breast cancer. The evidence for a potential benefit of raloxifene comes from studies that were primarily designed to look at osteoporosis. The participants in the study were chosen because of their bone problems, not their breast cancer risk, and most were at relatively low risk of breast cancer. Since the raloxifene study was primarily intended for other purposes, its findings with regard to breast cancer should be regarded only as suggestive rather than conclusive. Because of the limited nature of the evidence, the FDA has not yet approved raloxifene for breast cancer prevention. Physicians may still prescribe raloxifene for this purpose, but they must discuss with the patient the fact that this drug has not yet been FDA-approved for this indication.

To determine whether raloxifene is truly effective in breast cancer chemoprevention, researchers will need to conduct controlled trials similar to those already completed for tamoxifen. One such major study, called "STAR" (for "Study of Tamoxifen and Raloxifene"), is already in progress. In this study, postmenopausal women at high risk of breast cancer will be randomly assigned to receive either raloxifene or tamoxifen, and the outcomes of the two groups will be compared.

Until the STAR trial is completed, the value of raloxifene in breast cancer chemoprevention will remain uncertain. Women who are starting chemoprevention now would be well advised to note that the benefits of tamoxifen have been clearly established.

Individual Decision Making

Because the use of tamoxifen for breast cancer chemoprevention involves a complex mix of potential benefits and risks, decisions about its use should be made on an individual basis. A woman and her physician should begin by assessing her personal risk of breast cancer on the basis of her family, reproductive, and medical history. During this evaluation, some women may be surprised to learn that their risk is not as high as they had believed. For example, some women think that they are at increased risk of breast cancer because they have had breast injuries, breast augmentation surgery, or abortions, or because a distant relative had breast cancer. In actuality, however, none of these factors is known to be associated with a significant increase in risk.

If a woman's history indicates that she truly is at increased risk of breast cancer, the physician must then ask about a variety of other issues that will influence the decision whether or not to use tamoxifen. Some of these issues include:

- **Age:** Tamoxifen is approved for all women aged sixty or more, and for high-risk women aged thirty-five to fifty-nine.

- **History of blood clots requiring medical treatment:** Women with such a history should not take tamoxifen.

- **Use of anticoagulant ("blood thinner") medication:** Women who are taking this type of drug should not take tamoxifen.

- **Previous hysterectomy:** A woman who has had a hysterectomy is not at risk of endometrial cancer. Therefore, the balance of benefits and risks of tamoxifen is more favorable for her than for a woman with an intact uterus.

- **Use of hormone replacement therapy or raloxifene:** For women who are using hormone replacement therapy or raloxifene, taking tamoxifen is not advisable. Depending on their individual risks of the various diseases involved, some women may be better off taking hormone replacement therapy to reduce their risks of heart disease and osteoporosis, or using raloxifene to prevent or treat osteoporosis, than taking tamoxifen to reduce their risk of breast cancer.

- **Plans for contraception among premenopausal women:** Women should not become pregnant while taking tamoxifen or for two months after they stop taking it. Sexually active premenopausal women should have a pregnancy test before starting tamoxifen and should use a reliable form of contraception.

After all of this information has been collected, the physician will be able to tell whether a woman is a suitable candidate for breast cancer chemoprevention. The final decision, however, must be the woman's, and subjective factors, such as her fear of breast cancer and the degree to which she is willing to tolerate side effects of medication, may influence her decision.

The Future of Chemoprevention

It is likely that future improvements in chemoprevention will lead to a greater reduction in breast cancer risk than is possible today.

Scientists are currently using molecular targeting approaches to develop new selective estrogen-receptor modulator drugs that will be more therapeutically effective, having equivalent or greater protective effects and fewer risks and side effects. Researchers are also investigating other agents that may reduce breast cancer risk in other ways, including isoflavones, monoterpenes, vitamin D analogues, difluoromethylornithine, dehydroepiandrosterone, oltipraz, and retinoids. In the future, it may be possible to use two or more chemoprevention agents in combination to provide even greater protection against breast cancer, with even fewer side effects and risks.

Recommended Reading

Chlebowski, R. T., D. E. Collyar, and M. R. Somerfield, et al., American Society of Clinical Oncology. "Technology Assessment on Breast Cancer Risk Reduction Strategies: Tamoxifen and Raloxifene." *J Clin Oncol* 17 (1999): 1939–55.

Cummings, S. R., S. Eckert, and K. A. Krueger, et al., "The Effect of Raloxifene on Risk of Breast Cancer in Postmenopausal Women," *JAMA* 281 (1999): 2189–97.

Fisher, B., J. P. Costantino, and D. L. Wickerham, et al., "Tamoxifen for Prevention of Breast Cancer: Report of the National Surgical Adjuvant Breast and Bowel Project P-1 Study," *J Natl Cancer Inst* 90 (1998): 1371–88.

Fisher, B., J. Dignam, and N. Wolmark, et al., "Tamoxifen in Treatment of Intraductal Breast Cancer: National Surgical Adjuvant Breast and Bowel Project B-24 Randomised Controlled Trial," *Lancet* 353 (1999): 1993–2000.

Gail, M. H., J. P. Costantino, and J. Bryant, et al., "Weighing the Risks and Benefits of Tamoxifen Treatment for Preventing Breast Cancer," *J Natl Cancer Inst* 91 (1999): 1829–46.

Lippman, S. M., and P. H. Brown, "Tamoxifen Prevention of Breast Cancer: An Instance of the Fingerpost," *J Natl Cancer Inst* 91 (1999): 1809–19.

Morgan, J. W., J. E. Gladson, and K. S. Rau, "Position Paper of the American Council on Science and Health on Risk Factors for Breast Cancer: Established, Speculated, and Unsupported," *Breast Journal* 4 (1998): 177–97.

Phillips, K. A., G. Glendon, and J. A. Knight, "Putting the Risk of Breast Cancer in Perspective," *N Engl J Med* 340 (1999): 141–44.

Chapter 36

The Study of Tamoxifen and Raloxifene (STAR): Questions and Answers

What is the Study of Tamoxifen and Raloxifene (STAR)?

The Study of Tamoxifen and Raloxifene (STAR) is a clinical trial (a research study conducted with people) designed to see how the drug raloxifene (Evista®) compares with the drug tamoxifen (Nolvadex®) in reducing the incidence of breast cancer in women who are at an increased risk of developing the disease. Researchers with the National Surgical Adjuvant Breast and Bowel Project (NSABP) are conducting the study at more than four hundred centers across the United States, Puerto Rico, and Canada. The study is primarily funded by the National Cancer Institute (NCI), the U.S. government's main agency for cancer research.

What is tamoxifen?

Tamoxifen is a drug, taken by mouth as a pill. It has been used for more than twenty years to treat patients with breast cancer. Tamoxifen works against breast cancer, in part, by interfering with the activity of estrogen, a female hormone that promotes the growth of breast cancer cells. In October 1998, the U.S. Food and Drug Administration (FDA) approved tamoxifen to reduce the incidence of breast cancer in women at high risk of the disease based on the results of the Breast Cancer Prevention Trial (BCPT). The BCPT is a study of more than thirteen thousand pre- and postmenopausal high-risk women ages thirty-five and older who took either tamoxifen or a

Cancer Facts, National Cancer Institute, May 2002.

249

placebo (an inactive pill that looked like tamoxifen) for up to five years. The NSABP conducted the BCPT, which also showed that tamoxifen works like estrogen to preserve bone strength, decreasing fractures of the hip, wrist, and spine in the women who took the drug. Findings from the BCPT were reported in the September 16, 1998, issue of the *Journal of the National Cancer Institute.*

What is raloxifene?

Raloxifene is a drug, taken by mouth as a pill. In December 1997 it was approved by the FDA for the prevention of osteoporosis in postmenopausal women. Raloxifene is being studied because large studies testing its effectiveness against osteoporosis have shown that women taking the drug developed fewer breast cancers than women taking a placebo. One of these studies was the Multiple Outcomes of Raloxifene Evaluation (MORE) trial. The MORE trial was designed to study the effects of raloxifene on osteoporosis in postmenopausal women. Researchers also tracked rates of breast cancer and observed a reduction in the risk of breast cancer among the women who took raloxifene. The results of this study were reported in the June 16, 1999, issue of the *Journal of the American Medical Association.*

Who is eligible to participate in STAR?

Women at increased risk for developing breast cancer, who have gone through menopause and are at least thirty-five years old, can participate in STAR. All women must have an increased risk of breast cancer equivalent to or greater than that of an average sixty- to sixty-four-year-old woman. At that age, about seventeen of every one thousand women are expected to develop breast cancer within five years.

Why can't premenopausal women participate in STAR?

STAR is limited to postmenopausal women because the drug raloxifene has yet to be adequately tested for long-term safety in premenopausal women. NCI recently launched a separate study to evaluate the safety of raloxifene in premenopausal women.

What factors are used to determine increased risk of breast cancer for the participants?

For most women, the risk is determined by a computer calculation, which takes into account the following factors:

- Current age;

- Number of first-degree relatives (mother, daughters, or sisters) diagnosed with breast cancer;

- Whether a woman has had any children, and her age at her first delivery;

- The number of breast biopsies a woman has had, especially if the tissue showed a condition known as atypical hyperplasia; and

- The woman's age at her first menstrual period.

In addition, women diagnosed as having lobular carcinoma in situ (LCIS), a condition that is not cancer but indicates an increased chance of developing invasive breast cancer, are eligible based on that diagnosis alone, as long as their treatment for the condition was limited to local excision. Mastectomy, radiation, or systemic therapy would disqualify a woman with LCIS from the study.

How will a potential participant's risk of breast cancer be determined?

Each potential participant will complete a one-page questionnaire (risk assessment form), which will be forwarded to NSABP by the local STAR clinical staff. The NSABP will use computer software to generate an individualized risk profile based on the information provided and will return the profile to the local STAR site so that it can be given to the potential participant. The profile will estimate the woman's chance of developing breast cancer over the next five years and will also present the potential risks and benefits of the study drugs. The woman can then use this information to help her decide whether or not she is interested in participating in STAR.

What other factors affect eligibility for the study?

Certain existing health conditions affect eligibility for the study. Health professionals at the STAR site will discuss these with each potential participant. For example, women with a history of cancer (except basal or squamous cell skin cancer), blood clots, stroke, or certain types of heartbeat irregularities cannot participate. Women whose high blood pressure or diabetes is not controlled also cannot participate. Also, women taking hormone replacement therapy (estrogen or an estrogen/progesterone combination) cannot take part in the trial unless they stop taking this medication. Those who stop taking these hormones are eligible for the study three months after they discontinue the drugs. Women who have taken tamoxifen or raloxifene for no more than three months are eligible for the study, but they also must stop the medication for three months before joining STAR.

What are the common side effects of tamoxifen and raloxifene?

Like most medications, including over-the-counter medications, prescription drugs, or drugs in clinical trials, tamoxifen and raloxifene cause adverse effects in some women. The effects experienced most often by women taking either drug are hot flashes and vaginal symptoms, including discharge, dryness, or itching. It is possible that some women may experience leg cramps, constipation, pain with intercourse, sinus irritation or infection, or problems controlling the bladder upon exertion. Treatments that may minimize or eliminate most of these side effects will be available to the participants.

Does tamoxifen cause cancers of the uterus?

Tamoxifen increases the risk of two types of cancer that can develop in the uterus: endometrial cancer, which arises in the lining of the uterus, and uterine sarcoma, which arises in the muscular wall of the uterus. Like all cancers, endometrial cancer and uterine sarcoma are potentially life-threatening. Women who have had a hysterectomy (surgery to remove the uterus) and are taking tamoxifen are not at increased risk for these cancers.

Endometrial cancer: In the BCPT, women who took tamoxifen had more than twice the chance of developing endometrial cancer compared with women who took a placebo (an inactive substance that looks the same as, and is administered in the same way as, tamoxifen). The risk of endometrial cancer in women taking tamoxifen was in the same range as (or less than) the risk in postmenopausal women taking single-agent estrogen replacement therapy. This risk is about two cases of endometrial cancer per one thousand women taking tamoxifen each year.

Most of the endometrial cancers that have occurred in women taking tamoxifen have been found in the early stages, and treatment has usually been effective. However, for some breast cancer patients who developed endometrial cancer while taking tamoxifen, the disease was life-threatening.

Uterine sarcoma: Information collected by the U.S. Food and Drug Administration indicates that women who have used tamoxifen for breast cancer treatment or prevention have an increased risk of developing uterine sarcoma. Review of all the NSABP clinical trials using tamoxifen confirmed an increased risk of this rare cancer. In the BCPT, there are about two cases per ten thousand women taking tamoxifen each year. Research to date indicates that uterine sarcomas are more likely to be diagnosed at later stages than endometrial cancers, and may therefore be harder to control and more life-threatening than endometrial cancer.

Abnormal vaginal bleeding and lower abdominal (pelvic) pain are symptoms of cancers of the uterus. Women who are taking tamoxifen should talk with their doctor about having regular pelvic examinations, and should be checked promptly if they have any abnormal vaginal bleeding or pelvic pain between scheduled exams.

Does tamoxifen cause other serious side effects?

Women taking tamoxifen in the BCPT had three times the chance of developing a pulmonary embolism (blood clot in the lung) as women who took the placebo (eighteen women taking tamoxifen versus six on placebo). Three women taking tamoxifen died from these embolisms. Women in the tamoxifen group were also more likely to have a deep vein thrombosis (a blood clot in a major vein) than women on placebo (thirty-five women on tamoxifen versus twenty-two on placebo). Women taking tamoxifen also appeared to have an increased chance of stroke (thirty-eight women on tamoxifen versus twenty-four on placebo).

Does raloxifene have any serious side effects?

Information about raloxifene is limited compared with the data available on tamoxifen because of the shorter time it has been studied (about five years) and the smaller number of women who have been studied. Studies of raloxifene have generally involved women who received the drug to determine its effect on osteoporosis, and the duration of both therapy and follow-up have been short. Women taking raloxifene in clinical trials have about three times the chance of developing a deep vein thrombosis or pulmonary embolism as women on a placebo. In osteoporosis studies of raloxifene, the drug did not increase the risk of endometrial cancer. An important part of STAR will be to assess the long-term safety of raloxifene versus tamoxifen in women at increased risk of breast cancer.

Who will get which drug?

Participants in STAR will be randomized (assigned by chance) to receive either tamoxifen or raloxifene. In a process known as "double blinding," neither the participant nor her physician will know which pill she is receiving. Setting up a study in this way allows the researchers to directly compare the true benefits and side effects of each drug without the influence of other factors. All women in the study will take two pills a day for five years: half will take active tamoxifen and a raloxifene placebo (an inactive pill that looks like raloxifene); the other half will take active raloxifene and a tamoxifen placebo (an inactive pill that looks like tamoxifen). All women will receive one of the active drugs; no one in STAR will receive only the placebo. The dosages are 20 mg of tamoxifen and 60 mg of raloxifene.

Why does everyone have to take two pills?

Tamoxifen and raloxifene have different shapes. The trial would not be double blinded if participants or physicians could tell which drug they were receiving because of its shape. The maker of tamoxifen, AstraZeneca in Wilmington, Delaware, and the maker of raloxifene, Eli Lilly and Company in Indianapolis, Indiana, are providing the active pills and the look-alike placebos without charge.

Are participants required to have any medical exams? Who will pay for these exams?

Participants are required to have blood tests, a mammogram, a breast exam, and a gynecologic exam before they are accepted into the study. These tests will be repeated at intervals during the trial. Physicians' fees and the costs of medical tests will be charged to the participant in the same fashion as if she were not part of the trial; however, the costs for these tests generally are covered by insurance. Every effort is made to contain the costs specifically associated with participation in this trial, and financial assistance is available for some women.

How can a woman enroll in the trial?

Postmenopausal women who are interested in participating in STAR should contact the center nearest to them. To locate the nearest center in the United States (including Puerto Rico) by phone, a woman can call the NCI's Cancer Information Service at 1-800-4-CANCER

(1-800-422-6237). The number for deaf and hard of hearing callers with TTY equipment is 1-800-332-8615. In Canada, participating centers can be located by calling the Canadian Cancer Society's Cancer Information Service at 1-888-939-3333. To locate the nearest STAR center, visit NSABP's website at http://www.nsabp.pitt.edu or the Study of Tamoxifen and Raloxifene (STAR) Trial Digest Page on the NCI's website at http://cancer.gov/star on the internet.

How is the safety of participants ensured? Is the trial monitored?

The safety of participants is of primary importance to STAR investigators. There are strict requirements about who can join the trial as well as frequent monitoring of participants' health status. An independent Data Safety and Monitoring Committee (DSMC) will provide oversight of the trial. The DSMC includes medical and cancer specialists, biostatisticians, and bioethicists who have no other connection to NSABP. The DSMC will meet semiannually and review unblinded data from all participants. Two other committees will also provide oversight. The Participant Advisory Board (PAB) is made up of sixteen women from the BCPT. As women join STAR, board membership will change to include STAR participants. The PAB meets semiannually with professionals from NSABP and NCI and provides feedback on many study-related functions such as informed consent, participant recruitment, and communications issues. The STAR Steering Committee is made up of NSABP investigators, breast cancer advocates, experts from other medical disciplines, as well as NCI and NSABP personnel. The committee, which also meets semiannually, is charged with providing overall administrative oversight of the trial. In addition, NSABP provides the FDA, NCI, AstraZeneca, and Eli Lilly and Company with annual reports on STAR that summarize the overall data collected to date (only the DSMC receives unblinded data).

What is the National Surgical Adjuvant Breast and Bowel Project?

The NSABP is a cooperative group with a forty-year history of designing and conducting clinical trials, the results of which have changed the way breast cancer is treated and, now, prevented. Results of clinical trials conducted by NSABP researchers have been the dominant force in altering the standard surgical treatment of breast cancer from radical mastectomy to lumpectomy plus radiation. This group was also the first to demonstrate that adjuvant therapy could alter the natural history of breast cancer, thus increasing survival rates.

References

Cummings, S. R., S. Eckert, and K. A. Krueger, et al. "The Effect of Raloxifene on Risk of Breast Cancer in Postmenopausal Women: Results from the MORE Randomized Trial." *Journal of the American Medical Association* 281, no. 23 (1999): 2189–97.

Fisher B., J. P. Constantino, and D. L. Wickerham, et al. "Tamoxifen for Prevention of Breast Cancer: Report of the National Surgical Adjuvant Breast and Bowel Project P-1 Study." *Journal of the National Cancer Institute* 90, no. 18 (1998): 1371–88.

Chapter 37

Breast Cancer Prevention Studies

Breast cancer prevention studies are clinical trials that explore ways of reducing the risk, or chance, of developing breast cancer. Prevention studies are usually conducted with healthy women who have not had breast cancer, but have a high risk for this disease. Through such studies, scientists hope to determine what steps are effective in reducing the risk of breast cancer in women of all races and ethnic backgrounds.

Most breast cancer prevention research is based on evidence that the development of this disease is linked to exposure to the hormone estrogen. Many breast cancer prevention studies are testing the effectiveness of drugs called selective estrogen receptor modulators (SERMs). SERMs are drugs that have some estrogen-like properties and some anti-estrogen properties. For example, their estrogen-like properties may help prevent the loss of bone density in postmenopausal women, and may cause some premenopausal women to become more fertile. Their anti-estrogen activity may help reduce the risk of breast cancer by blocking the effects of estrogen on breast tissue.

The Breast Cancer Prevention Trial (BCPT)

The Breast Cancer Prevention Trial (BCPT) was a clinical trial funded by the National Cancer Institute (NCI) and conducted by the National Surgical Adjuvant Breast and Bowel Project (NSABP). The

Cancer Facts, National Cancer Institute, May 13, 2002.

BCPT was designed to see whether tamoxifen, a SERM, can prevent breast cancer in women who are at an increased risk of developing this disease. The study began recruiting participants in April 1992 and closed enrollment in September 1997. This study involved 13,388 premenopausal and postmenopausal women at more than three hundred centers across the United States and Canada and is one of the largest breast cancer prevention studies to date.

Results of the BCPT, reported in the September 16, 1998, *Journal of the National Cancer Institute,* showed 49 percent fewer diagnoses of invasive breast cancer in women who were randomized to take tamoxifen compared with women who were randomized to take a placebo (an inactive substance that looks the same as, and is administered in the same way as, a drug in a clinical trial). Women on tamoxifen also had 50 percent fewer diagnoses of noninvasive breast tumors, such as ductal or lobular carcinoma in situ. Nine women died of breast cancer: three women in the tamoxifen group and six women in the placebo group.

In the BCPT, most of the side effects associated with tamoxifen were temporary. However, there were some long-term risks, including several serious health problems: endometrial cancer (cancer of the lining of the uterus), uterine sarcoma (cancer of the muscular wall of the uterus), pulmonary embolism (blood clot in the lung), deep vein thrombosis (blood clot in a large vein), and stroke. Because of these risks, women taking tamoxifen should be monitored by their doctors for any sign of serious side effects. All BCPT participants have been asked to undergo regular follow-up examinations.

BCPT participants who were randomized to the tamoxifen group and had not completed five years of tamoxifen therapy when the study ended were given the opportunity to continue on therapy. Postmenopausal women who had been taking the placebo were invited to participate in another trial, the Study of Tamoxifen and Raloxifene (STAR). (See the following section for a description of this trial.) Women in the BCPT placebo group also have the option of seeking tamoxifen from their doctor.

The Study of Tamoxifen and Raloxifene (STAR)

The NSABP is conducting the Study of Tamoxifen and Raloxifene, known as STAR, which is seeking about twenty-two thousand participants. STAR will involve postmenopausal women who are at least thirty-five years old and are at increased risk for developing breast cancer. The study will determine whether raloxifene, another SERM, is also effective in reducing the risk of developing breast cancer in women who have not had the disease, and whether the drug has benefits over tamoxifen, such as fewer side effects. As with tamoxifen, most of the known side effects of raloxifene are temporary, but women taking raloxifene are at increased risk for pulmonary embolism and deep vein thrombosis. For people in the United States, information on STAR is available from the NCI's Cancer Information Service (CIS) at 1-800-4-CANCER (1-800-422-6237); people in Canada may call the Canadian Cancer Society's Cancer Information Service toll-free at 1-888-939-3333. Information about this study is also available at http://cancer.gov/star on the internet.

Capital Area SERM Study

The NCI is conducting the Capital Area SERM Study to evaluate the safety of raloxifene in premenopausal women between the ages of twenty-three and forty-seven who are at increased risk for breast cancer. This study is in progress at the National Institutes of Health's Warren Grant Magnuson Clinical Center and the National Naval Medical Center, both in Bethesda, Maryland. Women who are interested in participating in this study or who would like to have additional information may call the NCI Clinical Studies Support Center at 1-888-624-1937.

Other Breast Cancer Prevention Studies

Studies are being conducted with other drugs to determine if they may help to reduce the risk of breast cancer. Also, researchers are looking at the effect of a low-fat diet on breast cancer risk. More information on these studies is available from the CIS at 1-800-4-CANCER (1-800-422-6237).

A paper published in the January 14, 1999, issue of the *New England Journal of Medicine* described a study of women who had undergone surgery to remove their breasts (double mastectomy) because they were at high risk of breast cancer due to a family history of this disease. In this study, prophylactic (preventive) mastectomy was associated with a significant reduction in the number of cases of breast cancer.

Another study of prophylactic mastectomy in women with an increased risk of breast cancer was published in the November 7, 2001, issue of the *Journal of the National Cancer Institute*. The participants included women with a high risk of breast cancer due to alterations in their BRCA1 or BRCA2 genes. (Certain alterations in these genes are known to increase a person's risk of breast cancer and several other types of cancer.) The researchers found that prophylactic mastectomy was associated with a substantial reduction in the number of cases of breast cancer not only in women with a family history of the disease, but also in women with BRCA1 or BRCA2 alterations.

NCI Priorities for Breast Cancer Prevention Research

Recognizing the impact of breast cancer on our society, in 1997 the NCI convened a Breast Cancer Progress Review Group of experts and advocates to analyze the NCI's breast cancer research activities and develop recommendations for the future. Based on its assessment of the status of breast cancer research, the review group recommended research priorities to accelerate progress in breast cancer prevention and treatment. In August 1998, the group published its report, *Charting the Course: Priorities for Breast Cancer Research*. This report is available at http://prg.nci.nih.gov/breast/finalreport.html on the internet.

The review group identified key areas that need to be addressed. New strategies are needed to help researchers take discoveries from the laboratory and effectively study them with people. One of the recommendations in the report is that the NCI devote more funding to prevention research and increase the number of high-quality prevention studies. It is also important to encourage participation in studies, and seek suggestions about the types of studies in which women would be willing to participate. In addition, the review group recommended that researchers focus on increasing minority participation in prevention studies.

Estimating Breast Cancer Risk

No one knows why some women develop breast cancer and others do not. However, it is clear that breast cancer occurs more often in older women, and researchers have identified other risk factors that increase a woman's chance of getting the disease. Still, most women who develop breast cancer have no known risk factors (other than growing older), and most women who have known risk factors do not get breast cancer.

Scientists at the NCI and the NSABP have developed a computer program called the Breast Cancer Risk Assessment Tool. This tool can help women and their health care providers estimate a woman's chances of developing breast cancer based on several recognized risk factors. The Breast Cancer Risk Assessment Tool also provides information on tamoxifen. A copy of the computer program may be ordered by calling the NCI's Cancer Information Service (CIS) at 1-800-4-CANCER (1-800-422-6237), or from the NCI Publications Locator at http://cancer.gov/publications on the internet.

Doctors generally suggest that high-risk women be closely monitored and have regular medical checkups so that if breast cancer develops it is likely to be detected at an early stage. These women may also consider participating in prevention studies, taking tamoxifen, or undergoing preventive mastectomy. The decision is an individual one. With any medical procedure or intervention, both the benefits and the risks of the therapy must be considered. The balance of these factors will vary depending on a woman's personal and family health history and how she weighs the benefits and risks. Women who are considering taking steps to reduce the risk of breast cancer should discuss their personal risk factors with their doctor.

References

Fisher, B, J. P. Costantino, and D. L. Wickerham, et al. "Tamoxifen for Prevention of Breast Cancer: Report of the National Surgical Adjuvant Breast and Bowel Project P-1 Study." *Journal of the National Cancer Institute* 90, no. 18 (1998): 1371–88.

Hartmann, L. C., D. J. Schaid, and J. E. Woods, et al. "Efficacy of Bilateral Prophylactic Mastectomy in Women with a Family History of Breast Cancer." *New England Journal of Medicine* 340, no. 2 (1999): 77–84.

Hartmann, L. C., T. A. Sellers, and D. J. Schaid, et al. "Efficacy of Bilateral Prophylactic Mastectomy in BRCA1 and BRCA2 Gene Mutation Carriers." *Journal of the National Cancer Institute* 93, no. 21 (2001): 1633–37.

Chapter 38

Prophylactic Mastectomy

What is prophylactic mastectomy?

Prophylactic mastectomy (also called preventive mastectomy) is the surgical removal of both breasts to help prevent breast cancer. Prophylactic mastectomy is a controversial procedure among members of the medical community. Many physicians do not believe that surgically removing a woman's breast is appropriate unless it is performed as a treatment for breast cancer. However, based on recent scientific findings that show prophylactic mastectomy to be effective at preventing breast cancer, other physicians believe that certain individuals at especially high risk of breast cancer who are very worried about developing the disease may benefit from having prophylactic mastectomy. According to a statement from the American Cancer Society Board of Directors, "only very strong clinical and/or pathological indications warrant doing this type of 'preventive operation.'"

A woman's decision to have prophylactic mastectomy should be made carefully with physicians and counselors and should be a decision comfortable to the woman. Women considering the procedure should discuss their decision with close family members, friends, or other women who have previously undergone prophylactic mastectomy, if possible.

The information in this chapter is reprinted with permission from www.Imaginis.com. © 2004 Imaginis Corporation. All rights reserved. Complete information about Imaginis is included at the end of this chapter.

During a prophylactic mastectomy, the surgeon removes the entire breast, with its skin and nipple. This is called a simple or total mastectomy. Because the operation is not being performed for cancer treatment, lymph node removal is not necessary. Prophylactic mastectomy can usually be followed by immediate or delayed breast reconstruction.

Who is a candidate for prophylactic mastectomy?

Women should be aware that prophylactic mastectomy is an irreversible procedure and the decision to have the surgery should be made very carefully. Women considering the procedure should consult several physicians (preferably breast cancer specialists) who can provide specific information on the woman's individual risk of breast cancer. Physicians should also provide information on side effects, complications, and options for breast reconstruction (and the associated risks of reconstruction). It is also recommended that women who are considering prophylactic mastectomy discuss the procedure with a professional counselor who has experience dealing with patients who are considering this preventive option.

Women who are at high risk of breast cancer who may wish to consider prophylactic mastectomy after weighing other preventive options for breast cancer include:

- Those with a strong family history of breast cancer (especially if the breast cancer was diagnosed among several first-degree relatives, mother or sisters, before age fifty)

- Those who have tested positive for the BRCA1 or BRCA2 gene mutations

- Those who have a personal history of breast cancer and are at high risk for a recurrence

- In some cases, those who have been diagnosed with lobular carcinoma in situ (a marker for increased breast cancer risk)

- Less commonly, those at risk of breast cancer who also have breast microcalcifications (tiny calcium deposits) or who have very dense breast tissue that makes it difficult to detect breast cancer with imaging exams, such as mammography.

Also, some women who have had multiple breast biopsies revealing noncancerous conditions, which have caused scar tissue and other complications that may make it difficult to detect breast cancer in the future, may wish to consider prophylactic mastectomy.

Is prophylactic mastectomy effective?

Since most of the breast tissue is removed during prophylactic mastectomy, the chances that a woman will develop breast cancer are significantly reduced. A study conducted by Lynn C. Hartman, M.D., of the Mayo Clinic in Rochester, Minnesota, and her colleagues found that prophylactic mastectomy can reduce the likelihood that a woman will develop breast cancer by at least 90 percent.[1]

However, having a prophylactic mastectomy does not guarantee that a woman will never develop breast cancer. It is impossible for surgeons to remove every breast cell during mastectomy, and therefore, some breast tissue cells will remain. According to Dr. Hartman, if only three cells are left, cancer could develop from those three cells. In the Mayo Clinic study, 3 of the 214 women who had prophylactic mastectomy developed breast cancer within fourteen years of having the surgery.

While prophylactic mastectomy reduces the chances of developing breast cancer, some women identified to be at high risk of breast cancer will never develop the disease, and thus, prophylactic mastectomy is not necessary for these women. However, a recent study published in the *Journal of the American Medical Association* found that the majority of women who opt for prophylactic mastectomy to lower their risk of breast cancer are satisfied with their decision.[2]

In the study, Marlene H. Frost, R.N., Ph.D., of the Mayo Clinic, and her colleagues studied 572 women with a family history of breast cancer who had prophylactic mastectomy between 1960 and 1993. The researchers found that 70 percent of the women were satisfied with the procedure, 11 percent were neutral, and 19 percent were dissatisfied. The majority of women also reported no change or favorable effects on their emotional stability, level of stress, self-esteem, sexual relationships, feelings of femininity, and satisfaction with their body appearance.

What are alternatives to prophylactic mastectomy to help lower breast cancer risk?

For women at high risk of breast cancer, there are a number of options available besides prophylactic mastectomy to reduce the chances of developing the disease.

Frequent monitoring: Many women at high risk for breast cancer are closely monitored by physicians, with frequent clinical breast exams and mammograms (at an interval determined by the physician). All women should also practice monthly breast self-exams and see a physician immediately if they notice any changes or abnormalities. The earlier breast cancer is detected, the greater the chances for successful treatment and survival.

Guidelines for all women: Because breast cancer affects approximately one in eight women, all women should follow recommended screening guidelines to help detect breast cancer in its earliest stages, when the chances for survival are the greatest. The American Cancer Society, the American College of Radiology, the American College of Surgeons and the American Medical Association recommend the following:

- All women between twenty and thirty-nine years of age should practice monthly breast self-exams and have a physician-performed clinical breast exam at least every three years.

- All women forty years of age and older should have annual screening mammograms, practice monthly breast self-exams, and have yearly clinical breast exams.

- Women with a family history of breast cancer or those who test positive for the BRCA1 or BRCA2 gene mutations may want to talk to their physicians about beginning annual screening mammograms earlier than age forty, as early as age twenty-five in some cases.

Tamoxifen: In 1998, the U.S. Food and Drug Administration (FDA) approved the use of the drug tamoxifen (brand name: Nolvadex) for women who are at high risk of developing breast cancer. In a National Adjuvant Breast and Bowel Project (NSABP) study of 13,388 women at high risk of breast cancer (determined by family history, etc.), researchers found that the use of tamoxifen for a period of five years reduced the incidence of breast cancer by 49 percent. Most physicians who prescribe tamoxifen to help prevent breast cancer recommend that women take it for a period of five years. Tamoxifen has been shown to cause a number of side effects in some women, most commonly hot flashes, and poses a slight increase in the risk for endometrial cancer (cancer of the lining of the uterus), blood clotting, and other conditions.

STAR clinical trial: The NSABP is currently running its second major breast cancer prevention trial, the STAR trial. STAR (Study of Tamoxifen and Raloxifene) is designed to determine whether the drug raloxifene (brand name: Evista) is as effective as tamoxifen in preventing breast cancer. The researchers hope to recruit twenty-two thousand postmenopausal women at high risk of breast cancer over the next few years to participate in STAR.

References

1. The study, "Efficacy of Bilateral Prophylactic Mastectomy in Women with a Family History of Breast Cancer," was published in the January 14, 1999, issue of the *New England Journal of Medicine.* An abstract of the study is available at http://www.ncbi.nlm.nih.gov/entrez/query.fcgi?cmd=Retrieve &db=PubMed&list_uids=9887158&dopt=Abstract.

2. The study, "Long-Term Satisfaction and Psychological and Social Function following Bilateral Prophylactic Mastectomy," was published in the July 19, 2000, issue of the *Journal of the American Medical Association.* An abstract of the study is available at http://www.ncbi.nlm.nih.gov/entrez/query.fcgi ?cmd=Retrieve&db=PubMed&list_uids=10891963&dopt=Abstract

About Imaginis

Imaginis.com is an independent, award-winning, comprehensive resource for news and information on breast cancer prevention, screening, diagnosis, and treatment and related women's health topics such as hormone replacement therapy (HRT), multiple sclerosis, osteoporosis, and ovarian cancer. Imaginis.com also contains extensive information about medical procedures such as angiography, biopsy, CT, MR, nuclear medicine, ultrasound, x-ray imaging, and radiotherapy.

The goal of Imaginis.com is to provide women and their physicians with the most comprehensive and relevant information on breast health and related women's health issues. Imaginis content is created by an independent team of breast health specialists to ensure that it is up-to-date and accurate. Complicated medical terms are explained in everyday language to help individuals understand their options, make informed decisions, and achieve optimal health.

Part Five

Breast Cancer Screening

Chapter 39

Guidelines for the Early Detection of Breast Cancer

American Cancer Society Recommendations

The American Cancer Society recommendations for breast cancer screening are presented here.

Women at Average Risk

Begin mammography at age forty.

For women in their twenties and thirties, it is recommended that clinical breast examination (CBE) be part of a periodic health examination, preferably at least every three years. Asymptomatic women aged forty and over should continue to receive a clinical breast examination as part of a periodic health examination, preferably annually.

Beginning in their twenties, women should be told about the benefits and limitations of breast self-examination (BSE). The importance of prompt reporting of any new breast symptoms to a health professional should be emphasized. Women who choose to do BSE should receive instruction and have their technique reviewed on the occasion

Reprinted with permission from Robert A. Smith, Debbie Saslow, Kimberly Andrews Sawyer, Wylie Burke, Mary E. Costanza, W. Phil Evans III, Roger S. Foster Jr., Edward Hendrick, Harmon J. Eyre, and Steven Sener, "American Cancer Society Guidelines for Breast Cancer Screening: Update 2003," *CA: A Cancer Journal for Clinicians* 53, no. 3 (May/June 2003): 141–69; and from "Breast Cancer Screening," Summary of Recommendations from the U.S. Preventive Services Task Force, February 2002.

of a periodic health examination. It is acceptable for women to choose not to do BSE or to do BSE irregularly.

Women should have an opportunity to become informed about the benefits, limitations, and potential harms associated with regular screening.

Older Women

Screening decisions in older women should be individualized by considering the potential benefits and risks of mammography in the context of current health status and estimated life expectancy. As long as a woman is in reasonably good health and would be a candidate for treatment, she should continue to be screened with mammography.

Women at Increased Risk

Women at increased risk of breast cancer might benefit from additional screening strategies beyond those offered to women of average risk, such as earlier initiation of screening, shorter screening intervals, or the addition of screening modalities other than mammography and physical examination, such as ultrasound or magnetic resonance imaging. However, the evidence currently available is insufficient to justify recommendations for any of these screening approaches.

U.S. Preventative Services Task Force Recommendations

Mammography

The U.S. Preventive Services Task Force (USPSTF) recommends screening mammography, with or without clinical breast examination (CBE), every one to two years for women aged forty and older.

The USPSTF found fair evidence that mammography screening every twelve to thirty-three months significantly reduces mortality from breast cancer. Evidence is strongest for women aged fifty to sixty-nine, the age group generally included in screening trials. For women aged forty to forty-nine, the evidence that screening mammography reduces mortality from breast cancer is weaker, and the absolute benefit of mammography is smaller, than it is for older women. Most, but not all, studies indicate a mortality benefit for women undergoing mammography at ages forty to forty-nine, but the delay in observed benefit in women younger than fifty makes it difficult to determine the incremental benefit of beginning screening at age forty rather than at age fifty.

The absolute benefit is smaller because the incidence of breast cancer is lower among women in their forties than it is among older women. The USPSTF concluded that the evidence is also generalizable to women aged seventy and older (who face a higher absolute risk for breast cancer) if their life expectancy is not compromised by comorbid disease. The absolute probability of benefits of regular mammography increases along a continuum with age, whereas the likelihood of harms from screening (false-positive results and unnecessary anxiety, biopsies, and cost) diminishes from ages forty to seventy. The balance of benefits and potential harms, therefore, grows more favorable as women age. The precise age at which the potential benefits of mammography justify the possible harms is a subjective choice. The USPSTF did not find sufficient evidence to specify the optimal screening interval for women aged forty to forty-nine.

Clinical Breast Exam (CBE)

The USPSTF concludes that the evidence is insufficient to recommend for or against routine CBE alone to screen for breast cancer.

No screening trial has examined the benefits of CBE alone (without accompanying mammography) compared to no screening, and design characteristics limit the generalizability of studies that have examined CBE. The USPSTF could not determine the benefits of CBE alone or the incremental benefit of adding CBE to mammography. The USPSTF therefore could not determine whether potential benefits of routine CBE outweigh the potential harms.

Breast Self-Exam (BSE)

The USPSTF concludes that the evidence is insufficient to recommend for or against teaching or performing routine breast self-examination (BSE).

The USPSTF found poor evidence to determine whether BSE reduces breast cancer mortality. The USPSTF found fair evidence that BSE is associated with an increased risk for false-positive results and biopsies. Due to design limitations of published and ongoing studies of BSE, the USPSTF could not determine the balance of benefits and potential harms of BSE.

273

Chapter 40

Screening for Breast Cancer

What Is Screening?

Screening is looking for cancer before a person has any symptoms. This can help find cancer at an early stage. When abnormal tissue or cancer is found early, it may be easier to treat. By the time symptoms appear, cancer may have begun to spread.

Scientists are trying to better understand which people are more likely to get certain types of cancer. They also study the things we do and the things around us to see if they cause cancer. This information helps doctors recommend who should be screened for cancer, which screening tests should be used, and how often the tests should be done.

It is important to remember that your doctor does not necessarily think you have cancer if he or she suggests a screening test. Screening tests are given when you have no cancer symptoms.

If a screening test result is abnormal, you may need to have more tests done to find out if you have cancer. These are called diagnostic tests.

General Information about Breast Cancer

Breast cancer is a disease in which malignant (cancer) cells form in the tissues of the breast. The breast is made up of lobes and ducts.

PDQ® Cancer Information Summary. National Cancer Institute, Bethesda, MD. Breast Cancer (PDQ®): Screening-Patient. Updated September 2003. Available at: http://cancer.gov. Accessed April 2004.

Each breast has fifteen to twenty sections called lobes, which have many smaller sections called lobules. Lobules end in dozens of tiny bulbs that can produce milk. The lobes, lobules, and bulbs are linked by thin tubes called ducts.

Each breast also contains blood vessels and lymph vessels. The lymph vessels carry an almost colorless fluid called lymph. Lymph vessels lead to organs called lymph nodes. Lymph nodes are small, bean-shaped structures that are found throughout the body. They filter substances in lymph and help fight infection and disease. Clusters of lymph nodes are found near the breast in the axilla (under the arm), above the collarbone, and in the chest.

Breast cancer is the second leading cause of death from cancer in American women. Women in the United States get breast cancer more than any other type of cancer except for skin cancer. Breast cancer is second only to lung cancer as a cause of cancer death in women. Breast cancer occurs in men also, but the number of cases is small.

Risk Factors for Breast Cancer

Age and health history can affect the risk of developing breast cancer. Anything that increases your chance of getting a disease is called a risk factor. Risk factors for breast cancer include:

- Older age
- Early age at menarche (menstruation)
- Older age at first birth or never having given birth
- A personal history of breast cancer or benign (noncancer) breast disease
- A mother or sister with breast cancer
- Treatment with radiation therapy to the breast or chest
- Breast tissue that is dense on a mammogram
- Hormone use (such as estrogen and progesterone)
- Drinking alcoholic beverages
- Caucasian race

Breast Cancer Screening

A variety of tests are used to screen for cancer. Some screening tests are used because they have been shown to be helpful both in finding cancers early and in decreasing the chance of dying from these cancers.

Other tests are used because they have been shown to find cancer in some people; it is not yet known if use of these tests will decrease the risk of dying from cancer.

Scientists study screening tests to find those with the fewest risks and most benefits. Cancer screening trials also are meant to show whether early detection (finding cancer before it causes symptoms) decreases a person's chance of dying from the disease. For some types of cancer, finding and treating the disease at an early stage may result in a better chance of recovery.

Clinical trials that study cancer screening methods are taking place in many parts of the country. Information about ongoing clinical trials is available from the NCI website at www.cancer.gov.

Standard Screening Tests

Three tests are commonly used to screen for breast cancer:

Breast Self-Exam (BSE)

Breast self-exam is a way to check your own breasts for lumps or anything else that seems unusual.

Clinical Breast Exam (CBE)

A clinical breast exam is an exam of the breast by a doctor or other health professional. The doctor will carefully feel the breasts and under the arms for lumps or anything else that seems unusual.

Mammogram

A mammogram is an x-ray of the breast. This test may find tumors that are too small to feel. The ability of this test to find breast cancer may depend on the size of the tumor, the density of the breast tissue, and the skill of the radiologist.

If a lump or other abnormality is found using one of these three tests, ultrasound may be used to learn more. It is not used by itself as a screening test for breast cancer. Ultrasound is a procedure in which high-energy sound waves (ultrasound) are bounced off internal tissues or organs and make echoes. The echoes form a picture of body tissues called a sonogram.

Other Screening Tests

Other screening tests are being studied in clinical trials.

Magnetic Resonance Imaging (MRI)

MRI is a procedure that uses a magnet, radio waves, and a computer to make a series of detailed pictures of areas inside the body. This procedure is also called nuclear magnetic resonance imaging (NMRI). MRI tests are used to make decisions about breast masses that have been found by a clinical breast exam or a breast self-exam. MRI also can help show the difference between cancer and scar tissue. MRI does not use any x-rays. Scientists are studying MRI to find out how helpful it is in screening for breast cancer.

Screening clinical trials are taking place in many parts of the country. Information about ongoing clinical trials is available from the NCI web site at www.cancer.gov.

Risks of Breast Cancer Screening

Decisions about screening tests can be difficult. Not all screening tests are helpful, and most have risks. Before having any screening test, you may want to discuss the test with your doctor. It is important to know the risks of the test and whether it has been proven to reduce the risk of dying from cancer.

The risks of breast cancer screening tests include the following:

- *Finding breast cancer may not improve health* or help a woman live longer. Screening may not help you if you have fast-growing breast cancer or if it has already spread to other places in your body. Also, some breast cancers never cause symptoms or become life-threatening, but cancer may be found on a screening mammogram and treated. It is not known if treatment of these cancers would help you live longer than if no treatment were given, and treatments for cancer may have serious side effects.

- *False-negative test results can occur.* Screening test results may appear to be normal even though breast cancer is present. A woman who receives a false-negative test result (one that shows there is no cancer when there really is) may delay seeking medical care even if she has symptoms.

One in five cancers may be missed by mammography. False-negatives occur more often in younger women than in older women because the breast tissue of younger women is more dense. The size of the tumor, the rate of tumor growth, the level of hormones, such as estrogen and progesterone, in the woman's body, and the skill of the radiologist can also affect the chance of a false-negative result.

- *False-positive test results can occur.* Screening test results may appear to be abnormal even though no cancer is present. A false-positive test result (one that shows there is cancer when there really isn't) can cause anxiety and is usually followed by more tests (such as biopsy), which also have risks.

  Most abnormal test results turn out not to be cancer. False-positives are more common in younger women, women who have had previous breast biopsies, women with a family history of breast cancer, and women who take hormones, such as estrogen and progesterone. The skill of the doctor also can affect the chance of a false-positive result.

- *Mammograms expose the breast to radiation.* Being exposed to radiation is a risk factor for breast cancer. The risk of developing breast cancer from screening mammograms is greater with higher doses of radiation and in younger women. For women older than forty years of age, the benefits of an annual screening mammogram may be greater than the risks from radiation exposure. No matter how old you are, if you have risk factors for breast cancer you should ask for medical advice about when to begin having mammograms and how often to be screened.

Chapter 41

What to Expect during a Clinical Breast Exam

What Can You Expect during a Clinical Breast Exam?

- The exam is done in a private room.

- You will need to remove all clothing above your waist.

- You may want someone else to be in the room with you for the exam. Ask one of the female staff, a friend, or a family member to be present.

During the Exam

While Sitting

The doctor or nurse looks at your breasts to see if there are any changes in the shape, skin, or the nipple. You may be asked to put your arms in any of the following positions:

- Arms relaxed at side

- Arms above head

- Hands on hips

Reprinted with permission from the State of California Department of Health Services Cancer Detection Section brochure *What to Expect during a Clinical Breast Exam,* revised July 2003. © 2003 State of California. All rights reserved.

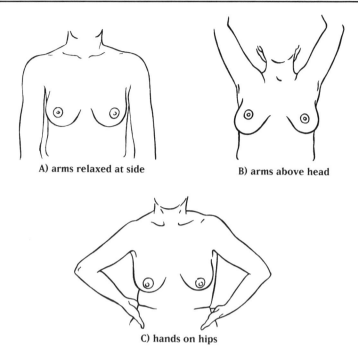

Figure 41.1. Clinical breast exam positions: arms relaxed at side; arms above head; and hands on hips.

The doctor or nurse checks the lymph nodes above and below your collarbone and under your arm area for any swelling.

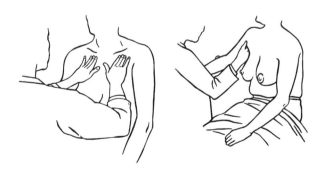

Figure 41.2. Examining the lymph nodes.

While Lying Down

The doctor or nurse feels your breast tissue by using the pads of the three middle fingers. This will help the doctor to feel all of your breast tissue.

The breast tissue covers a large area—from your collarbone to the bra line and from the breastbone to the middle of your underarm.

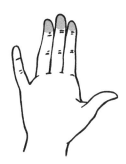

Pads of fingers

Figure 41.3. Parts of fingers used for clinical breast exam.

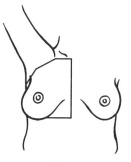

Area of breast tissue

Figure 41.4. Area covered by breast tissue.

The doctor or nurse performs a clinical breast exam (CBE) using a pattern of search. A good pattern is the vertical strip. This pattern moves up and down the breast in even rows. It will cover every part of the breast, including the nipple.

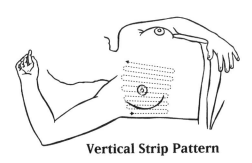

Vertical Strip Pattern

Figure 41.5. Vertical strip pattern.

The doctor or nurse feels your breast tissue using three levels of pressure—light, medium, and deep. These three pressures help to feel all the layers of the breast tissue where lumps may be found. Sometimes feeling the deep tissue may cause some discomfort, but feeling this deep tissue is very important.

End of the Exam

Your doctor or nurse may show you how to feel your own breast so that you can learn what is normal breast tissue for you.

You and your doctor or nurse will talk about a plan of regular screening and follow-up that is best for you.

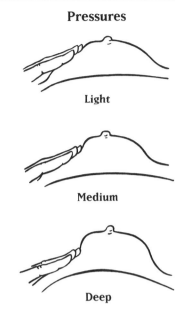

Pressures

Light

Medium

Deep

Figure 41.6. *Pressures: light, medium, deep.*

Chapter 42

Mammography

What is a mammogram?

A mammogram is a test that is done to look for any abnormalities, or problems, with a woman's breasts. The test uses a special x-ray machine to take pictures of both breasts. The results are recorded on film that your health care provider can examine.

Mammograms look for breast lumps and changes in breast tissue that may develop into problems over time. They can find small lumps or growths that a health care provider or woman can't feel when doing a physical breast exam. Breast lumps or growths can be benign (not cancer) or malignant (cancer). If a lump is found, a health care provider will order a biopsy, a test where a small amount of tissue is taken from the lump and area around the lump. The tissue is sent to a lab to look for cancer or changes that may mean cancer is likely to develop. Finding breast cancer early means that a woman has a better chance of surviving the disease. There are also more choices for treatment when breast cancer is found early.

Are there different types of mammograms?

There are two reasons mammograms are taken. Screening mammograms are done for women who have no symptoms of breast cancer. Diagnostic mammograms are done when a woman has symptoms of breast cancer or a breast lump. Diagnostic mammograms take longer

"Mammograms," National Women's Health Information Center, March 2002.

than screening mammograms because more pictures of the breast are taken.

In January 2000, the FDA approved a new way of doing mammograms, called digital mammography. This technique records x-ray images on a computer, rather than film. It can reduce exposure to radiation, allow the person taking the x-ray to make adjustments without having to take another mammogram, and takes pictures of the entire breast even if the denseness of the breast tissue varies.

Are mammograms safe?

A mammogram is a safe, low-dose x-ray of the breast. A high-quality mammogram, along with a clinical breast exam (an exam done by a professional health care provider) is the most effective tool for detecting breast cancer early.

How is a mammogram done?

You stand in front of a special x-ray machine. The person who takes the x-rays (always a woman) places your breasts (one at a time) between two plastic plates. The plates press your breast and make it flat. You will feel pressure on your breast for a few seconds. It may cause you some discomfort, feeling like squeezing or pinching. But, the flatter your breasts, the better the picture. Most often, two pictures are taken of each breast—one from the side and one from above. The whole thing takes only a few minutes.

How is a mammogram done in a woman with breast implants?

If you have breast implants, be sure to tell your mammography facility that you have them. You will need an x-ray technician who is trained in x-raying patients with implants. This is important because breast implants can hide some breast tissue, which could make if difficult for the radiologist to see breast cancer when looking at your mammograms. For this reason, to take a mammogram of a breast with an implant, the x-ray technician might gently lift the breast tissue slightly away from the implant.

How often should I get a mammogram?

Women over forty should get a mammogram every one to two years. This guideline was just re-issued by the federal government's U.S.

Preventive Services Task Force, and it is also the position of the secretary of the U.S. Department of Health and Human Services. Women who have had breast cancer or breast problems, or with a family history of breast cancer, may need to start having mammograms at a younger age or more often. Talk to your health care provider about how often you should get a mammogram. Be aware that mammograms don't take the place of getting breast exams from a health care provider and examining your own breasts.

If you find a lump or see changes in your breast, talk to your health care provider right away, no matter what your age. Your health care provider may order a mammogram in order to get a better look at your breast changes.

Where can I get a mammogram?

Be sure to get a mammogram from a facility certified by the Food and Drug Administration (FDA). These places must meet high standards for their x-ray machines and staff. Check out the FDA's website on the internet at: http://www.fda.gov/cdrh/mammography/certified.html for a list of FDA-certified mammography facilities. Some of these facilities also offer digital mammograms.

Your health care provider, local medical clinic, or local or state health department can tell you where to get no-cost or low-cost mammograms. Also, call the National Cancer Institute's toll free number (1-800-422-6237) for information on no-cost or low-cost mammograms.

How can I get ready for my mammogram?

First, check with the place you are having the mammogram done for any special things you may need to do before you go. Here are some general guidelines to follow:

- Make your mammogram appointment for one week after your period. Your breasts hurt less after your period.

- Wear a shirt with shorts, pants, or a skirt. That way you can undress from the waist up and leave your shorts, pants, or skirt on when you get your mammogram.

- Don't wear any deodorant, perfume, lotion, or powder under your arms or on your breasts on the day of your mammogram appointment. These things can make shadows show up on your mammogram.

Are there any problems with mammograms?

As with any medical test, mammograms can have limits. These limits include:

- Mammograms are only part of a complete breast exam. If they show abnormalities your health care provider will follow up with other tests.

- False negatives can happen. This means everything may look normal, but cancer is actually present. False negatives don't happen often. Younger women are more likely to have a false negative mammogram than are older women. This is because the breast tissue is denser, making cancer harder to spot.

- False positives can happen. This is when the mammogram results look like cancer is present, even though it is not. False positives are more common in younger women than older women.

Chapter 43

What Mammograms Show

Most standard mammographic workups include two views of each breast taken from different angles. Even if you have a lump in only one breast, pictures will be taken of both breasts. This is so the breasts can be compared, and so that the other breast can be checked for abnormalities. If you've had a mammogram before, the radiologist will compare your old mammogram to the new one to look for changes.

While they're looking for possible cancer, your doctors may also come across other masses or structures in the breast that deserve further investigation, including calcifications, cysts, and fibroadenomas.

Calcifications

Calcifications are tiny flecks of calcium—like grains of salt—in the soft tissue of the breast that can sometimes indicate the presence of an early breast cancer. Calcifications usually can't be felt, but they appear on a mammogram. Depending on how they're clustered and their shape, size, and number, your doctor may want to do further tests. Big calcifications—"macrocalcifications"—are usually not associated with cancer. Groups of small calcifications huddled together, called "clusters of microcalcifications," are associated with extra breast cell activity. Most of the time this is noncancerous extra cell growth, but sometimes clusters of microcalcifications can occur in areas of early cancer.

Cysts

Unlike cancerous tumors, which are solid, cysts are fluid-filled masses in the breast. Cysts are very common, and are rarely associated with cancer. Ultrasound is the best way to tell a cyst from a cancer, because sound waves pass right through a liquid-filled cyst. Solid lumps, on the other hand, bounce the waves right back to the film.

Fibroadenomas

Fibroadenomas are movable, solid, rounded lumps made up of normal breast cells. While not cancerous, these lumps may grow, and any solid lump that's getting bigger is usually removed to make sure that it's not a cancer. Fibroadenomas are the most common kind of breast mass, especially in young women.

Chapter 44

Breast Implant Imaging

Mammography Guidelines for Women with Breast Implants

Women with breast implants should follow the same American Cancer Society (ACS) program of recommended mammograms as women without breast implants. However, due to the implant, several special mammography views must be taken to allow visualization of both the breast tissue and the implant. For this reason, diagnostic mammography is usually performed on patients with breast implants (as opposed to the screening mammography that is typically performed on asymptomatic women without implants).

Examination of the augmented breasts is more time consuming; therefore, the imaging location performing the mammography should be informed of the presence of implants when the mammogram is scheduled. Patients with implants should also inform the physician and the technologist performing the exam that they have implants. We are unaware of any documented cases where mammography has been the direct cause of implant rupture.

The x-rays used for mammographic imaging of the breasts cannot penetrate silicone or saline implants well enough to image the overlying or underlying breast tissue. Therefore, some breast tissue (approximately 25 percent) will not be seen on the mammogram, as it

The information in this chapter is reprinted with permission from www.imaginis.com. © 2004 Imaginis Corporation. All rights reserved. Complete information about Imaginis is included at the end of this chapter.

will be covered up by the implant. In order to visualize as much breast tissue as possible, women with implants undergo four additional views as well as the four standard images taken during diagnostic mammography. In these additional x-ray pictures, called Eklund views or implant displacement (ID) views, the implant is pushed back against the chest wall and the breast is pulled forward over it. This allows better imaging of the forwardmost part of each breast. The implant displacement views are not as successful in women who have contractures (formation of hard scar tissue around the implants). The ID views are easiest to obtain in women whose implants are placed underneath (behind) the chest muscle.

Mammography Guidelines for Following Breast Reduction Surgery

Women who have had breast contouring or breast reduction (also called mastopexy or reduction mammaplasty) should also receive annual mammograms once they reach forty years of age. It is important for the radiologist to be aware of the patient's surgical history. This will help the radiologist when they interpret the mammogram images.

Magnetic Resonance (MR) Imaging of Breast Implants

Magnetic resonance (MR) imaging of the breasts (also called MR mammography or Breast MRI) can be used to image breast implants to check for ruptures or leaks. MR imaging may also be used as an adjunctive tool to conventional mammography for women with implants.

MR imaging gives radiologists significant freedom in acquiring direct views of the breasts in any plane or orientation. This is because the MR system switches magnetic fields and radio waves to achieve the acquisition of different views while x-ray mammography requires reorientation of the breast and mammography system for each view desired. MR also allows the doctors to easily visualize the muscle and chest wall in the vicinity of the breast, which may be important to check for the spread of cancer.

MR imaging can also be used to image breast tissue and cosmetic implants. Implants can obscure some of the breast tissue on conventional x-ray mammography images. This is because x-rays used for mammographic imaging of the breasts cannot penetrate silicone or saline implants well enough to image the overlying or underlying breast tissue. MR imaging does not have this limitation.

MR mammography can image the breast tissue that is compressed by an implant. However, x-ray mammography is still the best tool for evaluating breast tissue and for screening and diagnosing breast cancer. MR mammography requires intravenous contrast (gadolinium), is much more expensive than conventional mammography, and has limitations in sensitivity and specificity. There is no routine recommendation for using MR imaging as a cancer screening tool in women with implants, although it can be helpful in selected cases.

Magnetic resonance is the imaging method of choice to evaluate breast implants and to check for ruptures or leaks. MR imaging provides very good spatial resolution (detail) and excellent contrast resolution and enables MR to clearly visualize implant condition.

Ultrasound Imaging of Breast Implants

Breast ultrasound may also be used as a screening tool for the detection of implant rupture or leak. However, the sensitivity and specificity of ultrasound is lower than that of magnetic resonance imaging since ultrasound typically provides lower spatial resolution and less contrast resolution than MR. Ultrasound imaging is usually less expensive than MR imaging. MR imaging can also be more time consuming than ultrasound. Some patients may also prefer ultrasound over MR imaging, which some find to cause claustrophobia and mild anxiety.

Breast Biopsy for Women with Implants

Vacuum-assisted biopsy (brand names Mammotome or MIBB) allows physicians to perform accurate breast biopsies on women with breast implants. Prior to the advent of vacuum-assisted biopsy, women with implants typically had to undergo open surgical biopsy if breast cancer was suspected.

Unlike surgical biopsy, vacuum-assisted biopsy is a percutaneous ("through the skin") procedure. Vacuum-assisted biopsy relies on stereotactic mammography or ultrasound imaging for guidance. Stereotactic mammography involves using computers to pinpoint the exact location of a breast mass based on mammograms (x-rays) taken from two different angles. The computer coordinates will help the physician to guide the needle to the correct area in the breast. With ultrasound, the radiologist or surgeon will watch the needle on the ultrasound monitor to help guide it to the area of concern.

The precision and directional abilities of vacuum-assisted biopsy make it the most viable percutaneous ("through the skin") biopsy option for women with breast implants. Conventional core needle biopsy is typically less precise in locating breast abnormalities (lesions) and requires multiple needle insertions in order to obtain adequate breast tissue samples. Due to these limitations, core needle biopsy has been problematic in the past for women with breast implants.

Vacuum-assisted breast biopsy provides a safer approach for women with implants. Unlike core needle biopsy, the vacuum-assisted biopsy probe is inserted just once into the breast through a small nick in the skin. Multiple tissue samples may be taken by rotating the sampling needle aperture (opening) and using vacuum assistance. The vacuum-assisted biopsy needle is carefully manually positioned between the implant and the breast abnormality (lesion).

About Imaginis

Imaginis.com is an independent, award-winning, comprehensive resource for news and information on breast cancer prevention, screening, diagnosis, and treatment and related women's health topics such as hormone replacement therapy (HRT), multiple sclerosis, osteoporosis, and ovarian cancer. Imaginis.com also contains extensive information about medical procedures such as angiography, biopsy, CT, MR, nuclear medicine, ultrasound, x-ray imaging, and radiotherapy.

The goal of Imaginis.com is to provide women and their physicians with the most comprehensive and relevant information on breast health and related women's health issues. Imaginis content is created by an independent team of breast health specialists to ensure that it is up-to-date and accurate. Complicated medical terms are explained in everyday language to help individuals understand their options, make informed decisions, and achieve optimal health.

Chapter 45

The Effects of Age, Breast Density, and Hormone Therapy on the Accuracy of Screening Mammograms

What is the problem and what is known about it so far?

Mammograms are special x-rays of the breast that can identify breast cancers before a woman or her doctor can feel a lump in the breast. However, mammograms are not totally accurate. They sometimes suggest a cancer when it is not present (a false-positive result). Other times, mammograms look normal even though a cancer is present (a false-negative result). Younger women's breasts contain less fat and are denser than older women's breasts. In addition to age, breast density is affected by hormones, such as combinations of progestin and estrogen or estrogen alone. When a woman takes these hormones, her breasts become less fatty and denser. Mammograms of dense breasts are harder to read than mammograms of fatty breasts. However, the way that breast density, age, and hormone therapy influence the accuracy of mammograms (alone and in combination) is not well understood.

Why did the researchers do this particular study?

To learn how breast density, age, and hormone therapy (alone and in combination) affect the accuracy of screening mammograms.

Reprinted from "Summaries for Patients: The Effects of Age, Breast Density, and Hormone Therapy on the Accuracy of Screening Mammograms," by P. A. Carney, D. L. Miglioretti, B. C. Yankaskas, K. Kerlikowske, R. Rosenberg, C. M. Rutter, B. M. Geller, L. A. Abraham, S. H. Taplin, M. Dignan, G. Cutter, and R. Ballard-Barbash, *Annals of Internal Medicine* 138, no. 3 (February 4, 2003): 1–28. © 2003 American College of Physicians. Reprinted with permission.

Who was studied?

329,495 women between forty and eighty-nine years of age who had mammograms from 1996 to 1998 in several U.S. cities and states.

How was the study done?

The researchers looked at the results of the women's mammograms and whether the breast cancer was eventually diagnosed. They then looked at the accuracy of the mammogram in relation to a woman's age, breast density, and whether she was taking hormone therapy.

What did the researchers find?

The accuracy of mammograms increased as women's breasts became more fatty and less dense. Mammograms were also more accurate as women aged. The accuracy of mammograms was the same for users and nonusers of hormone therapy, as long as the researchers accounted for breast density and age. Hormone therapy by itself did not affect the accuracy of mammograms; however, by its effect on breast density, it affected mammogram accuracy.

What were the limitations of the study?

The study used information from a mammogram registry; thus, information on some women was missing.

What are the implications of the study?

Mammograms are less accurate in young women than in older women and in women with dense breasts than in women with fatty breasts. While hormone therapy may increase breast density, it will not affect the ability of mammography to detect cancer if it is present. However, women with dense breasts may need additional imaging studies to confirm the presence of cancer.

Chapter 46

Digital Mammography

One of the most recent advances in x-ray mammography is digital mammography. Digital (computerized) mammography is similar to standard mammography in that x-rays are used to produce detailed images of the breast. Digital mammography uses essentially the same mammography system as conventional mammography, but the system is equipped with a digital receptor and a computer instead of a film cassette. Several studies have demonstrated that digital mammography is at least as accurate as standard mammography.

Digital spot view mammography allows faster and more accurate stereotactic biopsy. This results in shorter examination times and significantly improved patient comfort and convenience, since the time the patient must remain still is much shorter. With digital spot-view mammography, images are acquired digitally and displayed immediately on the system monitor. Spot-view digital systems have been approved by the U.S. Food and Drug Administration (FDA) for use in guiding breast biopsy. Traditional stereotactic biopsy requires a mammogram film be exposed, developed, and then reviewed, greatly increasing the time before the breast biopsy can be completed.

In addition to spot-view digital mammography, the FDA has recently approved a "full-field" digital mammography system to screen for and diagnose breast cancer. With continued improvements, the

---

"full-field" mammography systems may eventually replace traditional mammography.

How Does Digital Mammography Differ from Standard Mammography?

In standard mammography, images are recorded on film using an x-ray cassette. The film is viewed by the radiologist using a "light box" and then stored in a jacket in the facility's archives. With digital mammography, the breast image is captured using a special electronic x-ray detector, which converts the image into a digital picture for review on a computer monitor. The digital mammogram is then stored on a computer. With digital mammography, the magnification, orientation, brightness, and contrast of the image may be altered after the exam is completed to help the radiologist more clearly see certain areas.

To date, studies of digital mammography and standard film mammography have shown that digital mammography is "comparable" to film mammography in terms of detecting breast cancer. Small studies have shown that digital mammography may provide additional benefits, such as lower radiation doses and higher sensitivity to abnormalities. For example, a study reported in the March 2001 issue of *Radiology* found that the use of digital mammography can lead to fewer "recalls" (repeat mammograms) than film mammography. Other data from German researchers suggest that the radiation dose can be reduced by up to 50 percent with digital mammography and still detect breast cancer as well as the standard radiation dose of film mammography. However, the radiation dose of standard film mammography is still extremely low and does not pose a risk to women.

The largest U.S. federally funded clinical trial on medical imaging will soon be under way to determine whether digital mammography is equal or superior to standard film mammography in helping to detect breast cancer. While the first digital mammography system has already gained U.S. Food and Drug Administration (FDA) approval and others are awaiting approval, researchers need a large-scale study to thoroughly investigate the benefits and limitations of the new technology. The study, called the Digital Mammographic Screening Trial (DMIST), will be conducted at several locations throughout the United States.

Digital mammography systems cost approximately four to five times as much as standard film mammography systems. While procedural time saved by using digital mammography over standard film mammography justifies part of the cost for facilities that perform several thousand mammograms each year, the study will determine whether the high cost of digital mammography is justifiable in terms of its benefits in detecting breast cancer.

From the patient's perspective, a digital mammogram is the same as a standard film-based mammogram in that breast compression and radiation are necessary to create clear images of the breast. The time needed to position the patient is the same for each method. However, conventional film mammography requires several minutes to develop the film while digital mammography provides the image on the computer monitor in less than a minute after the exposure/data acquisition. Thus, digital mammography provides a shorter exam for the woman and may possibly allow mammography facilities to conduct more mammograms in a day. Digital mammography can also be manipulated to correct for under- or overexposure after the exam is completed, eliminating the need for some women to undergo repeat mammograms before leaving the facility.

With digital mammography, the magnification, orientation, brightness, and contrast of the mammogram image may also be altered after the exam is completed to help the radiologist more clearly see certain areas of the breast.

In the near future, digital mammography may provide many benefits over standard film mammography. These benefits include:

- Improved contrast between dense and non-dense breast tissue

- Faster image acquisition (less than a minute)

- Shorter exam time (approximately half that of film-based mammography)

- Easier image storage

- Physician manipulation of breast images for more accurate detection of breast cancer

- Ability to correct under- or overexposure of films without having to repeat mammograms

- Transmittal of images over phone lines or a network for remote consultation with other physicians

Promising Developments in Digital Mammography

The FDA approved the first "full-field" digital mammography scanner to screen for and diagnose breast cancer in February 2000. Before applying for FDA certification, data was gathered from 662 patients at four institutions: the University of Colorado, the University of Massachusetts Medical Center, Massachusetts General Hospital, and the Hospital of the University of Pennsylvania. The data compared hard copies of digital breast images on film to conventional mammography films, finding that digital mammography is as effective at detecting breast cancer as standard film mammograms. A separate study revealed that the digital mammography scanner showed a slight advantage in the visibility of breast tissue at the skin line.

In November 2000, the FDA approved soft-copy reading of digital mammogram images that are produced by the GE Senographe 2000D digital mammography system. The Senographe 2000D system is currently installed at approximately thirty-five locations in the United States. Other manufacturers, such as Siemens Medical Systems and Fischer Imaging, are also developing digital mammography systems.

Disadvantages to Digital Mammography

While digital mammography is quite promising, it still has additional hurdles to overcome before it replaces conventional mammography. Digital mammography must:

- provide higher detail resolution (as standard mammography does)

- become less expensive (digital mammography is currently several times more costly than conventional mammography)

- provide a method to efficiently compare digital mammogram images with existing mammography films on computer monitors

Standard mammography using film cassettes has the benefit of providing very high detail resolution (image sharpness), which is especially useful for imaging microcalcifications (tiny calcium deposits) and very small abnormalities that may indicate early breast cancer. While full-field digital mammography may lack the spatial resolution of film, clinical trials have shown digital mammography to be at least equivalent to standard film screening mammography. This is because digital mammography has the benefit of providing improved contrast resolution, which may make abnormalities easier to see. Various manufacturers are trying to develop digital mammography systems with detail resolution equivalent to standard film mammography while also providing the benefits of digital mammography noted previously.

The high cost of digital mammography is a major obstacle. Digital mammography systems cost roughly four to five times as much as standard mammography equipment. Standard mammography systems are currently installed in over ten thousand locations across the United States. It may take years for this current equipment to be updated or replaced and for digital mammography to become widespread.

About Imaginis

Imaginis.com is an independent, award-winning, comprehensive resource for news and information on breast cancer prevention, screening, diagnosis, and treatment and related women's health topics such as hormone replacement therapy (HRT), multiple sclerosis, osteoporosis, and ovarian cancer. Imaginis.com also contains extensive information about medical procedures such as angiography, biopsy, CT, MR, nuclear medicine, ultrasound, x-ray imaging, and radiotherapy.

The goal of Imaginis.com is to provide women and their physicians with the most comprehensive and relevant information on breast health and related women's health issues. Imaginis content is created by an independent team of breast health specialists to ensure that it is up-to-date and accurate. Complicated medical terms are explained in everyday language to help individuals understand their options, make informed decisions, and achieve optimal health.

Chapter 47

Improving Methods for Breast Cancer Detection

The National Cancer Institute (NCI) is funding numerous research projects to improve conventional mammography (an x-ray technique to visualize the internal structure of the breast) and develop other imaging technologies to detect, diagnose, and characterize breast tumors.

High-quality mammography is the most effective technology presently available for breast cancer screening. Efforts to improve mammography focus on refining the technology and improving how it is administered and x-ray films are interpreted. NCI is funding research to reduce the already low radiation dosage of mammography; enhance mammogram image quality; develop statistical techniques for computer-assisted interpretation of images; enable long-distance, electronic image transmission technology (telemammography/teleradiology) for clinical consultations; and improve image-guided techniques to assist with breast biopsies. (A breast biopsy is the removal of cells or tissues to look at under a microscope to check for signs of disease). NCI also supports research on technologies that do not use x-rays, such as magnetic resonance imaging (MRI), ultrasound, and breast-specific positron emission tomography (PET) to detect breast cancer. The following information describes the latest imaging techniques that are in use or being studied.

Cancer Facts, National Cancer Institute, April 2002. For more information from the National Cancer Institute, visit the website at www.cancer.gov or call 1-800-4CANCER.

303

Ultrasound

Ultrasound, also called sonography, is an imaging technique in which high-frequency sound waves that cannot be heard by humans are bounced off tissues and internal organs. Their echoes produce a picture called a sonogram. Ultrasound imaging of the breast is used to distinguish between solid tumors and fluid-filled cysts. Ultrasound can also be used to evaluate lumps that are hard to see on a mammogram. Sometimes, ultrasound is used as part of other diagnostic procedures, such as fine needle aspiration (also called needle biopsy). Fine needle aspiration is the removal of tissue or fluid with a needle for examination under a microscope to check for signs of disease.

During an ultrasound examination, the clinician spreads a thin coating of lubricating jelly over the area to be imaged to improve conduction of the sound waves. A hand-held device called a transducer directs the sound waves through the skin toward specific tissues. As the sound waves are reflected back from the tissues within the breast, the patterns formed by the waves create a two-dimensional image of the breast on a computer.

Ultrasound is not used for routine breast cancer screening because it does not consistently detect certain early signs of cancer such as microcalcifications (tiny deposits of calcium in the breast that can not be felt but can be seen on a conventional mammogram). A cluster of microcalcifications may indicate that cancer is present.

Digital Mammography

Digital mammography is a technique for recording x-ray images in computer code instead of on x-ray film, as with conventional mammography. The images are displayed on a computer monitor and can be enhanced (lightened or darkened) before they are printed on film. Images can also be manipulated; the radiologist (a doctor who specializes in creating and interpreting pictures of areas inside the body) can magnify or zoom in on an area. From the patient's perspective, the procedure for a mammogram with a digital system is the same as for conventional mammography.

Digital mammography may have some advantages over conventional mammography. The images can be stored and retrieved electronically, which makes long-distance consultations with other mammography specialists easier. Because the images can be adjusted by the radiologist, subtle differences between tissues may be noted. The improved accuracy of digital mammography may reduce the number of follow-up procedures. Despite these benefits, studies have not yet shown that digital mammography is more effective in finding cancer than conventional mammography.

The first digital mammography system received U.S. Food and Drug Administration (FDA) approval in 2000. An example of a digital mammography system is the Senographe® 2000D. Women considering digital mammography should talk with their doctor or contact a local FDA-certified mammography center to find out if this technique is available at that location. Only facilities that have been certified to practice conventional mammography and have FDA approval for digital mammography may offer the digital system. A list of conventional mammography facilities is available by calling the Cancer Information Service at 1–800–4–CANCER (1-800-422-6237), or by visiting the FDA website at http://www.accessdata.fda.gov/scripts/cdrh/cfdocs/cfmqsa/search.cfm on the internet.

Computer-Aided Detection

Computer-aided detection (CAD) involves the use of computers to bring suspicious areas on a mammogram to the radiologist's attention. It is used after the radiologist has done the initial review of the mammogram. In 1998, the FDA approved a breast-imaging device that uses CAD technology. Others are in development. An example of a breast-imaging device that uses CAD technology is the ImageChecker®. This device scans the mammogram with a laser beam and converts it into a digital signal that is processed by a computer. The image is then displayed on a video monitor, with suspicious areas highlighted for the radiologist to review. The radiologist can compare the digital image with the conventional mammogram to see if any of the highlighted areas were missed on the initial review and require further evaluation. CAD technology may improve the accuracy of screening mammography. The incorporation of CAD technology with digital mammography is under evaluation.

Magnetic Resonance Imaging (MRI)

In magnetic resonance imaging (MRI), a magnet linked to a computer creates detailed pictures of areas inside the body without the use of radiation. Each MRI produces hundreds of images of the breast from side-to-side, top-to-bottom, and front-to-back. The images are then interpreted by a radiologist.

During an MRI of the breast, the patient lies on her stomach on the scanning table. The breast hangs into a depression or hollow in the table, which contains coils that detect the magnetic signal. The table is moved into a tube-like machine that contains the magnet. After an initial series of images has been taken, the patient may be given a contrast agent intravenously (by injection into a vein). The contrast agent is not radioactive; it is sometimes used to improve the visibility of a tumor. Additional images are then taken. The entire imaging session takes about one hour.

Breast MRI is not used for routine breast cancer screening, but clinical trials (research studies with people) are being performed to determine if MRI is valuable for screening certain women, such as young women at high risk for breast cancer. MRI cannot always accurately distinguish between cancer and benign (noncancerous) breast conditions. Like ultrasound, MRI cannot detect microcalcifications.

MRI is used primarily to evaluate breast implants for leaks or ruptures, and to assess abnormal areas that are seen on a mammogram or are felt after breast surgery or radiation therapy. It can be used after breast cancer is diagnosed to determine the extent of the tumor in the breast. MRI is also sometimes useful in imaging dense breast tissue, which is often found in younger women, and in viewing breast abnormalities that can be felt but are not visible with conventional mammography or ultrasound.

PET Scan

The positron emission tomography (PET) scan creates computerized images of chemical changes that take place in tissue. The patient is given an injection of a substance that consists of a combination of a sugar and a small amount of radioactive material. The radioactive sugar can help in locating a tumor, because cancer cells take up or absorb sugar faster than other tissues in the body.

After receiving the radioactive drug, the patient lies still for about forty-five minutes while the drug circulates throughout the body. If a tumor is present, the radioactive sugar will accumulate in the tumor. The patient then lies on a table, which gradually moves through the PET scanner six to seven times during a forty-five-minute period. The PET scanner is used to detect the radiation. A computer translates this information into the images that are interpreted by a radiologist.

PET scans may play a role in determining whether a breast mass is cancerous. However, PET scans are more accurate in detecting larger and more aggressive tumors than they are in locating tumors that are smaller than 8 mm or less aggressive. They may also detect cancer when other imaging techniques show normal results. PET scans may be helpful in evaluating and staging recurrent disease (cancer that has come back).

An NCI-sponsored clinical trial is evaluating the usefulness of PET scan results in women who have breast cancer compared with the findings from other imaging and diagnostic techniques. This trial is also studying the effectiveness of PET scans in tracking the response of a tumor to treatment.

Electrical Impedance Scanning

Different types of tissue have different electrical impedance levels (electrical impedance is a measurement of how fast electricity travels through a given material). Some types of tissue have high electrical impedance, while others have low electrical impedance. Breast tissue that is cancerous has a much lower electrical impedance (conducts electricity much better) than normal breast tissue. Electrical impedance scanning devices are used along with conventional mammography to detect breast cancer. The T-Scan 2000, also known as the T-Scan, is an example of such a device. The FDA approved the T-Scan 2000 in 1999.

The electrical impedance scanning device, which does not emit any radiation, consists of a hand-held scanning probe and a computer screen that displays two-dimensional images of the breast. An electrode patch, similar to that used for an electrocardiogram, is placed on the patient's arm. A very small amount of electric current, about the same amount used by a small penlight battery, is transmitted through the patch and into the body. The current travels through the breast, where it is measured by the scanning probe placed over the breast. An image is generated from the measurements of electrical impedance. Because breast cancer cells conduct electricity better than normal breast cells and tend to have lower electrical impedance, breast tumors may appear as bright white spots on the computer screen.

This device can confirm the location of abnormal areas that were detected by a conventional mammogram. The scanner sends the image directly to a computer, allowing the radiologist to move the probe around the breast to get the best view of the area being examined. The device may reduce the number of biopsies needed to determine whether a mass is cancerous. It may also improve the identification of women who should have a biopsy.

The scanner is not approved as a screening device for breast cancer, and is not used when mammography or other findings clearly indicate the need for a biopsy. This device has not been studied with patients who have implanted electronic devices, such as pacemakers. It is not recommended for use on such patients.

Image-Guided Breast Biopsy Techniques

Imaging techniques play an important role in helping doctors perform breast biopsies, especially of abnormal areas that cannot be felt but can be seen on a conventional mammogram or with ultrasound. One type of needle biopsy, the stereotactic-guided biopsy, involves the precise location of the abnormal area in three dimensions using conventional mammography. (Stereotactic refers to the use of a computer and scanning devices to create three-dimensional images.) A needle is then inserted into the breast and a tissue sample is obtained. Additional samples can be obtained by moving the needle within the abnormal area.

Another type of needle biopsy uses a different system, known as the Mammotome® breast biopsy system. The FDA approved Mammotome in 1996; the hand-held version of the Mammotome received FDA clearance in September 1999. A large needle is inserted into the suspicious area using ultrasound or stereotactic guidance. The Mammotome is then used to gently vacuum tissue from the suspicious area. Additional tissue samples can be obtained by rotating the needle. This procedure can be performed with the patient lying on her stomach on a table. If the hand-held device is used, the patient may lie on her back or in a seated position.

There have been no reports of serious complications resulting from the Mammotome breast biopsy system. Women interested in this procedure should talk with their doctor.

Ductal Lavage

Ductal lavage is an investigational technique for collecting samples of cells from breast ducts for analysis under a microscope. A saline (saltwater) solution is introduced into a milk duct through a catheter (a thin, flexible tube) that is inserted into the opening of the duct on the surface of the nipple. Fluid, which contains cells from the duct, is withdrawn through the catheter. The cells are checked under a microscope to identify changes that may indicate cancer or changes that may increase the risk for breast cancer. The usefulness of ductal lavage is still under study.

Imaging Clinical Trials

In March 1999, the NCI began funding the American College of Radiology Imaging Network (ACRIN) as part of the NCI's Clinical Trials Cooperative Group Program. (A cooperative group is a group of physicians, hospitals, or both that works with the NCI to identify important questions in cancer research and design clinical trials to answer these questions.) The Cooperative Group program is designed to promote and support clinical trials of new cancer treatments, explore methods of cancer prevention and early detection, and study quality of life issues and rehabilitation during and after treatment. ACRIN is dedicated to increasing the number and quality of clinical trials that involve imaging technologies to detect and diagnose cancer. The NCI actively participates in the planning, review, and monitoring of clinical trials that are organized by ACRIN.

People interested in taking part in a clinical trial should talk with their doctor. Information about clinical trials is available from the Cancer Information Service (CIS) at 1-800-4-CANCER. Information specialists at the CIS use PDQ®, NCI's cancer information database, to identify and provide detailed information about specific ongoing clinical trials. Patients also have the option of searching for clinical trials on their own. The clinical trials page of the NCI's Cancer.gov website provides general information about clinical trials and links to PDQ. This page is located at http://www.cancer.gov/clinical_trials on the internet.

Part Six

Diagnosis and Treatment Options

Chapter 48

Diagnostic Mammography

What is diagnostic mammography?

Diagnostic mammography is an x-ray exam of the breasts that is performed in order to evaluate a breast complaint or abnormality detected by physical exam or routine screening mammography. Diagnostic mammography is different from screening mammography in that additional views of the breast are usually taken, as opposed to two views typically taken with screening mammography. Thus, diagnostic mammography is usually more time-consuming and costly than screening mammography.

The goal of diagnostic mammography is to pinpoint the exact size and location of breast abnormality and to image the surrounding tissue and lymph nodes. In many cases, diagnostic mammography will help show that the abnormality is highly likely to be benign (noncancerous). When this occurs, the radiologist may recommend that the woman return at a later date for a follow-up mammogram, typically in six months. However, if an abnormality seen with diagnostic mammography is suspicious, additional breast imaging (with exams such as ultrasound) or a biopsy may be ordered. Biopsy is the only definitive way to determine whether a woman has breast cancer.

The information in this chapter is reprinted with permission from www.imaginis.com. © 2004 Imaginis Corporation. All rights reserved. Complete information about Imaginis is included at the end of this chapter.

What types of views are taken with diagnostic mammography?

Typical views for diagnostic mammograms include the cranio-caudal view (CC), the mediolateral oblique view (MLO), and supplemental views tailored to the specific problem. These can include views from each side (latero medial, LM: from the side toward the center of the chest, and mediolateral view, ML: from the center of the chest out), exaggerated cranial-caudal, and other special mammography views such as spot compression and magnification views.

What types of abnormalities can diagnostic mammography detect?

Mammography is used to detect a number of abnormalities, the two main ones being calcifications and masses. Calcifications are tiny mineral deposits within the breast tissue that appear as small white regions on the mammogram films. There are two types of calcifications: microcalcifications and macrocalcifications. A mass is any group of cells clustered together more densely than the surrounding tissue. A cyst (pocket of fluid) may also appear as a mass on mammography. Radiologists may often use ultrasound to help differentiate between a solid mass and a cyst.

Calcifications, masses and other conditions that may appear on a mammogram:

- Microcalcifications are tiny (less than 1/50 of an inch or ½ of a millimeter) specks of calcium in the breast. When many microcalcifications are seen in one area, they are referred to as a cluster and may indicate a small cancer. About half of the cancers detected by mammography appear as a cluster of microcalcifications. Microcalcifications are the most common mammographic sign of ductal carcinoma in situ (an early cancer confined to the breast ducts). Almost 90 percent of cases of ductal carcinoma in situ are associated with microcalcifications. An area of microcalcifications seen on a mammogram does not always indicate that cancer is present. The shape and arrangement of microcalcifications help the radiologist judge the likelihood of cancer. In some cases, the microcalcifications do not indicate a need for a biopsy. Instead, a physician may advise a follow-up mammogram, typically within six months. In other cases, the microcalcifications are more suspicious and a stereotactic biopsy is recommended.

Only approximately 17 percent of calcifications requiring biopsy are cancerous. The radiologist may describe the shape of suspicious microcalcifications on the mammogram report as "pleomorphic" or "polymorphic."

- Macrocalcifications are coarse (large) calcium deposits that are often associated with benign fibrocystic change or with degenerative changes in the breasts, such as aging of the breast arteries, old injuries, or inflammation. Macrocalcification deposits are associated with benign (noncancerous) conditions and do not usually require a biopsy. Macrocalcifications are found in approximately 50 percent of women over the age of fifty.

- Masses: Another important change seen on a mammogram is the presence of a mass, which may occur with or without associated calcifications. A mass is any group of cells clustered together more densely than the surrounding tissue. A cyst (a noncancerous collection of fluid in the breast) may appear as a mass on a mammogram film. A cyst cannot be diagnosed by physical exam alone nor can it be diagnosed by mammography alone, although certain signs can suggest the presence of a cyst or cysts. To confirm that a mass is a cyst, either breast ultrasound or aspiration with a needle is required. If a mass is not a cyst, then further imaging may be ordered. As with calcifications, a mass can be caused by benign breast conditions or by breast cancer. Some masses can be monitored with periodic mammography while others may require biopsy. The size, shape, and margins (edges) of the mass help the radiologist in evaluating the likelihood of cancer. Prior mammograms may help show that a mass is unchanged for many years, indicating a benign condition and helping to avoid unnecessary biopsy. Therefore, it is important for women to bring their previous mammogram films with them if they change mammogram facilities.

- Density: The glandular tissue of the breasts, or breast density, shows up as white areas on a mammogram film. In general, younger women have denser breasts than older women. Breast density can make it more difficult to detect microcalcifications and other masses with mammography, since breast abnormalities also show up as white areas on the mammogram. After menopause, the glandular tissue of the breasts is replaced with fat, typically making abnormalities easier to detect with mammography. Therefore, most physicians do not recommend that women begin receiving annual screening mammograms until they reach forty years of age unless they are at high risk of developing breast cancer.

By law, the mammography facility is required to provide the woman with a written summary of the mammogram findings within thirty days of the mammogram. This letter is not a copy of the official radiologist's report, but rather it is a separate document that clearly explains whether an abnormality was detected and provides general information about that abnormality. Women who are self-referred should also receive a copy of the formal radiologist's report. The letter will also indicate whether additional imaging or biopsy is recommended. Women should contact the mammography facility if they do not receive this letter within thirty days of their mammogram.

What other exams or procedures may be ordered to evaluate a breast abnormality?

Mammography alone cannot prove that an abnormal area is cancerous, although some abnormalities may be very characteristic of malignancy. If mammography raises a significant suspicion of cancer, additional breast imaging or biopsy may be ordered. A breast biopsy involves removing samples of tissue for examination under the microscope. This is the only way breast cancer can be definitively diagnosed. Between 65 and 80 percent of breast biopsies reveal benign (noncancerous) conditions. Other breast imaging exams that may be ordered include:

- Ultrasound (especially beneficial for distinguishing cysts from masses)

- Breast MRI (especially beneficial for imaging breast implants)

- Other exams, such as nuclear medicine imaging or T-scan

- Ductography (also called a galactogram)

Ductography is a special type of contrast-enhanced mammography used for imaging the breast ducts. Ductography can aid in diagnosing the cause of an abnormal nipple discharge and is valuable in diagnosing intraductal papillomas.

About Imaginis

Imaginis.com is an independent, award-winning, comprehensive resource for news and information on breast cancer prevention, screening, diagnosis, and treatment and related women's health topics such as hormone replacement therapy (HRT), multiple sclerosis, osteoporosis, and ovarian cancer. Imaginis.com also contains extensive information about medical procedures such as angiography, biopsy, CT, MR, nuclear medicine, ultrasound, x-ray imaging, and radiotherapy.

The goal of Imaginis.com is to provide women and their physicians with the most comprehensive and relevant information on breast health and related women's health issues. Imaginis content is created by an independent team of breast health specialists to ensure that it is up-to-date and accurate. Complicated medical terms are explained in everyday language to help individuals understand their options, make informed decisions, and achieve optimal health.

Chapter 49

The Diagnostic Biopsy

A biopsy is a test that establishes the precise diagnosis when a breast lump or other abnormality is discovered. With this procedure, cells or tissue are removed and examined under a microscope by a specially trained doctor called a pathologist. Of the approximately half-million breast biopsies performed each year, as many as 80 percent turn out to be benign.

What Happens when a Lump Is Found or an Abnormal Mammogram Report Occurs? (Diagnostic Alternatives)

Cyst Aspiration

Cyst aspiration uses a narrow-gauge needle attached to a hypodermic syringe to remove fluid from a "cyst" (a fluid-filled mass). The mass may be palpable or detected by mammography. If fluid appears, the growth is a cyst that will break down and disappear from the monitor. If the physician is unable to draw out any fluid, the growth is solid, making it necessary to perform a biopsy.

Fine Needle Aspiration Biopsy (FNAB)

Fine needle aspiration biopsy (FNAB) uses a narrow-gauge needle, under vacuum pressure (similar to or smaller than the type used to draw blood), attached to a hypodermic syringe to remove cells from a palpable mass or thickening for pathologic study. The gauge of the needle is based on the size of the patient's breast and the profile of the suspicious lump.

Needle Localization Biopsy

When nonpalpable mammographic findings warrant biopsy to determine the presence or absence of malignancy, a needle localization biopsy can be performed. This mammographic procedure localizes the abnormality by placing a special needle or wire through the skin to guide the surgeon. An x-ray of the problem area is usually taken during surgery to ensure accurate tissue removal.

Stereotactic Biopsy

Another way to localize a nonpalpable lesion is by stereotactic guidance. This is most commonly used to biopsy microcalcifications or indiscriminate mammographic shadows. Stereotactic biopsy uses radiation to produce double-image (stereo views) mammography of the suspicious area. The two stereo images are viewed next to each other on the same film. Computer-generated coordinates are then created from the two images. The abnormal area is targeted and a needle is "shot" into the breast to remove a sample of tissue.

Core Needle Biopsy

Core needle biopsy uses a larger bore-cutting needle to withdraw a sample of tissue from a palpable or mammographically detected mass. The gauge of the needle is based on the size of the patient's breast and the profile of the suspicious lump.

Incisional Biopsy

An incisional biopsy surgically removes a portion of the lump for microscopic examination of tissue, after making an incision in the skin. This technique involves either a local or a general anesthesia.

Excisional Biopsy

An excisional biopsy surgically removes (excises) the entire lump through a skin incision. This technique also involves either a local or a general anesthesia.

Ultrasound-Guided Biopsy

Ultrasound-guided biopsies can be useful for patients with lesions that show up on only one view or that show up only in an ultrasound image, for pregnant women or nursing mothers who need to avoid exposure to x-rays, and for patients with multiple lesions in one or both breasts. High-resolution ultrasound uses high-frequency sound waves, or echoes, to project the internal anatomy of the breast onto the screen of a monitor. A transducer, functioning like a microphone, is placed on the breast after a special gel has been applied to the skin. The transducer both sends and receives sound waves that produce the internal imaging of the breast.

1. **Ultrasound-Guided Fine Needle Aspiration:** The radiologist or sonographer performing the ultrasound can locate the growth with the help of a transducer to direct a fine gauge needle into the area of the growth. With the needle functioning under vacuum pressure, the physician is then able to drain away any fluid. If fluid appears, the growth is a cyst that will break down and disappear from the monitor. If the physician is unable to draw out any fluid, the growth is solid, making it necessary to perform a biopsy.

2. **Ultrasound-Guided Fine Needle Aspiration Biopsy:** An ultrasound-guided fine needle aspiration biopsy is like an ultrasound-guided fine needle aspiration. A local anesthetic may be used to numb an area of skin on the breast. Once the physician locates the suspicious area, he can then guide a needle to the area with the use of the ultrasound equipment. Once the needle is in place, a vacuum is created within the syringe and cells are drawn into the needle. It is common for the doctor to make several insertions (passes) of the needle into the growth to make sure that an adequate sampling of cells is obtained.

3. **Ultrasound-Guided Core Needle Biopsy:** An ultrasound-guided core needle biopsy is similar to an ultrasound-guided fine needle biopsy. A transducer is placed on the patient's breast, where it will receive and send the sound waves that will produce the internal breast image. A local anesthetic is used to numb the patient's breast(s), after which a fourteen- or eighteen-gauge core needle is injected. Due to the size of

the needle, the physician will need to make a small incision (nick) in the skin to insert the wider core needle. The size of the needle is the main difference between a fine needle and a core needle biopsy.

Future Techniques Currently under Investigation

Ultrasound Computed Tomography (CT)

Ultrasound CT is currently being tested at the University of California, San Diego, California. It does not involve radiation to get inside the breast for cross-sectional pictures or image "slices" called tomograms. The images are projected onto a computer screen for viewing via ultrasound equipment. It takes about twenty minutes for a full screening that requires seven or eight images to get a complete picture of the breast. Researchers are hopeful that this technique will provide clinicians with better-defined images of solid masses that are particularly difficult to identify in dense breasts.

Positron Emission Tomography (PET Scan)

In a PET scan tomogram, a patient receives an injection of a radioisotope that releases a nuclear substance (positron). Concentrations of the isotope are absorbed by breast cells that can form "hot spots." A rapid film sequence creates image "slices" (tomograms) that, when put together, create a complete picture of the breast. A radiologist can then zero in on the "hot spots" to detect a small cancer growth and the spread of cancer to the lymph nodes. The PET scan also allows clinicians to get a good view of very dense breasts. False-positive results can occur because the images produced make it difficult to distinguish between infections and cancer.

Chapter 50

Sentinel Lymph Node Biopsy: What Breast Cancer Patients Need to Know

Introduction

When discussing the surgical treatment of your breast cancer with you, your surgeon will discuss whether or not your breast cancer is invasive. Breast cancers can be confined within the lining of the endothelial cells along the breast duct (in-situ cancers); or it can start to spread beyond the breast duct (invasive cancers). This is important because the blood vessels and lymph vessels that potentially spread the cancer beyond the breast run along this area. If the cancer has spread beyond the lining of the breast duct, and is picked up by the blood vessels or lymph vessels, then it can potentially spread elsewhere in the body, or "metastasize." Lymph vessels are small channels that drain all the tissues of the body. Lymph vessels drain excess fluid back into your circulation. As lymph fluid drains back into your circulation, it goes through lymph nodes. Lymph nodes are collections of lymph tissue that have a high concentration of white blood cells, the cells in your body that fight infection and cancer. The lymph vessels of the breast drain into the lymph nodes in your axilla (underneath your arm), and sometimes into the lymph nodes along your sternum (or breastbone) and above your clavicle (collarbone).

"Sentinal Lymph Node Biopsy: What Breast Cancer Patients Need to Know," by Kathleen M. Diehl, M.D. and Alfred E. Chang, M.D., Division of Surgical Oncology, University of Michigan Comprehensive Cancer Center, February 2002. Reprinted with permission from Cancer news on the Net®, www.cancernews.com. © Cancernews.com. All rights reserved.

Axillary Lymph Node Dissection

Traditionally, if your breast cancer is invasive, an axillary lymph node dissection is recommended by your surgeon in order to see if the cancer has spread to the lymph nodes underneath the arm. During an axillary lymph node dissection, the surgeon makes an incision underneath your arm and removes the bulk of the lymph node tissue that drains from the breast. The lymph node tissue is then sent to the laboratory, and a pathologist looks at the lymph nodes under a microscope and determines if any of them contain cancer. On average, approximately ten to fifteen lymph nodes are removed with this operation. An axillary lymph node dissection usually requires an overnight stay in the hospital. Since the remaining tissues underneath the arm tend to "leak" some lymph fluid when the lymph nodes are removed, a drain is left in place for the first two to three weeks after the operation until the area heals. The drain is a flexible plastic tube that exits the skin and is connected to a plastic collection bulb. When the drainage diminishes to a certain amount, the drain is removed in the clinic. After you go home you are given physical therapy exercises to maintain strength and flexibility in your shoulder while this area heals. Approximately 5 to 10 percent of the patients who undergo an axillary lymph node dissection experience chronic problems related to the dissection, such as arm swelling (lymphedema) or pain or discomfort in the area of the dissection. Almost all women will have some residual numbness under the inside of the arm.

Sentinel Lymph Node Biopsy

A sentinel lymph node biopsy is a new technique. This was developed as a test to determine if breast cancer has spread to the lymph ducts or lymph nodes in the axilla without having to do a traditional axillary lymph node dissection. Experience has shown us that the lymph ducts of the breast usually drain to one lymph node first, before draining through the rest of the lymph nodes underneath the arm. That first lymph node is called the sentinel lymph node. That is the lymph node that helps sound the warning that the cancer has spread. Lymph node mapping helps identify that lymph node, and a sentinel lymph node biopsy removes only that lymph node. The sentinel lymph node is identified in one of two ways, either by a weak radioactive dye (technetium-labeled sulfur colloid) that can be measured by a hand-held probe, or by a blue dye (isosulfan blue) that stains the lymph tissue a bright blue so it can be seen. Most breast cancer surgeons use a combination of both dyes. This procedure is new. The "best" way to administer the dye, which dye to use, and the benefits and risks of the procedure in various situations are still being studied. A traditional axillary lymph node dissection is the "tried and true" method, and is still considered the "gold standard."

Advantages to Sentinal Lymph Node Biopsy

The advantages to the sentinel lymph node procedure are many. There is no need to stay overnight in the hospital. There is no need for a drain or physical therapy exercises. Your recuperation from the procedure is faster. You are typically doing your regular activities within a few days, and the incision is well healed within a few weeks. A sentinel lymph node biopsy can lead to a more accurate assessment of whether the cancer has spread to the lymph nodes. In a traditional axillary dissection, the pathologist receives at least ten lymph nodes; there is no way of telling which one is the sentinel lymph node. So the pathologist makes one cut in each lymph node and looks for cancer. When the pathologist receives only one, or a few, lymph nodes from a sentinel lymph node procedure, he or she can make many cuts through that lymph node to look for cancer. A negative sentinel lymph node(s) indicates a greater than 95 percent chance that the remaining lymph nodes in the axilla are also cancer-free. Therefore, there is no need to undergo a full axillary lymph node dissection, or to risk the long-term complications and side effects from an axillary dissection.

What to Expect

If you decide to undergo the procedure, the morning of your operation you will see a nuclear medicine specialist who is a physician specifically trained in injecting the radioactive dye used for the procedure. The injections are done into the area of the breast where the tumor is, and around the nipple areolar complex of the breast. You will then return to the nuclear medicine department a few hours later, and pictures will be taken that show the pathways the dye takes as it leaves the breast. This will help guide your surgeon in identifying the sentinel lymph node. Then you will proceed to the operating room. At the beginning of the operation, your surgeon will inject the blue dye. The surgeon then makes an incision underneath your arm in the area of the axillary lymph tissue. A hand-held sterile probe measures areas that have the radioactive dye. The lymph nodes that have taken up the radioactive dye, or are stained with the blue dye, are removed. Usually one to three nodes are removed. These nodes are sent to the pathologist, who then looks at them under a microscope to see if the sentinel node contains cancer. Your incision is closed, and there is no need for a drain. There is no need for physical therapy exercises. Unless you are having another operation done that requires you to stay overnight, you can go home from the hospital that day. The sentinel lymph node biopsy can be done in combination with a lumpectomy or a mastectomy. The procedure is successful in more than 90 percent of those patients whom we think are good candidates for the procedure. If the procedure is unsuccessful in identifying the sentinel node, a full axillary dissection is done.

Who Shouldn't Undergo the Procedure

Unfortunately, the sentinel lymph node biopsy procedure can't be performed on everyone with an invasive breast cancer. People who have had radiation therapy or surgery in their breast or axilla should not undergo the technique, as changes in the breast and axilla from the radiation therapy or surgery may make the results inaccurate. People who have enlarged lymph nodes underneath their arm, or people whom we know already have breast cancer metastatic to their axillary lymph nodes should undergo a traditional axillary lymph node dissection. People who already have had a mastectomy can't undergo the procedure because there is no accurate way to inject the dye to identify the lymph node. People with large tumors (greater then 5 cm) have a higher incidence of lymph node spread of their cancer, and may be better served by a traditional lymph node dissection. They should discuss this with their surgeon. People in whom it will be difficult to accurately inject the dye would likely be better served by a full axillary lymph node dissection. This includes those people in whom we are unable to find the primary breast tumor (an "occult" malignancy), and people in whom the tumor is dispersed through more then one area of the breast (a multifocal tumor).

If the Sentinel Lymph Node Is Positive

If the pathology results show that the breast cancer has spread to the sentinel lymph node, then typically you will need to return to the operating room to undergo a complete axillary lymph node dissection. This is done to remove the remaining lymph nodes, which may contain cancer. Since the majority of patients with breast cancer involving lymph nodes receive chemotherapy, the new question for breast cancer specialists has been whether or not it matters if there is cancer in any of the other lymph nodes within the axilla. The answer is that we don't know yet. There is currently a large national clinical trial called Z0011, which is evaluating exactly that question. In this trial some patients are chosen (randomized) to receive a full axillary lymph node dissection if their sentinel lymph node is positive. Some patients are chosen to not undergo any further lymph node dissection, and they are carefully watched. All of these patients will receive chemotherapy. The two groups of patients will be compared to see if there is a benefit to doing the full axillary dissection if the sentinel lymph node is positive. Or, alternatively, they will be compared to see if there is a detriment to not doing a full axillary dissection if the sentinel lymph node is positive. This is still experimental, and should be done only under controlled circumstances after being enrolled in this trial by a participating breast cancer surgeon. Doing a full axillary lymph node dissection if the sentinel lymph node is positive is still considered "the standard of care" with which all patients should be treated. To do otherwise risks undertreating your breast cancer.

Who Should Do the Procedure

One of the factors that influences the results obtained with the procedure is the qualification of the breast surgeon doing the procedure. Initial studies have shown that most surgeons need to do twenty to thirty sentinel lymph node biopsy procedures before obtaining accurate results using the technique. Surgeons can perform these cases during an accredited residency or fellowship at an institution that does a large number of these cases a year. Alternatively, surgeons can attend a conference to learn the technique, then acquire these twenty to thirty cases as part of a training protocol. During the training period, the surgeon will perform the sentinel lymph node biopsy and then complete a full axillary lymph node dissection at the same operation. After obtaining the pathology results, the surgeon can then determine if the sentinel lymph node was correctly identified. In addition, the surgeon can determine that the cancer was found in the sentinel node, and not in the lymph nodes that would otherwise have been left behind (false negative rate). After a surgeon has done twenty to thirty cases in which the sentinel lymph node is identified in greater than 90 percent of the cases, and the false negative rate is less then 5 percent, then the surgeon "goes off protocol," and does sentinel lymph node biopsies without a full axillary dissection. Until the surgeon has completed a large number of cases and determined his or her accuracy for doing the technique, any cases done "off protocol" may inaccurately determine if there has been spread of cancer to the axillary lymph nodes. It is therefore important to ask your surgeon if he or she has done a large number of cases during an accredited residency or fellowship, or if he or she has completed the learning protocol for the technique. No matter how the training for doing the procedure was acquired, there is some evidence to show that the surgeons who continue to perform this procedure on a regular basis will have more accurate results from the technique.

Summary

Invasive breast cancer can spread through the lymph ducts and blood vessels to other areas of the body. The sentinel lymph node is the first lymph node that the lymph ducts drain into. Whether or not the cancer has spread to the sentinel lymph node indicates whether the cancer has started to spread beyond the breast. A new technique called sentinel lymph node biopsy identifies this lymph node and allows only this lymph node to be removed. Removing only the sentinel lymph node can allow breast cancer patients to avoid many of the complications and side effects associated with a traditional axillary lymph node dissection. Patients with invasive breast cancer should discuss sentinel lymph node biopsy with their surgeon.

References

American Society of Breast Surgeons Revised Consensus Statement on Guidelines for Performance of Sentinel Lymphadenectomy for Breast Cancer. August 25, 2000. http://www.breastsurgeons.org/sentinel.htm.

Arnold, D. K., K. N. Tran, et al. "Lessons Learned from 500 Cases of Lymphatic Mapping for Breast Cancer." *Ann Surg* 229, no. 4 (1999): 528–35.

Cox, C. E., C. J. Salud, et al. "Learning Curves for Breast Cancer Sentinel Lymph Node Mapping Based on Surgical Volume Analysis." *J Am Coll Surg* 193 (2001): 593–600.

Edwards, M. J., P. Whitworth, L. Tafra, and K. M. McMasters. "The Details of Successful Sentinel Lymph Node Staging for Breast Cancer." *Am J Surg* 180, no. 4 (2000): 257–61.

McMasters, K.M., S. L. Wong, et al. "Defining the Optimal Surgeon Experience for Breast Cancer Sentinel Lymph Node Biopsy: A Model for Implementation of New Surgical Techniques." *Ann Surg* 234, no. 3 (2001): 292–300.

Surgical Clinics of North America: Breast Cancer Management. W. B. Saunders Co., Ismail Jatoi, ed. "Management of the Axilla in Primary Breast Cancer." 79, no. 5 (October 1999): 1061–73.

Chapter 51

A Guide to Your Pathology Report

Wait for the Whole Picture

Waiting is so hard! But just one test can lead to several different reports. Some tests take longer than others. Not all tests are done by the same lab. Most information comes within one to two weeks after surgery, and you will usually have all the results within a few weeks. Your doctor can let you know when the results come in. If you don't hear from your doctor, give her or him a call.

Get All the Information You Need

Be sure that you have all the test information you need before you make a final decision about your treatment. Also, don't focus too much on any one piece of information by itself. Try to look at the whole picture as you think about your options.

Different labs and hospitals may use different words to describe the same thing. If there are words in your pathology report that are not explained in this chapter, don't be afraid to ask your doctor what they mean.

Breast Cancer Stage

The pathology report will help your doctor decide the stage of your breast cancer. It could be:

From "A Guide to Your Pathology Report," © 2003 breastcancer.org. Reprinted with permission from the nonprofit organization breastcancer.org, dedicated to providing the most reliable, complete, and up-to-date information about breast cancer.

- Stage 0
- Stage I (1)
- Stage II (2)
- Stage IIIA (3A)
- Stage IIIB (3B) or
- Stage IV (4)

Staging is based on the size of the tumor, whether lymph nodes are involved, and whether the cancer has spread beyond the breast. Your doctors use all parts of the pathology report as well as the breast cancer stage to shape your treatment plan.

How to Start

First, check the top of the report for your name, the date you had your operation, and the type of operation you had. Make sure they are right for you.

Parts of Your Report

- **Specimen.** This section describes where the tissue samples came from. Tissue samples could be taken from the breast, from the lymph nodes under your arm (axilla), or both.

- **Clinical history.** This is a short description of you and how the breast abnormality was found. It also describes the kind of surgery that was done.

- **Clinical diagnosis.** This is the diagnosis the doctors were expecting before your tissue sample was tested.

- **Gross description.** This section describes the tissue sample or samples. It talks about the size, weight, and color of each sample.

- **Microscopic description.** This section describes the way the cancer cells look under the microscope.

- **Special tests or markers.** This section reports the results of tests for proteins, genes, and how fast the cells are growing.

- **Summary or final diagnosis.** This section is the short description of all the important findings in each tissue sample.

The Breast Cancer

Is the tumor a cancer?

A tumor is an overgrowth of cells. It can be made of normal cells or cancer cells. Cancer cells are cells that grow in an uncontrolled way. They may stay in the place where they started to grow. Or they may grow into the normal tissue around them. The pathology report will tell you what kind of cells are in the tumor.

Is the breast cancer invasive?

The single most important fact about any breast cancer is whether it has grown beyond the milk ducts or lobules of the breast where it first started. Noninvasive cancers stay within the milk ducts or milk lobules in the breast. They do not grow into or invade normal tissues within or beyond the breast. These are sometimes called in situ or pre-cancers. If the cancer has grown beyond where it started, it is called invasive. Most cancers are invasive. Sometimes cancer cells can also spread to other parts of the body through the blood or lymph system.

You may see these descriptions of cancer in your report:

- **DCIS (Ductal Carcinoma In Situ).** This is a cancer that is not invasive. It stays inside the milk ducts.

- **LCIS (Lobular Carcinoma In Situ).** This is a tumor that is an overgrowth of cells that stay inside the milk-making part of the breast (called lobules). LCIS is not a true cancer. It is a warning sign for an increased risk of having an invasive cancer in the future, in either breast.

- **IDC (Invasive Ductal Carcinoma).** This is a cancer that begins in the milk duct but grows into the surrounding normal tissue inside the breast. This is the most common kind of breast cancer.

- **ILC (Invasive Lobular Carcinoma).** This is a cancer that starts inside the milk-making glands (called lobules), but grows into the surrounding normal tissue inside the breast.

How different are the cancer cells from normal cells?

Experts call this "grade." They compare cancer cells to normal breast cells. Based on these comparisons, they give a "grade" to the cancer.

There are three cancer grades:

- **Grade 1 (Low Grade or Well Differentiated):** Grade 1 cancer cells still look a lot like normal cells. They are usually slow growing.

- **Grade 2 (Intermediate/Moderate Grade or Moderately Differentiated):** Grade 2 cancer cells do not look like normal cells. They are growing somewhat faster than normal cells.

- **Grade 3 (High Grade or Poorly Differentiated):** Grade 3 cancer cells do not look at all like normal cells. They are fast growing.

How big is the cancer?

Doctors measure cancers in centimeters (cm). The size of the cancer helps to determine its stage.

Size doesn't tell the whole story. Lymph node status is also important. A small cancer can be very fast growing. A larger cancer can be a "gentle giant."

Has the whole cancer been removed?

When cancer cells are removed from the breast, the surgeon tries to take out the whole cancer with an extra area or "margin" of normal tissue around it. This is to be sure that all of the cancer is removed.

The tissue around the very edge of what was removed is called the margin of resection. It is looked at very carefully to see if it is clear of cancer cells.

The pathologist also measures the distance between the cancer cells and the outer edge of the tissue.

Note: What is called "negative" (or "clean") margins can be different from hospital to hospital. In some places, doctors want at least two millimeters (mm) of normal tissue beyond the edge of the cancer. In other places, just one healthy cell is called a negative margin.

Margins around a cancer are described in three ways:

- **Negative:** No cancer cells can be seen at the outer edge. Usually, no more surgery is needed.

- **Positive:** Cancer cells come right out to the edge of the tissue. More surgery may be needed.

- **Close:** Cancer cells are close to the edge of the tissue, but not right at the edge. More surgery may be needed.

Are there cancer cells in your lymph or blood vessels?

The breast has a network of blood vessels and lymph channels that connect breast tissue to other parts of the body. These are the "highways" that bring in nourishment and remove waste products.

There is an increased risk of cancer coming back when cancer cells are found in the fluid channels of the breast. In these cases, your doctor may recommend treatment to your whole body, not just the breast area.

This test result will look like this:

Lymphatic/vascular invasion:

Present (yes, it has been found) or
Absent (no, invasion not found).

How fast are the cancer cells growing?

There are two tests that may be used to see how fast the cancer is growing: S-phase fraction test and Ki-67 test. Both tests measure if the cells are growing at a normal rate or faster than normal.

Even in very experienced labs, these tests are hard to do reliably. That's why many doctors depend on other information to make the best treatment decisions.

Do the cancer cells have hormone receptors?

Hormone receptors are like ears on breast cells that listen to signals from hormones. These signals "turn on" growth in breast cells that have receptors.

A cancer is called "ER-positive" if it has receptors for the hormone estrogen. It is called "PR-positive" if it has receptors for the hormone progesterone. Breast cells that do not have receptors are "negative" for these hormones.

Breast cancers that are either ER-positive or PR-positive or both tend to respond well to hormone therapy. These cancers can be treated with medicine that reduces the estrogen in your body. They can also be treated with medicine that keeps estrogen away from the receptors.

If the cancer has no hormone receptors, there are still very effective treatments available.

You will see the results of your hormone receptor test written in one of these three ways:

1. The number of cells that have receptors out of one hundred cells tested. You will see a number between 0% (no receptors) and 100% (all have receptors).

2. A number between 0 and 3. You will see the number

    *   0 (no receptors),

    *   1+ (a small number),

    *   2+ (a medium number), or

    *   3+ (a large number of receptors).

3. The word "positive" or "negative."

Note: If your report just says "negative," ask your doctor or lab to give you a number. This is important because sometimes a low number may be called "negative." But even cancers with low numbers of receptors may respond to hormone therapy.

Does the cancer have genes that are not normal?

HER-2 (also called HER-2/neu) is a gene that helps control how cells grow, divide, and repair themselves. About one out of four breast cancers has too many copies of the HER-2 gene. The HER-2 gene directs the production of special proteins, called HER-2 receptors, in cancer cells.

Cancers with too many copies of the HER-2 gene or too many HER-2 receptors tend to grow fast. They are also associated with an increased risk of spread. But they do respond very well to treatment that works against HER-2. This treatment is called anti-HER-2 antibody therapy.

There are two tests for HER-2:

1. IHC test (IHC stands for ImmunoHistoChemistry)

    *   The IHC test shows if there is too much HER-2 receptor protein in the cancer cells.

    *   The results of the IHC test can be 0 (negative), 1+ (negative), 2+ (borderline), or 3+ (positive).

2. FISH test (FISH stands for Fluorescence In Situ Hybridization)

    *   The FISH test shows if there are too many copies of the HER-2 gene in the cancer cells.

- The results of the FISH test can be "positive" (extra copies) or "negative" (normal number of copies).

Find out which test for HER-2 you had. This is important. Only cancers that test IHC "3+" or FISH "positive" will respond well to therapy that works against HER-2. An IHC 2+ test result is called borderline. If you have a 2+ result, you can and should ask to have the tissue tested with the FISH test.

The Lymph Nodes

Are there breast cancer cells in your lymph nodes?

Having cancer cells in the lymph nodes under your arm is associated with an increased risk of the cancer spreading.

Lymph nodes are filters along the lymph fluid channels. Lymph fluid leaves the breast and goes back into the bloodstream. The lymph nodes try to catch and trap cancer cells before they reach other parts of the body.

When lymph nodes are free or "clear" of cancer, the test results are called "negative." If lymph nodes have some cancer cells in them, they are called "positive."

How many lymph nodes are involved?

The more lymph nodes have cancer cells in them, the more serious the cancer might be. For this reason, doctors use the number of involved lymph nodes to help make treatment decisions. Doctors also look at the amount of cancer in the lymph nodes.

You may see these words describing how much cancer is in each lymph node:

- **Microscopic:** Only a few cancer cells are in the node. A microscope is needed to find them.

- **Gross:** There is a lot of cancer in the node. You can see or feel the cancer without a microscope.

- **Extracapsular extension:** Cancer has spread outside the wall of the node.

Key Questions

Here are important questions to be sure you understand, with your doctor's help:

1. Is this breast cancer invasive or noninvasive?

2. Are any lymph nodes involved with cancer? If so, how many?

3. What did the hormone receptor test show? Can you take a medicine that lowers or blocks your estrogen?

4. Were the margins negative, close, or positive?

5. Was the HER-2 test normal or abnormal?

6. Is this a slow-growing or a fast-growing breast cancer?

7. What other lab tests were done on the tumor tissue?

8. What did these tests show?

9. Is any further surgery recommended based on these results?

10. What types of treatment are most likely to work for this specific cancer?

Chapter 52

Breast Cancer Treatment

There are different types of treatment available for patients with breast cancer. Some treatments are standard (the currently used treatment) and some are being tested in clinical trials. Before starting treatment, patients may want to think about taking part in a clinical trial. A treatment clinical trial is a research study meant to help improve current treatments or obtain information on new treatments for patients with cancer. When clinical trials show that a new treatment is better than the "standard" treatment, the new treatment may become the standard treatment.

Clinical trials are taking place in many parts of the country. Information is available from the National Cancer Institute (NCI) website at www.cancer.gov. Choosing the most appropriate cancer treatment is a decision that ideally involves the patient, family, and health care team.

Standard Treatment for Breast Cancer

Four types of standard treatment are used: surgery, radiation therapy, chemotherapy, and hormone therapy.

Surgery

Most patients with breast cancer have surgery to remove the cancer from the breast. Some of the lymph nodes under the arm are usually

PDQ® Cancer Information Summary. National Cancer Institute, Bethesda, MD. Breast Cancer (PDQ®): Treatment - Patient. Updated October 2003. Available at http://cancer.gov. Accessed April 2004.

taken out and looked at under a microscope to see if they contain cancer cells.

Breast-conserving surgery, an operation to remove the cancer but not the breast itself, includes the following:

- **Lumpectomy:** A surgical procedure to remove a tumor (lump) and a small amount of normal tissue around it.

- **Partial mastectomy:** A surgical procedure to remove the part of the breast that contains cancer and some normal tissue around it. This procedure is also called a segmental mastectomy.

Patients who are treated with breast-conserving surgery may also have some of the lymph nodes under the arm removed for biopsy. This procedure is called lymph node dissection. It may be done at the same time as the breast-conserving surgery or after. Lymph node dissection is done through a separate incision.

Other types of surgery include the following:

- **Total mastectomy:** A surgical procedure to remove the whole breast that contains cancer. This procedure is also called a simple mastectomy. Some of the lymph nodes under the arm may be removed for biopsy at the same time as the breast surgery or after. This is done through a separate incision.

- **Modified radical mastectomy:** A surgical procedure to remove the whole breast that contains cancer, many of the lymph nodes under the arm, the lining over the chest muscles, and sometimes part of the chest wall muscles.

- **Radical mastectomy:** A surgical procedure to remove the breast that contains cancer, chest wall muscles under the breast, and all of the lymph nodes under the arm. This procedure is sometimes called a Halsted radical mastectomy.

Even if the doctor removes all of the cancer that can be seen at the time of surgery, the patient may be given radiation therapy, chemotherapy, or hormone therapy after surgery to try to kill any cancer cells that may be left. Treatment given after surgery to increase the chances of a cure is called adjuvant therapy.

If a patient is going to have a mastectomy, breast reconstruction (surgery to rebuild a breast's shape after a mastectomy) may be considered. Breast reconstruction may be done at the time of the mastectomy or at a future time. The reconstructed breast may be made with the patient's own (nonbreast) tissue or by using implants filled with saline or silicone gel. The Food and Drug Administration (FDA) has decided that breast implants filled with silicone gel may be used only in clinical trials. Before the decision to get an implant is made, patients can call the FDA's Center for Devices and Radiologic Health at 1-888-INFO-FDA (1-888-463-6332) for more information.

Radiation Therapy

Radiation therapy is a cancer treatment that uses high-energy x-rays or other types of radiation to kill cancer cells. There are two types of radiation therapy. External radiation therapy uses a machine outside the body to send radiation toward the cancer. Internal radiation therapy uses a radioactive substance sealed in needles, seeds, wires, or catheters that are placed directly into or near the cancer. The way the radiation therapy is given depends on the type and stage of the cancer being treated.

Chemotherapy

Chemotherapy is a cancer treatment that uses drugs to stop the growth of cancer cells, either by killing the cells or by stopping the cells from dividing. When chemotherapy is taken by mouth or injected into a vein or muscle, the drugs enter the bloodstream and can reach cancer cells throughout the body (systemic chemotherapy). When chemotherapy is placed directly in the spinal column, a body cavity such as the abdomen, or an organ, the drugs mainly affect cancer cells in those areas. The way the chemotherapy is given depends on the type and stage of the cancer being treated.

Hormone Therapy

Hormone therapy is a cancer treatment that removes hormones or blocks their action and stops cancer cells from growing. Hormones are substances produced by glands in the body and circulated in the bloodstream. The presence of some hormones can cause certain cancers to grow. If tests show that the cancer cells have places where hormones can attach (receptors), drugs, surgery, or radiation therapy are used to reduce the production of hormones or block them from working.

Hormone therapy with tamoxifen is often given to patients with early stages of breast cancer and those with metastatic breast cancer (cancer that has spread to other parts of the body). Hormone therapy with tamoxifen or estrogens can act on cells all over the body and may increase the chance of developing endometrial cancer. Women taking tamoxifen should have a pelvic examination every year to look for any signs of cancer. Any vaginal bleeding, other than menstrual bleeding, should be reported to a doctor as soon as possible.

Clinical Trials

Other types of treatment are being tested in clinical trials. These include the following:

Sentinel Lymph Node Biopsy Followed by Surgery

Sentinel lymph node biopsy is the removal of the sentinel lymph node (the first lymph node the cancer is likely to spread to from the tumor) during surgery. A radioactive substance or blue dye is injected near the tumor. The substance or dye flows through the lymph ducts to the lymph nodes. The first lymph node to receive the substance or dye is removed for biopsy. A pathologist views the tissue under a microscope to look for cancer cells. If cancer cells are not found, it may not be necessary to remove more lymph nodes. After the sentinel lymph node biopsy, the surgeon removes the tumor (breast-conserving surgery or mastectomy).

High-Dose Chemotherapy with Bone Marrow or Peripheral Blood Stem Cell Transplantation

This is a method of giving very high doses of chemotherapy and replacing blood-forming cells destroyed by the cancer treatment. Stem cells (immature blood cells) are removed from the bone marrow or blood of the patient or a donor and are frozen for storage. After the chemotherapy is completed, the stored stem cells are thawed and given back to the patient through an infusion. Over a short time, these reinfused stem cells grow into (and restore) the body's blood cells.

Studies have shown that high-dose chemotherapy followed by bone marrow transplantation or peripheral blood stem cell transplantation does not work better than standard chemotherapy in the treatment of breast cancer. Doctors have decided that, for now, high-dose chemotherapy should only be tested in clinical trials. Before taking part in such a trial, women should talk with their doctors about the serious side effects, including death, that may be caused by high-dose chemotherapy.

Treatment Options by Stage

Ductal Carcinoma In Situ (DCIS)

Treatment of ductal carcinoma in situ (DCIS) may include the following:

- Breast-conserving surgery with or without radiation therapy or hormone therapy.
- Total mastectomy with or without hormone therapy.
- Clinical trials testing breast-conserving surgery and hormone therapy with or without radiation.

Lobular Carcinoma In Situ (LCIS)

Treatment of lobular carcinoma in situ (LCIS) may include the following:

- Biopsy to diagnose the LCIS followed by regular examinations and regular mammograms to find any changes as early as possible. This is referred to as observation.
- Tamoxifen to reduce the risk of developing breast cancer.
- Bilateral prophylactic mastectomy. This treatment choice is sometimes used in women who have a high risk of getting breast cancer. Most surgeons believe that this is a more aggressive treatment than is needed.
- Clinical trials testing cancer prevention drugs.

Stage I, Stage II, and Stage IIIA Breast Cancer

Treatment of stage I, stage II, and stage IIIA breast cancer that is confined to the breast and lymph nodes under the arm may include the following:

- Breast-conserving surgery to remove only the cancer and some surrounding breast tissue, followed by lymph node dissection and radiation therapy.
- Modified radical mastectomy with or without breast reconstruction surgery.
- A clinical trial evaluating sentinel lymph node biopsy followed by surgery.

341

Adjuvant therapy (treatment given after surgery to increase the chances of a cure) may include the following:

- Radiation therapy to the lymph nodes near the breast and to the chest wall after a modified radical mastectomy.

- Systemic chemotherapy with or without hormone therapy.

- Hormone therapy.

Stage IIIB, Stage IIIC, Stage IV, and Metastatic Breast Cancer

Treatment of stage IIIB and advanced stage IIIC breast cancer (early stage IIIC breast cancer is treated as Stage I, stage II, and stage IIIA breast cancer) may include the following:

- Systemic chemotherapy.

- Systemic chemotherapy followed by surgery (breast-conserving surgery or total mastectomy), with lymph node dissection followed by radiation therapy. Additional systemic therapy (chemotherapy, hormone therapy, or both) may be given.

- Clinical trials testing new anticancer drugs, new drug combinations, and new ways of giving treatment.

Treatment of stage IV or metastatic breast cancer may include the following:

- Hormone therapy and/or chemotherapy with or without trastuzumab (Herceptin).

- Radiation therapy and/or surgery for relief of pain and other symptoms.

- Clinical trials testing new chemotherapy or hormone therapy. Clinical trials are also studying new combinations of trastuzumab (Herceptin) with anticancer drugs.

- Clinical trials testing other approaches, including high-dose chemotherapy with bone marrow transplantation or peripheral blood stem cell transplantation.

Treatment Options for Inflammatory Breast Cancer

Treatment of inflammatory breast cancer may include the following:

- Systemic chemotherapy.

- Systemic chemotherapy followed by surgery (breast-conserving surgery or total mastectomy), with lymph node dissection followed by radiation therapy. Additional systemic therapy (chemotherapy, hormone therapy, or both) may be given.

- Clinical trials testing new anticancer drugs, new drug combinations, and new ways of giving treatment.

Treatment Options for Recurrent Breast Cancer

Treatment of recurrent breast cancer (cancer that has come back after treatment) in the breast or chest wall may include the following:

- Surgery (radical or modified radical mastectomy), radiation therapy, or both.

- Systemic chemotherapy or hormone therapy.

This chapter refers to specific treatments under study in clinical trials, but it may not mention every new treatment being studied. Information about ongoing clinical trials is available from the NCI website at www.cancer.gov.

Chapter 53

Mastectomy vs. Lumpectomy: Issues to Consider

Today, many women with breast cancer are given the opportunity to choose between total removal of a breast (mastectomy) and breast-conserving surgery (lumpectomy) followed by radiation.

For women with only one site of cancer in their breast, and a tumor under four centimeters that was removed with clear margins (no cancer cells in the tissue surrounding the tumor), lumpectomy followed by radiation is likely to be equally as effective as mastectomy.

Factors in the Decision

Although most women who have a choice prefer the less invasive lumpectomy, what you choose will depend on many factors, including:

- Whether or not radiation therapy is as good an option for you relative to mastectomy.

- Whether you are interested in reconstructive surgery.

- How important keeping your breast is to you.

- How much you think that removing the entire breast would help you worry less about the possibility of the breast cancer coming back.

The main advantage of lumpectomy is that it can preserve much of the appearance and sensation of your breast. It is a less invasive surgery, so your recovery time is shorter and easier than with mastectomy.

Drawbacks of Lumpectomy

Lumpectomy followed by radiation has several drawbacks:

- After surgery, you are likely to have five to seven weeks of radiation therapy, five days per week, to make sure the cancer is gone.

- You are at a somewhat higher risk of developing a local recurrence of the cancer than are women who undergo mastectomy. However, recurrence can be treated successfully with mastectomy.

- Your breast cannot safely tolerate additional radiation if cancer occurs in the same breast after lumpectomy. This is true for either a recurrence of the same cancer, or for a new cancer. If you have a second cancer in the same breast, your doctor will usually recommend that your breast be removed.

For some women, removing the entire breast provides greater peace of mind ("just get the whole thing out of there!"). Radiation therapy may still be needed, depending on the results of the pathology.

Drawbacks of Mastectomy

Mastectomy has three main drawbacks:

- The surgery is longer and more extensive, with more postsurgery side effects and a longer recuperation time.

- The surgery means a permanent loss of your breast.

- If, like most women, you pursue reconstruction after mastectomy, you are likely to face additional surgeries in a multistep cosmetic procedure.

Making Your Own Decision

Your breasts may be such an important part of your identity—your sense of who you are—that you'll go to great lengths to preserve them. That's a completely acceptable approach to take, no matter what your age or figure, as long as it doesn't endanger your overall health and chances for a full recovery.

Lumpectomy Plus Radiation as Effective as Mastectomy

Long-term studies have found that lumpectomy plus radiation is as effective as mastectomy for small and early-stage breast cancer.

Background and Importance of the Studies

When you get hit with a diagnosis of breast cancer, your first instinct may be: "The more treatment, the better." For this reason, when it comes to surgery, you may think that mastectomy is better than lumpectomy plus radiation. But when you and your doctor evaluate the options, you may find out—depending on the type of cancer you have—that more radical treatment may not offer any extra advantage.

Years ago, before breast preservation therapy (lumpectomy plus radiation) was an option, researchers began to look at whether more radical mastectomy was any better than less radical mastectomy. In September 2002, breastcancer.org reported on the conclusion of that twenty-five-year study. The results showed no difference in disease-free survival between women who had radical mastectomy (removing the entire breast, underlying chest muscles, and the lymph nodes) and those who had total mastectomy (removing the whole breast) plus radiation.

Those long-term results were not surprising. Early results of the study had been reported after ten and fifteen years, giving doctors enough evidence to gradually stop using radical mastectomy. The final results confirmed that even twenty-five years after surgery, radical mastectomy has no extra benefit over total mastectomy.

Once lumpectomy became available, researchers carried out studies to compare its effectiveness to mastectomy. As a result of these studies, in the past twenty years many women with small cancers (less than four centimeters) that are at an early stage (Stage I or II) have been able to choose lumpectomy plus radiation instead of mastectomy.

Breast preservation therapy got its biggest boost after 1990, when the National Cancer Institute recommended this approach over mastectomy for women with early-stage disease. The NCI recommendation was based on the results of a number of major studies, including the early reports from the two studies reviewed here. The first study compared total mastectomy to lumpectomy with or without radiation. The second study compared radical mastectomy to lumpectomy plus radiation.

Data from these studies after five and ten years showed that women had the same survival rates whether they had mastectomy or breast-conserving surgery plus radiation. Now these two large studies have ended, and the final twenty-year results confirm the earlier findings. They

347

show that lumpectomy plus radiation is as effective as mastectomy for women with early-stage cancers that are under four centimeters.

Total Mastectomy vs. Lumpectomy with or without Radiation: Twenty-Year Results

Background

This study was started in 1976 by researchers from the U.S. National Surgical Adjuvant Breast and Bowel Project and the University of Pittsburgh. They wanted to find out whether lumpectomy with or without radiation was as effective as total mastectomy for treating invasive breast cancer.

Study Design

The researchers studied more than two thousand women with invasive Stage I or Stage II breast cancer. All of the women had one cancer that was four centimeters or less in diameter.

The women all had lymph node dissection:

- 62 percent had negative lymph nodes (no cancer cells found in the nodes),
- 26 percent had one or more positive lymph nodes (cancer cells found in the nodes), and
- 12 percent had four or more positive nodes.

The women were randomly assigned to one of three treatment groups:

- total mastectomy,
- lumpectomy, or
- lumpectomy plus radiation.

The women in all three groups were similar in terms of their age and diagnosis, tumor size, hormone receptor status, and lymph node involvement.

Results

The researchers gathered complete follow-up data for 1,851 of the women who first joined the study. They looked at the information in several different ways.

Looking at the two groups of women who had lumpectomies, researchers found that adding radiation significantly reduced a woman's chances of having a recurrence (the cancer coming back) in the same breast. Twenty years after surgery, the percentage of women who had a recurrence in the same breast was:

- 14.3 percent for women who had lumpectomy and radiation, and

- 39.2 percent for women who had lumpectomy alone.

But researchers also found that women in both lumpectomy groups fared equally well in terms of disease-free survival. This means that twenty years after surgery, similar numbers of women in both groups were alive and did not have any more breast cancer. The percentages of disease-free survival were:

- 36 percent for women treated with lumpectomy plus radiation, and

- 35 percent for women treated with lumpectomy alone.

Finally, researchers found no significant differences in overall survival among all three treatment groups. At twenty years after surgery, the overall survival rates were:

- 47 percent for women treated with total mastectomy,

- 46 percent for women treated with lumpectomy and radiation, and

- 46 percent for women treated with lumpectomy alone.

Conclusion

In terms of disease-free survival, this study found that total mastectomy, lumpectomy plus radiation, and lumpectomy alone (all with lymph node dissection) were equally effective.

But there was a significant difference in recurrence rates between the women treated with lumpectomy plus radiation and the women who had lumpectomy alone.

This is important because even if recurrence does not affect long-term survival, it often requires more treatment, including more disfiguring surgery. In addition, living with around a 40 percent risk of recurrence can seriously affect your peace of mind. Most women want to do what they can to get their risk as low as possible.

Radical Mastectomy vs. Lumpectomy and Radiation for Small Cancers

Background

This study was started in 1973 by researchers at the Milan Cancer Institute in Milan, Italy. They wanted to find out whether lumpectomy plus radiation was as effective as radical mastectomy in women with a small breast cancer (no more than two centimeters).

Study Design

Between 1973 and 1980, researchers assigned 701 women to one of two treatment groups:

- radical mastectomy, or
- lumpectomy plus radiation.

All of the women had lymph node dissection. After 1976, women in both groups who had positive lymph nodes (cancer cells found in the nodes) also received chemotherapy with cyclophosphamide, methotrexate, and fluorouracil (CMF).

Results

After twenty years of follow-up, researchers found that women who had radical mastectomies were significantly less likely than those treated with lumpectomy and radiation to have a recurrence (cancer coming back) in the same breast area. The percentages of recurrence in the same breast area were:

- 2.3 percent of the women who had radical mastectomy, and
- 8.8 percent of the women who had lumpectomy plus radiation.

But researchers found no significant differences in risk between the two groups in terms of:

- developing a new cancer in the same breast area,
- getting cancer in the other breast, or
- the cancer spreading to other parts of the body.

And the two groups showed no significant difference in rates of death from breast cancer. After twenty years of follow-up, the percentages of women who died of breast cancer were:

- 24.3 percent of the women who had radical mastectomy, and

- 26.1 percent of the women who had lumpectomy plus radiation.

Overall survival rates were:

- 41.2 percent of the women who had radical mastectomy, and

- 41.7 percent of the women who had lumpectomy plus radiation.

Conclusion

The long-term survival of women with small breast cancers who had mastectomy and women who had lumpectomy plus radiation was the same. This was true even though the women who had lumpectomy plus radiation had a higher risk of local recurrence (the cancer coming back in the same breast).

It might seem strange that survival could be the same, even though one group had more local recurrences. The explanation for this is that the few local recurrences in the lumpectomy group were treatable. In general, local recurrences have less impact on overall survival than recurrences beyond the breast.

Take-Home Message from the Two Studies

The message from both of these studies is that for early-stage breast cancer, lumpectomy plus radiation is just as effective as mastectomy. One study defined early-stage breast cancer as a tumor that was four centimeters or less. In the other study the tumor could be no more than two centimeters.

In terms of long-term survival, one of the studies showed that lumpectomy alone is also as effective as mastectomy (both with lymph node removal). But without radiation, there is a 40 percent greater chance that the cancer will come back in the same breast. This means that if you don't get radiation after lumpectomy, you'll need more follow-up, which means more tests and possibly more surgery and other treatments in the future.

Unfortunately, many women are still not benefiting from these two studies and others with similar findings. Surveys show that in the United States, only about 30 percent of women with cancers that can be treated with lumpectomy plus radiation hear about this option from their doctors.

Yet it's been over a decade since the National Cancer Institute issued its clear recommendation for breast-conserving surgery. This is an example of an important treatment option that is not being offered by all doctors. And it's an example of why getting accurate information about all your options is so important.

Still, it's also important to remember that no single treatment choice is right for everyone. Women with more than one cancer in the breast, or a cancer that's larger than four centimeters, or with skin involvement may be best treated with mastectomy.

Also don't forget that since the start of these studies, many more treatment options have become available. They include different types of chemotherapy, anti-estrogen (hormonal) therapy, and immune therapy. The long-term survival rates reported in these studies were achieved without most of these newer types of treatment. Today's many treatment options are likely to result in much improved survival.

Chapter 54

Chemotherapy for Breast Cancer

What Breast Cancer Patients Need to Know about Chemotherapy

What Is Chemotherapy?

In cancer treatment, chemotherapy refers to the use of drugs whose main effect is either to kill or slow the growth of rapidly multiplying cells.

Chemotherapy often includes a combination of drugs, since this is more effective than a single drug given alone. There are many drug combinations used to treat breast cancer. Ask your doctor for specific information and side effects you can expect from your chemotherapy medications.

How Is Chemotherapy Given?

Chemotherapy drugs are given intravenously (directly into the vein) or orally (by mouth). How it is received depends on the drugs being used; most are effective by only one route. Once the drugs enter

"What Breast Cancer Patients Need to Know about Chemotherapy" is from "Chemotherapy for Breast Cancer," © 2003 The Cleveland Clinic Foundation, 9500 Euclid Avenue, Cleveland, OH 44195, 800-223-2273 ext. 48950, www.clevelandclinic.org. Additional information is available from the Cleveland Clinic Health Information Center, 216-444-3771, or www.clevelandclinic.org/health. "A Practical Guide for Chemotherapy Patients" is excerpted from "Chemotherapy and You: A Guide to Self-Help during Cancer Treatment," National Institutes of Health, National Cancer Institute, NIH Pub. No. 99-1136, June 1999. Revised by David A. Cooke, M.D., on May 17, 2004.

the bloodstream, they reach all parts of the body to reach cancer cells that may have spread beyond the breast—therefore chemotherapy is considered a systemic form of breast cancer treatment.

Chemotherapy is given in cycles of treatment followed by a recovery period. When given after surgery, the entire chemotherapy treatment generally lasts three to six months, depending on the type of drugs given. When chemotherapy is being used to treat breast cancer that has spread to other organs, chemotherapy may be given for a longer period of time.

When Is Chemotherapy Given?

When breast cancer is localized only to the breast or to the lymph nodes, chemotherapy may be given after a lumpectomy or mastectomy. This is known as adjuvant treatment and may help reduce the chance of breast cancer recurrence. Chemotherapy is sometimes given before surgery (called neoadjuvant treatment) in order to shrink the tumor so it can be removed more easily or so that a lumpectomy can be performed instead of a mastectomy. Chemotherapy may also be given as the main treatment for women whose cancer has spread to other parts of the body outside of the breast and lymph nodes. This spread is known as metastatic breast cancer and occurs in a small number of women at the time of diagnosis or when the cancer recurs some time after initial treatment for localized breast cancer.

What Are the Potential Side Effects of Chemotherapy Drugs?

There are several dozen varieties of chemotherapy medications, and each one has different side effects. Some drugs have almost no side effects, while others can make a person very ill. Which drugs are used depends on the kind of cancer is being treated. Some medications are very effective against some types of cancers, but are useless against other kinds of cancer.

The side effects you may experience will depend mostly on which drugs are being used. The dose of the medications and the length of time you will receive them are also important factors. It is very hard to generalize about side effects of chemotherapy medications, since they vary so much from drug to drug. However, the following temporary side effects are the most common:

- Nausea and vomiting
- Loss of appetite

- Hair loss

- Mouth sores

- Changes in menstrual cycle

- Higher risk of infection (due to decreased white blood cells)

- Bruising or bleeding

- Fatigue

- Premature menopause (not having any more menstrual periods) and infertility (not being able to become pregnant) are potential permanent complications of chemotherapy.

Please contact your health care provider about specific side effects you can expect to experience from your chemotherapy medications. Also discuss troubling or unmanageable side effects with your provider.

Can I Still Work While Receiving Chemotherapy Treatments?

Yes. Most people are able to continue working while they are being treated with chemotherapy. It may be possible to schedule your treatments later in the day or right before the weekend so they don't interfere as much with your work schedule. You may have to adjust your work schedule while receiving chemotherapy, especially if you have side effects.

How Will I Know If the Chemotherapy Treatments Are Working?

Although some people may think that if they do not experience side effects, their chemotherapy treatment is not working, this is just a myth.

If you are receiving adjuvant chemotherapy (after surgery that removed all of the known cancer), it is not possible for your doctor to directly determine whether the treatment is working because there are no tumors left to assess. However, adjuvant chemotherapy treatments have been proven helpful in studies in which some women were given chemotherapy while others were not.

After completing adjuvant therapy, your doctor will evaluate your progress through periodic physical examinations, routine mammography, and appropriate testing if a new problem develops. If you are receiving chemotherapy for metastatic disease, the effects will be monitored by blood tests, scans, or x-rays.

A Practical Guide for Chemotherapy Patients

How Does Chemotherapy Work?

Normal cells grow and die in a controlled way. When cancer occurs, cells in the body that are not normal keep dividing and forming more cells without control. Anticancer drugs destroy cancer cells by stopping them from growing or multiplying. Healthy cells can also be harmed, especially those that divide quickly. Harm to healthy cells is what causes side effects. These cells usually repair themselves after chemotherapy.

Because some drugs work better together than alone, two or more drugs are often given at the same time. This is called combination chemotherapy.

Other types of drugs may be used to treat your cancer. These may include certain drugs that can block the effect of your body's hormones. Or doctors may use biological therapy, which is treatment with substances that boost the body's own immune system against cancer. Your body usually makes these substances in small amounts to fight cancer and other diseases. These substances can be made in the laboratory and given to patients to destroy cancer cells or change the way the body reacts to a tumor. They may also help the body repair or make new cells destroyed by chemotherapy.

What Can Chemotherapy Do?

Depending on the type of cancer and how advanced it is, chemotherapy can be used for different goals:

• To cure the cancer. Cancer is considered cured when the patient remains free of evidence of cancer cells.

• To control the cancer. This is done by keeping the cancer from spreading, slowing the cancer's growth, and killing cancer cells that may have spread to other parts of the body from the original tumor.

• To relieve symptoms that the cancer may cause. Relieving symptoms such as pain can help patients live more comfortably.

Is Chemotherapy Used with Other Treatments?

Sometimes chemotherapy is the only treatment a patient receives. More often, however, chemotherapy is used in addition to surgery, radiation therapy, or biological therapy to:

- Shrink a tumor before surgery or radiation therapy. This is called neo-adjuvant therapy.

- Help destroy any cancer cells that may remain after surgery or radiation therapy. This is called adjuvant chemotherapy.

- Make radiation therapy and biological therapy work better.

- Help destroy cancer if it recurs or has spread to other parts of the body from the original tumor.

Which Drugs Are Given?

Some chemotherapy drugs are used for many different types of cancer, while others might be used for just one or two types of cancer. Your doctor recommends a treatment plan based on:

- What kind of cancer you have.
- Where in the body the cancer is found.
- The effect of cancer on your normal body functions.
- Your general health.

Questions to Ask Your Doctor

About Chemotherapy

- Why do I need chemotherapy?
- What are the benefits of chemotherapy?
- What are the risks of chemotherapy?
- Are there any other possible treatment methods for my type of cancer?
- What is the standard care for my type of cancer?
- Are there any clinical trials for my type of cancer?

About Your Treatment

- How many treatments will I be given?
- What drug or drugs will I be taking?
- How will the drugs be given?
- Where will I get my treatment?
- How long will each treatment last?

About Side Effects

- What are the possible side effects of the chemotherapy? When are side effects likely to occur?

- What side effects are more likely to be related to my type of cancer?

- Are there any side effects that I should report right away?

- What can I do to relieve the side effects?

About Contacting Medical Staff

- How do I contact a health professional after hours, and when should I call?

Hints for Talking with Your Doctor

These tips might help you keep track of the information you learn during visits with your doctor:

- Bring a friend or family member to sit with you while you talk with your doctor. This person can help you understand what your doctor says during your visit and help refresh your memory afterward.

- Ask your doctor for printed information that is available on your cancer and treatment.

- You, or the person who goes with you, may want to take notes during your appointment.

- Ask your doctor to slow down when you need more time to write.

- You may want to ask if you can use a tape recorder during your visit. Take notes from the tape after the visit is finished. That way, you can review your conversation later as many times as you wish.

Where Will I Get Chemotherapy?

Chemotherapy can be given in many different places: at home, a doctor's office, a clinic, a hospital's outpatient department, or as an "inpatient" in a hospital. The choice of where you get chemotherapy depends on which drug or drugs you are getting, your insurance, and sometimes your own and your doctor's wishes. Most patients receive their treatment as an "outpatient" and are not hospitalized. Sometimes, a patient starting chemotherapy may need to stay at the hospital for a short time so that the medicine's effects can be watched closely and any needed changes can be made.

How Often and for How Long Will I Get Chemotherapy?

How often and how long you get chemotherapy depends on:

- The kind of cancer you have.
- The goals of the treatment.
- The drugs that are used.
- How your body responds to them.

You may get treatment every day, every week, or every month. Chemotherapy is often given in cycles that include treatment periods alternated with rest periods. Rest periods give your body a chance to build healthy new cells and regain its strength. Ask your health care provider to tell you how long and how often you may expect to get treatment.

Sticking with your treatment schedule is very important for the drugs to work right. Schedules may need to be changed for holidays and other reasons. If you miss a treatment session or skip a dose of the drug, contact your doctor.

Sometimes your doctor may need to delay a treatment based on the results of certain blood tests. Your doctor will let you know what to do during this time and when to start your treatment again.

How Will I Feel During Chemotherapy?

Most people receiving chemotherapy find that they tire easily, but many feel well enough to continue to lead active lives. Each person and treatment is different, so it is not always possible to tell exactly how you will react. Your general state of health, the type and extent of cancer you have, and the kind of drugs you are receiving can all affect how well you feel.

You may want to have someone available to drive you to and from treatment if, for example, you are taking medicine for nausea or vomiting that could make you tired. You may also feel especially tired from the chemotherapy as early as one day after a treatment and for several days. It may help to schedule your treatment when you can take off the day of and the day after your treatment. If you have young children, you may want to schedule the treatment when you have someone to help at home the day of and at least the day after your treatment. Ask your doctor when your greatest fatigue or other side effects are likely to occur.

Most people can continue working while receiving chemotherapy. However, you may need to change your work schedule for a while if your chemotherapy makes you feel very tired or have other side effects. Talk with your employer about your needs and wishes. You may be able to agree on a part-time schedule, find an area for a short nap during the day, or perhaps you can do some of your work at home.

Under federal and state laws, some employers may be required to let you work a flexible schedule to meet your treatment needs. To find out about your on-the-job protections, check with a social worker, or your congressional or state representative.

Can I Take Other Medicines While I Am Getting Chemotherapy?

Some medicines may interfere or react with the effects of your chemotherapy. Give your doctor a list of all the medicines you take before you start treatment. Include:

- the name of each drug
- the dosage
- the reason you take it
- how often you take it

Remember to tell your doctor about all over-the-counter remedies, including vitamins, laxatives, medicines for allergies, indigestion, and colds, aspirin, ibuprofen, or other pain relievers, and any mineral or herbal supplements. Your doctor can tell you if you should stop taking any of these remedies before you start chemotherapy. After your treatments begin, be sure to check with your doctor before taking any new medicines or stopping the ones you are already taking.

Questions to Ask about Side Effects

- What are the short-term side effects that may occur?
- What are the long-term side effects that may occur?
- How serious are the side effects likely to be?
- How long will the side effects last?
- What can I do to relieve or lessen the side effects?

- When should I call the doctor or nurse about side effects?
- What can I do to feel better emotionally while trying to cope with the side effects?

What Causes Side Effects?

Because cancer cells may grow and divide more rapidly than normal cells, many anticancer drugs are made to kill growing cells. But certain normal, healthy cells also multiply quickly, and chemotherapy can affect these cells, too. This damage to normal cells causes side effects. The fast-growing, normal cells most likely to be affected are blood cells forming in the bone marrow and cells in the digestive tract (mouth, stomach, intestines, esophagus), reproductive system (sexual organs), and hair follicles. Some anticancer drugs may affect cells of vital organs, such as the heart, kidney, bladder, lungs, and nervous system.

You may have none of these side effects or just a few. The kinds of side effects you have and how severe they are depend on the type and dose of chemotherapy you get and how your body reacts. Before starting chemotherapy, your doctor will discuss the side effects that you are most likely to get with the drugs you will be receiving. Before starting the treatment, you will be asked to sign a consent form. You should be given all the facts about treatment, including the drugs you will be given and their side effects, before you sign the consent form.

How Long Do Side Effects Last?

Normal cells usually recover when chemotherapy is over, so most side effects gradually go away after treatment ends and the healthy cells have a chance to grow normally. The time it takes to get over side effects depends on many things, including your overall health and the kind of chemotherapy you have been taking.

Most people have no serious long-term problems from chemotherapy. However, on some occasions, chemotherapy can cause permanent changes or damage to the heart, lungs, nerves, kidneys, or reproductive or other organs. Certain types of chemotherapy may have delayed effects, such as a second cancer, that show up many years later. Ask your doctor about the chances of any serious, long-term effects that can result from the treatment you are receiving (but remember to balance your concerns with the immediate threat of your cancer).

Great progress has been made in preventing and treating some of chemotherapy's common as well as rare serious side effects. Many new drugs and treatment methods destroy cancer more effectively while doing less harm to the body's healthy cells.

The side effects of chemotherapy can be unpleasant, but they must be measured against the treatment's ability to destroy cancer. Medicines can help prevent some side effects such as nausea. Sometimes people receiving chemotherapy become discouraged about the length of time their treatment is taking or the side effects they are having. If that happens to you, talk to your doctor or nurse. He or she may be able to suggest ways to make side effects easier to deal with or reduce them.

Following you will find suggestions for dealing with some of the more common side effects of chemotherapy.

Fatigue

Fatigue, feeling tired and lacking energy, is the most common symptom reported by cancer patients. The exact cause is not always known. It can be due to your disease, chemotherapy, radiation, surgery, low blood counts, lack of sleep, pain, stress, or poor appetite, along with many other factors.

Fatigue from cancer feels different from fatigue of everyday life. Fatigue caused by chemotherapy can appear suddenly. Patients with cancer have described it as a total lack of energy and have used words such as *worn out, drained,* and *wiped out* to describe their fatigue. And rest does not always relieve it. Not everyone feels the same kind of fatigue. You may not feel tired while someone else does, or your fatigue may not last as long as someone else's does. It can last days, weeks, or months. Yet severe fatigue does go away gradually as the tumor responds to treatment.

How Can I Cope with Fatigue?

- Plan your day so that you have time to rest.

- Take short naps or breaks, rather than one long rest period.

- Save your energy for the most important things.

- Try easier or shorter versions of activities you enjoy.

- Take short walks or do light exercise if possible. You may find this helps with fatigue.

- Talk to your health care provider about ways to save your energy and treat your fatigue.

- Try activities such as meditation, prayer, yoga, guided imagery, visualization, and so on. You may find that these help with fatigue.

- Eat as well as you can and drink plenty of fluids. Eat small amounts at a time, if that is helpful.

- Join a support group. Sharing your feelings with others can ease the burden of fatigue. You can learn how others deal with their fatigue. Your health care provider can put you in touch with a support group in your area.

- Limit the amount of caffeine and alcohol you drink.

- Allow others to do some things for you that you usually do.

- Keep a diary of how you feel each day. This will help you plan your daily activities.

- Report any changes in energy level to your doctor or nurse.

Nausea and Vomiting

Many patients fear that they will have nausea and vomiting while receiving chemotherapy. Yet new drugs have made these side effects far less common and, when they do occur, much less severe. These powerful new antiemetic or antinausea drugs are very effective, and can prevent or lessen nausea and vomiting in most patients. Different drugs work for different people, and you may need more than one drug to get relief. Do not give up. Continue to work with your doctor and nurse to find the drug or drugs that work best for you. Also, be sure to tell your doctor or nurse if you are very nauseated or have vomited for more than a day, or if your vomiting is so bad that you cannot keep liquids down.

What Can I Do If I Have Nausea and Vomiting?

- Drink liquids at least an hour before or after mealtime, instead of with your meals. Drink frequently and drink small amounts.

- Eat and drink slowly.

- Eat small meals throughout the day, instead of one, two, or three large meals.

- Eat foods cold or at room temperature so you won't be bothered by strong smells.

- Chew your food well for easier digestion.

- If nausea is a problem in the morning, try eating dry foods like cereal, toast, or crackers before getting up. (Do not try this if you have mouth or throat sores or are troubled by a lack of saliva.)

363

- Drink cool, clear, unsweetened fruit juices, such as apple or grape juice or light-colored sodas such as ginger ale that have lost their fizz and do not have caffeine.

- Suck on mints, or tart candies. (Do not use tart candies if you have mouth or throat sores.)

- Prepare and freeze meals in advance for days when you do not feel like cooking.

- Wear loose-fitting clothes.

- Breathe deeply and slowly when you feel nauseated.

- Distract yourself by chatting with friends or family members, listening to music, or watching a movie or TV show.

- Use relaxation techniques.

- Try to avoid odors that bother you, such as cooking smells, smoke, or perfume.

- Avoid sweet, fried, or fatty foods.

- Rest but do not lie flat for at least two hours after you finish a meal.

- Avoid eating for at least a few hours before treatment if nausea usually occurs during chemotherapy.

- Eat a light meal before treatment.

Pain

Certain chemotherapy drugs can cause some side effects that are painful. These drugs can damage nerves, leading to burning, numbness, tingling, or shooting pain, most often in the fingers or toes. Some drugs can also cause mouth sores, headaches, muscle pains, and stomach pains.

Not everyone with cancer or who receives chemotherapy experiences pain from the disease or its treatment. Yet if you do, it can be relieved. The first step to take is to talk with your doctor, nurse, and pharmacist about your pain. They need to know as many details about your pain as possible. You may want to describe your pain to your family and friends. They can help you talk to your caregivers about your pain, especially if you are too tired or in too much pain to talk to them yourself.

You need to tell your doctor, nurse, and pharmacist and family or friends:

- Where you feel pain.

- What it feels like—sharp, dull, throbbing, steady.

- How strong the pain feels.

- How long it lasts.

- What eases the pain, what makes the pain worse.

- What medicines you are taking for the pain and how much relief you get from them.

Using a pain scale is helpful in describing how much pain you are feeling. Try to assign a number from 0 to 10 to your pain level. If you have no pain, use a 0. As the numbers get higher, they stand for pain that is getting worse. A 10 means the pain is as bad as it can be. You may wish to use your own pain scale using numbers from 0 to 5 or even 0 to 100. Be sure to let others know what pain scale you are using and use the same scale each time, for example, "My pain is 7 on a scale of 0 to 10."

The goal of pain control is to prevent pain that can be prevented, and treat the pain that can't. To do this:

- If you have persistent or chronic pain, take your pain medicine on a regular schedule (by the clock).

- Do not skip doses of your scheduled pain medicine. If you wait to take pain medicine until you feel pain, it is harder to control.

- Try using relaxation exercises at the same time you take medicine for the pain. This may help to lessen tension, reduce anxiety, and manage pain.

- Some people with chronic or persistent pain that is usually controlled by medicine can have breakthrough pain. This occurs when moderate to severe pain "breaks through" or is felt for a short time. If you experience this pain, use a short-acting medicine ordered by your doctor. Don't wait for the pain to get worse. If you do, it may be harder to control.

There are many different medicines and methods available to control cancer pain. You should expect your doctor to seek all the information and resources necessary to make you as comfortable as possible. If you are in pain and your doctor has no further suggestions, ask to see a pain specialist or have your doctor consult with a pain specialist. A pain specialist may be an oncologist, anesthesiologist, neurologist, neurosurgeon, other doctor, nurse, or pharmacist.

Hair Loss

Hair loss (alopecia) is a common side effect of chemotherapy, but not all drugs cause hair loss. Your doctor can tell you if hair loss might occur with the drug or drugs you are taking. When hair loss does occur, the hair may become thinner or fall out entirely. Hair loss can occur on all parts of the body, including the head, face, arms and legs, underarms, and pubic area. The hair usually grows back after the treatments are over. Some people even start to get their hair back while they are still having treatments. Sometimes, hair may grow back a different color or texture.

Hair loss does not always happen right away. It may begin several weeks after the first treatment or after a few treatments. Many people say their head becomes sensitive before losing hair. Hair may fall out gradually or in clumps. Any hair that is still growing may become dull and dry.

How Can I Care for My Scalp and Hair during Chemotherapy?

- Use a mild shampoo.

- Use a soft hair brush.

- Use low heat when drying your hair.

- Have your hair cut short. A shorter style will make your hair look thicker and fuller. It also will make hair loss easier to manage if it occurs.

- Use a sunscreen, sun block, hat, or scarf to protect your scalp from the sun if you lose hair on your head.

- Avoid brush rollers to set your hair.

- Avoid dying, perming, or relaxing your hair.

Some people who lose all or most of their hair choose to wear turbans, scarves, caps, wigs, or hairpieces. Others leave their head uncovered. Still others switch back and forth, depending on whether they are in public or at home with friends and family members. There are no "right" or "wrong" choices; do whatever feels comfortable for you.

If you choose to cover your head:

- Get your wig or hairpiece before you lose a lot of hair. That way, you can match your current hairstyle and color. You may be able to buy a wig or hairpiece at a specialty shop just for cancer patients. Someone may even come to your home to help you. You also can buy a wig or hairpiece through a catalog or by phone.

- You may also consider borrowing a wig or hairpiece, rather than buying one. Check with the nurse or social work department at your hospital about resources for free wigs in your community.

- Take your wig to your hairdresser or the shop where it was purchased for styling and cutting to frame your face.

- Some health insurance policies cover the cost of a hairpiece needed because of cancer treatment. It is also a tax-deductible expense. Be sure to check your policy and ask your doctor for a "prescription."

Losing hair from your head, face, or body can be hard to accept. Feeling angry or depressed is common and perfectly all right. At the same time, keep in mind that it is a temporary side effect. Talking about your feelings can help. If possible, share your thoughts with someone who has had a similar experience.

Anemia

Some kinds of chemotherapy can reduce the bone marrow's ability to make red blood cells, which carry oxygen to all parts of your body. When there are too few red blood cells, body tissues do not get enough oxygen to do their work. This condition is called anemia. Anemia can make you feel short of breath, very weak, and tired. Call your doctor if you have any of these symptoms:

- Fatigue (feeling very weak and tired).

- Dizziness or feeling faint.

- Shortness of breath.

- Feeling as if your heart is "pounding" or beating very fast.

Your doctor will check your blood cell count often during your treatment. She or he may also prescribe a medicine that can boost the growth of your red blood cells. Discuss this with your doctor if you become anemic often. Unlike more common forms of anemia, anemia caused by chemotherapy is not due to deficiency of iron or other vitamins, and taking these supplements will not help. If your red count falls too low, you may need a blood transfusion or a medicine called erythropoietin to raise the number of red blood cells in your body.

Things You Can Do If You Are Anemic

- Get plenty of rest. Sleep more at night and take naps during the day if you can.

- Limit your activities. Do only the things that are essential or most important to you.

- Ask for help when you need it. Ask family and friends to pitch in with things like child care, shopping, housework, or driving.

- Eat a well-balanced diet.

- When sitting, get up slowly. When lying down, sit first and then stand. This will help prevent dizziness.

Central Nervous System Problems

Some kinds of chemotherapy can interfere with certain functions in your central nervous system (brain) causing tiredness, confusion, and depression. These feelings will go away once the chemotherapy dose is lowered or you finish chemotherapy. Call your doctor if these symptoms occur.

Infection

Some forms of chemotherapy make you more likely to get infections. This happens because many anticancer drugs affect the bone marrow, making it harder to make white blood cells (WBCs), the cells that fight many types of infections. Your doctor will check your blood cell count often while you are getting chemotherapy. There are medicines that help speed the recovery of white blood cells, shortening the time when the white blood count is very low. These medicines are called colony stimulating factors (CSF). Raising the white blood cell count greatly lowers the risk of serious infection.

Most infections come from bacteria normally found on your skin and in your mouth, intestines, and genital tract. Sometimes, the cause of an infection may not be known. Even if you take extra care, you still may get an infection. But there are some things you can do.

How Can I Help Prevent Infections?

- Wash your hands often during the day. Be sure to wash them before you eat, after you use the bathroom, and after touching animals.

- Clean your rectal area gently but thoroughly after each bowel movement. Ask your doctor or nurse for advice if the area becomes irritated or if you have hemorrhoids. Also, check with your doctor before using enemas or suppositories.

- Stay away from people who have illnesses you can catch, such as a cold, the flu, measles, or chicken pox.

- Try to avoid crowds. For example, go shopping or to the movies when the stores or theaters are least likely to be busy.

- Stay away from children who recently have received "live virus" vaccines such as chicken pox and oral polio, since they may be contagious to people with a low blood cell count. Call your doctor or local health department if you have any questions.

- Do not cut or tear the cuticles of your nails.

- Be careful not to cut or nick yourself when using scissors, needles, or knives.

- Maintain good mouth care.

- Do not squeeze or scratch pimples.

- Take a warm (not hot) bath, shower, or sponge bath every day. Pat your skin dry using a light touch. Do not rub too hard.

- Use lotion or oil to soften and heal your skin if it becomes dry and cracked.

- Clean cuts and scrapes right away and daily until healed with warm water, soap, and an antiseptic.

- Avoid contact with animal litter boxes and waste, bird cages, and fish tanks.

- Avoid standing water, for example, birdbaths, flower vases, or humidifiers.

- Wear protective gloves when gardening or cleaning up after others, especially small children.

- Do not get any immunizations, such as flu or pneumonia shots, without checking with your doctor first.

- Do not eat raw fish, seafood, meat, or eggs.

- Use an electric shaver instead of a razor to prevent breaks or cuts in your skin.

Symptoms of Infection

Call your doctor right away if you have any of these symptoms:

- Fever over 100° F or 38° C.
- Chills, especially shaking chills.
- Sweating.
- Loose bowel movements.
- Frequent urgency to urinate or a burning feeling when you urinate.
- A severe cough or sore throat.
- Unusual vaginal discharge or itching.
- Redness, swelling, or tenderness, especially around a wound, sore, ostomy, pimple, rectal area, or catheter site.
- Sinus pain or pressure.
- Earaches, headaches, or stiff neck.
- Blisters on the lips or skin.
- Mouth sores.

Report any signs of infection to your doctor right away, even if it is in the middle of the night. This is especially important when your white blood cell count is low. If you have a fever, do not take aspirin, acetaminophen, or any other medicine to bring your temperature down without checking with your doctor first.

Blood Clotting Problems

Some anticancer drugs can affect the bone marrow's ability to make platelets, the blood cells that help stop bleeding by making your blood clot. If your blood does not have enough platelets, you may bleed or bruise more easily than usual, even without an injury.

Call your doctor if you have any of these symptoms:

- unexpected bruising
- small, red spots under the skin
- reddish or pinkish urine
- black or bloody bowel movements
- bleeding from your gums or nose
- vaginal bleeding that is new or lasts longer than a regular period
- headaches or changes in vision
- warm to hot feeling of an arm or leg

Your doctor will check your platelet count often while you are having chemotherapy. If your platelet count falls too low, the doctor may give you a platelet transfusion to build up the count. There are also medicines called thrombopoietin or colony stimulating factors that help increase your platelets.

How to Help Prevent Problems If Your Platelet Count Is Low

- Check with your doctor or nurse before taking any vitamins or herbal remedies, including all over-the-counter medicines. Many of these products contain aspirin, which can affect platelets.
- Before drinking any alcoholic beverages, check with your doctor.
- Use a very soft toothbrush to clean your teeth.
- When cleaning your nose blow gently into a soft tissue.
- Take extra care not to cut or nick yourself when using scissors, needles, knives, or tools.
- Be careful not to burn yourself when ironing or cooking.
- Avoid contact sports and other activities that might result in injury.
- Ask your doctor if you should avoid sexual activity.
- Use an electric shaver instead of a razor.

Mouth, Gum, and Throat Problems

Good oral care is important during cancer treatment. Some anticancer drugs can cause sores in the mouth and throat, a condition called stomatitis or mucositis. Anticancer drugs also can make these tissues dry and irritated or cause them to bleed. Patients who have not been eating well since beginning chemotherapy are more likely to get mouth sores.

In addition to being painful, mouth sores can become infected by the many germs that live in the mouth. Every step should be taken to prevent infections, because they can be hard to fight during chemotherapy and can lead to serious problems.

How Can I Keep My Mouth, Gums, and Throat Healthy?

- Talk to your doctor about seeing your dentist at least several weeks before you start chemotherapy. You may need to have your teeth cleaned and to take care of any problems such as cavities, gum abscesses, gum disease, or poorly fitting dentures. Ask your dentist to show you the best ways to brush and floss your teeth during chemotherapy. Chemotherapy can make you more likely to get cavities, so your dentist may suggest using a fluoride rinse or gel each day to help prevent decay.

- Brush your teeth and gums after every meal. Use a soft toothbrush and a gentle touch. Brushing too hard can damage soft mouth tissues. Ask your doctor, nurse, or dentist to suggest a special toothbrush or toothpaste if your gums are very sensitive. Rinse with warm saltwater after meals and before bedtime.

- Rinse your toothbrush well after each use and store it in a dry place.

- Avoid mouthwashes that contain any amount of alcohol. Ask your doctor or nurse to suggest a mild or medicated mouthwash that you might use. For example, mouthwash with sodium bicarbonate (baking soda) is non-irritating.

If you develop sores in your mouth, tell your doctor or nurse. You may need medicine to treat the sores. If the sores are painful or keep you from eating, you can try these ideas:

- Ask your doctor if there is anything you can apply directly to the sores or to prescribe a medicine you can use to ease the pain.

- Eat foods cold or at room temperature. Hot and warm foods can irritate a tender mouth and throat.

- Eat soft, soothing foods, such as ice cream, milkshakes, baby food, soft fruits (bananas and applesauce), mashed potatoes, cooked cereals, soft-boiled or scrambled eggs, yogurt, cottage cheese, macaroni and cheese, custards, puddings, and gelatin. You also can puree cooked foods in the blender to make them smoother and easier to eat.

- Avoid irritating, acidic foods and juices, such as tomato and citrus (orange, grapefruit, and lemon); spicy or salty foods; and rough or coarse foods such as raw vegetables, granola, popcorn, and toast.

How Can I Cope with Mouth Dryness?

- Ask your doctor if you should use an artificial saliva product to moisten your mouth.

- Drink plenty of liquids.

- Ask your doctor if you can suck on ice chips, popsicles, or sugarless hard candy. You can also chew sugarless gum. (Sorbitol, a sugar substitute that is in many sugar-free foods, can cause diarrhea in many people. If diarrhea is a problem for you, check the labels of sugar-free foods before you buy them and limit your use of them.)

- Moisten dry foods with butter, margarine, gravy, sauces, or broth.

- Dunk crisp, dry foods in mild liquids.

- Eat soft and pureed foods.

- Use lip balm or petroleum jelly if your lips become dry.

- Carry a water bottle with you to sip from often.

Diarrhea

If the form of chemotherapy you are receiving affects the cells lining the intestine, it can cause diarrhea (watery or loose stools). If you have diarrhea that continues for more than twenty-four hours, or if you have pain and cramping along with the diarrhea, call your doctor. In severe cases, the doctor may prescribe a medicine to control the diarrhea. If diarrhea persists, you may need intravenous (IV)

373

fluids to replace the water and nutrients you have lost. Often these fluids are given on an outpatient basis and do not require hospitalization. Do not take any over-the-counter medicines for diarrhea without asking your doctor.

How Can I Help Control Diarrhea?

- Drink plenty of fluids. This will help replace those you have lost through diarrhea. Mild, clear liquids, such as water, clear broth, sports drinks such as Gatorade, or ginger ale, are best. If these drinks make you more thirsty or nauseous, try diluting them with water. Drink slowly and make sure drinks are at room temperature. Let carbonated drinks lose their fizz before you drink them.

- Eat small amounts of food throughout the day instead of three large meals.

- Unless your doctor has told you otherwise, eat potassium-rich foods. Diarrhea can cause you to lose this important mineral. Bananas, oranges, potatoes, and peach and apricot nectars are good sources of potassium.

- Ask your doctor if you should try a clear liquid diet to give your bowels time to rest. A clear liquid diet does not provide all the nutrients you need, so do not follow one for more than three to five days.

- Eat low-fiber foods. Low-fiber foods include white bread, white rice or noodles, creamed cereals, ripe bananas, canned or cooked fruit without skins, cottage cheese, yogurt without seeds, eggs, mashed or baked potatoes without the skin, pureed vegetables, chicken, or turkey without the skin, and fish.

- Avoid high-fiber foods, which can lead to diarrhea and cramping. High-fiber foods include whole grain breads and cereals, raw vegetables, beans, nuts, seeds, popcorn, and fresh and dried fruit.

- Avoid hot or very cold liquids, which can make diarrhea worse.

- Avoid coffee, tea with caffeine, alcohol, and sweets. Stay away from fried, greasy, or highly spiced foods, too. They are irritating and can cause diarrhea and cramping.

- Avoid milk and milk products, including ice cream, if they make your diarrhea worse.

Constipation

Some anticancer medicines, pain medicines, and other medicines can cause constipation. It can also occur if you are less active or if your diet lacks enough fluid or fiber. If you have not had a bowel movement for more than a day or two, call your doctor, who may suggest taking a laxative or stool softener. Do not take these measures without checking with your doctor, especially if your white blood cell count or platelets are low.

What Can I Do about Constipation?

- Drink plenty of fluids to help loosen the bowels. If you do not have mouth sores, try warm and hot fluids, including water, which work especially well.

- Check with your doctor to see if you can increase the fiber in your diet (there are certain kinds of cancer and certain side effects you may have for which a high-fiber diet is not recommended). High fiber foods include bran, whole-wheat breads and cereals, raw or cooked vegetables, fresh and dried fruit, nuts, and popcorn.

- Get some exercise every day. Go for a walk or you may want to try a more structured exercise program. Talk to your doctor about the amount and type of exercise that is right for you.

Nerve and Muscle Effects

Some anticancer drugs can cause problems with your body's nerves. One example of a condition affecting the nervous system is peripheral neuropathy, where you feel a tingling, burning, weakness, numbness, or pain in the hands or feet. Some drugs can also affect the muscles, making them weak, tired, or sore.

Sometimes these nerve and muscle side effects, though annoying, may not be serious. In other cases, nerve and muscle symptoms may be serious and need medical attention. Be sure to report any nerve or muscle symptoms to your doctor. Most of the time, these symptoms will get better; however, it may take up to a year after your treatment ends.

Some nerve and muscle-related symptoms include:

- tingling
- burning

- weakness or numbness in the hands or feet
- pain when walking
- weak, sore, tired, or achy muscles
- loss of balance
- clumsiness
- difficulty picking up objects and buttoning clothing
- shaking or trembling
- walking problems
- jaw pain
- hearing loss
- stomach pain
- constipation

How Can I Cope with Nerve and Muscle Problems?

- If your fingers are numb, be very careful when grasping objects that are sharp, hot, or otherwise dangerous.
- If your sense of balance or muscle strength is affected, avoid falls by moving carefully, using handrails when going up or down stairs, and using bath mats in the bathtub or shower.
- Always wear shoes with rubber soles (if possible).
- Ask your doctor for pain medicine.

Effects on Skin and Nails

You may have minor skin problems while you are having some forms of chemotherapy, such as redness, rashes, itching, peeling, dryness, acne, and increased sensitivity to the sun. Certain anticancer drugs, when given intravenously, may cause the skin all along the vein to darken, especially in people who have very dark skin. Some people use makeup to cover the area, but this can take a lot of time if several veins are affected. The darkened areas will fade a few months after treatment ends.

Your nails may also become darkened, yellow, brittle, or cracked. They also may develop vertical lines or bands.

While most of these problems are not serious and you can take care of them yourself, a few need immediate attention. Certain drugs given intravenously (IV) can cause serious and permanent tissue damage if they leak out of the vein. Tell your doctor or nurse right away if you feel any burning or pain when you are getting IV drugs. These symptoms do not always mean there is a problem, but they must always be checked at once. Don't hesitate to call your doctor about even the less serious symptoms.

Some symptoms may mean you are having an allergic reaction that may need to be treated at once. Call your doctor or nurse right away if:

- you develop sudden or severe itching.

- your skin breaks out in a rash or hives.

- you have wheezing or any other trouble breathing.

How Can I Cope with Skin and Nail Problems?

Acne:

- Try to keep your face clean and dry.

- Ask your doctor or nurse if you can use over-the-counter medicated creams or soaps.

Itching and dryness:

- Apply corn starch as you would a dusting powder.

- To help avoid dryness, take quick showers or sponge baths. Do not take long, hot baths. Use a moisturizing soap.

- Apply cream and lotion while your skin is still moist.

- Avoid perfume, cologne, or aftershave lotion that contains alcohol.

- Use a colloid oatmeal bath or diphenhydramine for generalized pruritus.

Nail problems:

- You can buy nail-strengthening products in a drugstore. Be aware that these products may bother your skin and nails.

- Protect your nails by wearing gloves when washing dishes, gardening, or doing other work around the house.

- Be sure to let your doctor know if you have redness, pain, or changes around the cuticles.

Sunlight sensitivity:

- Avoid direct sunlight as much as possible, especially between 10 AM and 4 PM when the sun's rays are the strongest.

- Use a sunscreen lotion with a skin protection factor (SPF) of fifteen or higher to protect against sun damage. A product such as zinc oxide, sold over the counter, can block the sun's rays completely.

- Use a lip balm with a sun protection factor.

- Wear long-sleeve cotton shirts, pants, and hats with a wide brim (particularly if you are having hair loss) to block the sun.

- Even people with dark skin need to protect themselves from the sun during chemotherapy.

Radiation Recall

Some people who have had radiation therapy develop "radiation recall" during their chemotherapy. During or shortly after certain anticancer drugs are given, the skin over an area that had received radiation turns red—a shade anywhere from light to very bright. The skin may blister and peel. This reaction may last hours or even days. Report radiation recall reactions to your doctor or nurse. You can soothe the itching and burning by:

- Placing a cool, wet compress over the affected area.

- Wearing soft, non-irritating fabrics. Women who have radiation for breast cancer following lumpectomy often find cotton bras the most comfortable.

Kidney and Bladder Effects

Some anticancer drugs can irritate the bladder or cause temporary or permanent damage to the bladder or kidneys. If you are taking one or more of these drugs, your doctor may ask you to collect a twenty-four-hour urine sample. A blood sample may also be obtained before you begin chemotherapy to check your kidney function. Some anticancer drugs cause the urine to change color (orange, red, green, or yellow) or take on a strong or medicine-like odor for twenty-four to seventy-two hours. Check with your doctor to see if the drugs you are taking may have any of these effects.

Always drink plenty of fluids to ensure good urine flow and help prevent problems. This is very important if you are taking drugs that affect the kidney and bladder. Water, juice, soft drinks, broth, ice cream, soup, popsicles, and gelatin are all considered fluids.

Tell your doctor if you have any of these symptoms:

- Pain or burning when you urinate (pass your water).
- Frequent urination.
- Not being able to urinate.
- A feeling that you must urinate right away ("urgency").
- Reddish or bloody urine.
- Fever.
- Chills, especially shaking chills.

Flu-Like Symptoms

Some people feel as though they have the flu for a few hours to a few days after taking certain chemotherapy drugs. This may be especially true if you are receiving chemotherapy in combination with biological therapy. Flu-like symptoms—muscle and joint aches, headache, tiredness, nausea, slight fever (usually less than 100°F), chills, and poor appetite—may last from one to three days. An infection or the cancer itself can also cause these symptoms. Check with your doctor if you have flu-like symptoms.

Fluid Retention

Your body may retain fluid when you are having chemotherapy. This may be due to hormonal changes from your therapy, to the drugs themselves, or to your cancer. Check with your doctor or nurse if you notice swelling or puffiness in your face, hands, feet, or abdomen. You may need to avoid table salt and foods that have a lot of salt. If the problem is severe, your doctor may prescribe a diuretic, medicine to help your body get rid of excess fluids.

Effects on Sexual Organs

Chemotherapy may—but does not always—affect sexual organs (testis in men, vagina and ovaries in women) and functioning in both men and women. The side effects that might occur depend on the drugs used and the person's age and general health.

- **Effects on the Ovaries:** Anticancer drugs can affect the ovaries and reduce the amount of hormones they produce. Some women find that their menstrual periods become irregular or stop completely while having chemotherapy. Related side effects may be temporary or permanent.

- **Infertility:** Damage to the ovaries may result in infertility, the inability to become pregnant. The infertility can be either temporary or permanent. Whether infertility occurs, and how long it lasts, depends on many factors, including the type of drug, the dosage given, and the woman's age.

- **Menopause:** A woman's age and the drugs and dosages used will determine whether she experiences menopause while on chemotherapy. Chemotherapy may also cause menopause-like symptoms such as hot flashes and dry vaginal tissues. These tissue changes can make intercourse uncomfortable and can make a woman more prone to bladder or vaginal infections. Any infection should be treated right away. Menopause may be temporary or permanent.

  - Help for hot flashes: dress in layers; avoid caffeine and alcohol; exercise; and try meditation or other relaxation methods.

  - Relieving vaginal symptoms and preventing infection: use a water or mineral oil-based vaginal lubricant at the time of intercourse; there are products that can be used to stop vaginal dryness (ask your pharmacist about vaginal gels that can be applied to the vagina); avoid using petroleum jelly, which is difficult for the body to get rid of and increases the risk of infection; wear cotton underwear and pantyhose with a ventilated cotton lining; avoid wearing tight slacks or shorts; ask your doctor about prescribing a vaginal cream or suppository to reduce the chances of infection; and ask your doctor about using a vaginal dilator if painful intercourse continues.

- **Pregnancy:** Although pregnancy may be possible during chemotherapy, it still is not advisable because some anticancer drugs may cause birth defects. Doctors advise women of childbearing age, from the teens through the end of menopause, to use some method of birth control throughout their treatment, such as condoms, spermicidal agents, diaphragms, or birth control pills. Birth control pills may not be appropriate for some women, such as those with breast cancer. Ask your doctor about these contraceptive options. If a woman is pregnant when her cancer is discovered, it may be possible to delay chemotherapy until after the baby is born. For a woman who needs treatment sooner, the possible effects of chemotherapy on the fetus need to be evaluated.

Eating Well during Chemotherapy

It is very important to eat well while you are getting chemotherapy. Eating well during chemotherapy means choosing a balanced diet that contains all the nutrients the body needs. Eating well also means having a diet high enough in calories to keep your weight up and high enough in protein to rebuild tissues that cancer treatment may harm. People who eat well can cope with side effects and fight infection better. Also, their bodies can rebuild healthy tissues faster.

What If I Don't Feel Like Eating?

On some days you may feel you just cannot eat. You can lose your appetite if you feel depressed or tired. Or, side effects such as nausea or mouth and throat problems may make it difficult or painful to eat. In some cases, if you cannot eat for a long period of time, your doctor may recommend that you be given nutrition intravenously until you are able to eat again.

When a poor appetite is the problem, try these suggestions:

- Eat frequent, small meals or snacks whenever you want, perhaps four to six times a day. You do not have to eat three regular meals each day.

- Keep snacks within easy reach, so you can have something whenever you feel like it.

- Even if you do not want to eat solid foods, try to drink beverages during the day. Juice, soup, and other fluids like these can give you important calories and nutrients.

- Vary your diet by trying new foods and recipes.

- When possible, take a walk before meals; this may make you feel hungrier.

- Try changing your mealtime routine. For example, eat in a different location.

- Eat with friends or family members. When eating alone, listen to the radio or watch TV.

- Ask your doctor or nurse about nutrition supplements.

- Speak with your dietitian about your specific nutrition needs.

Can I Drink Alcoholic Beverages?

Small amounts of alcohol can help you relax and increase your appetite. On the other hand, alcohol may interfere with how some drugs work or worsen their side effects. For this reason, some people must drink less alcohol or avoid alcohol completely during chemotherapy. Ask your doctor if and how much beer, wine, or other alcoholic beverages you can drink during treatment.

Can I Take Extra Vitamins and Minerals?

You can usually get all the vitamins and minerals you need by eating a healthy diet. Talk to your doctor, nurse, registered dietitian, or a pharmacist before taking any vitamin or mineral supplements. Certain vitamins or supplements interfere with chemotherapy drugs, and can cause chemotherapy to fail. Some vitamins and minerals are poisonous if taken in large doses; too much of vitamins and minerals can be just as dangerous as too little. Find out what is recommended for you.

Chapter 55

High-Dose Chemotherapy

Over the past twenty years, more than fifteen thousand women with breast cancer have been treated with an arduous yet largely unproven procedure: high doses of chemotherapy followed by blood cell transplants to replenish the bone marrow damaged by the chemotherapy.

In the early 1990s, after a few encouraging preliminary reports, breast cancer patients and advocates began demanding the treatment. Some state legislatures responded by mandating that insurance companies pay for the intensive procedure, which can cost up to $100,000 per case, much more than conventional treatments. By mid-decade, more people were receiving the treatment for breast cancer than for any other cancer.

However, the vast majority of the women who received the high-dose regimens did so outside of a clinical trial, which meant that the success or failure of the treatment could not be reliably established. Results from well-conducted, carefully monitored, randomized trials were urgently needed to figure out which breast cancer patients, if any, might benefit from high-dose therapy plus transplants, said Jeff Abrams, M.D., a breast cancer researcher at NCI.

So in the late 1990s, multiple randomized studies were begun. In early 2000, reports from three of these clinical trials were published. Two showed that high doses of chemotherapy were no more effective than standard chemotherapy for women with advanced or high-risk

Information in this chapter is reprinted from "High-Dose Chemotherapy for Breast Cancer: History," National Cancer Institute, reviewed January 2004; and "High-Dose Chemotherapy with Stem Cell Transplantation: Still No Clear Benefit," National Cancer Institute, July 2003.

breast cancer. Results from the third study contradicted these findings and came out in favor of the high-dose treatment. However, this study was later discounted after the lead South African researcher admitted fraud and misconduct.

These developments left the practice of high-dose chemotherapy for breast cancer in limbo. At that point, the American Society of Clinical Oncology (ASCO) recommended that women receive the treatment only if they were taking part in a "high-quality" clinical trial. Editorials in the March 18, 2000, issue of the *Lancet* and the April 13, 2000, *New England Journal of Medicine* made the same argument.

In another sign of support for the clinical trials approach, in early 2000 one of the nation's largest insurers, Aetna/U.S. Healthcare, announced that it will pay for high-dose chemotherapy plus transplants only for patients enrolled in federally sponsored clinical trials. The company previously had reimbursed expenses for women who were not in clinical trials.

Researchers at the National Cancer Institute (NCI) have long supported this approach. As of spring 2001, four large national trials sponsored by NCI had all completed enrollment, with results beginning to become available.

High-Dose Chemotherapy with Stem Cell Transplantation

Summary

Two studies examined the benefits of high-dose chemotherapy with stem-cell transplantation for women at high risk of a breast cancer relapse. In both studies, a subgroup of women who underwent the experimental procedure experienced a significant delay in recurrence compared to women who received standard therapy, but they did not ultimately live any longer.

While these studies reaffirm conventional treatment as the standard of care for high-risk breast cancer, they do provide a rationale for further research to refine the technique and determine whether a subset of women might benefit from the high-dose approach.

Background

Women with high-risk breast cancer have a strong chance of relapsing and dying from their disease within ten years. (High-risk breast cancer is generally defined as having cancer in four or more axillary lymph nodes.) Researchers have been investigating whether higher doses of chemotherapy drugs can do a better job of preventing or delaying the spread or return of breast cancer in these patients.

However, high-dose chemotherapy damages the bone marrow, which is then no longer able to produce needed blood cells. In the two studies highlighted here, researchers also performed stem cell transplantation to help repair the damage. Stem cells are able to become fully mature red blood cells.

Study 1 (Netherlands Cancer Institute)

The 885 patients in this phase III clinical trial consisted of women younger than fifty-six who had surgery for breast cancer, at least four cancer-positive axillary lymph nodes, and no cancer beyond the lymph nodes. Patients were randomly assigned either to receive the standard treatment (chemotherapy every three weeks for five courses, followed by radiation therapy and tamoxifen) or the same treatment but with the fifth course consisting of high-dose chemotherapy and stem cell transplantation. The study was led by Sjoerd Rodenhuis, M.D., of the Netherlands Cancer Institute in Amsterdam.

Study 1 Results

After a median follow-up time of fifty-seven months, the five-year, relapse-free survival rates for all patients were 59 percent for the conventional treatment group and 65 percent for the high-dose chemotherapy and stem-cell transplantation group. However, this difference was not statistically significant—that is, it could have occurred by chance.

The researchers took a closer look at two subgroups: women with four to nine cancer-positive axillary nodes, and women with ten or more positive nodes. Only women with ten or more positive nodes had significantly improved relapse-free survival: 51 percent of the subgroup treated conventionally survived without a recurrence for five years, compared to 61 percent of the experimentally treated subgroup.

However, overall survival rates for all patients, as well as for both subgroups, were not significantly improved for those receiving high-dose therapy with stem cell transplantation.

The authors concluded that while the results should be "interpreted with caution," they do justify future studies in which the experimental procedure itself can be refined and researchers can select patients who may be most likely to benefit.

Study 2 (U.S. Intergroup Study)

This phase III trial consisted of 511 women no older than sixty (median age: forty-four) whose breast cancer had spread to at least ten axillary lymph nodes but not beyond the lymph nodes. After surgery, the women were randomly assigned to receive six courses of standard chemotherapy or the same treatment followed by high-dose chemotherapy with stem cell transplantation. The study was led by Martin S. Tallman, M.D., of the Northwestern University Feinberg School of Medicine in Chicago, Illinois.

Study 2 Results

After a median follow-up of seventy-three months, 55 percent of the experimental group had survived without a recurrence of their breast cancer, compared to 48 percent of the conventional group. This difference, however, was not statistically significant.

But when the researchers looked at the data for the 417 patients who met the trial's strictest eligibility criteria, they found that relapse-free survival rates were significantly higher in the experimental group compared to those in the conventional group: 55 percent compared to 45 percent.

Nonetheless, overall survival rates between the two groups were not significantly different: 58 percent for the experimental group versus 62 percent for the conventional group. In addition, among those who received the high-dose chemotherapy treatment, nine died as a result of transplantation complications and nine developed preleukemia or acute myeloid leukemia.

According to the authors, these results suggest that conventional therapy for high-risk breast cancer patients should remain the standard of care.

Limitations

Jeffrey Abrams, M.D., coordinator of the NCI-sponsored U.S. Intergroup Study trial, comments that "based on the evidence from these two studies, high-dose chemotherapy with stem-cell transplantation for women with high-risk breast cancer remains an investigational treatment that should be limited to carefully controlled clinical trials."

While attempts to refine and improve high-dose treatments are worthy of further research, he says, all the studies to date indicate that this approach is not clearly better than standard-dose chemotherapy regimens, which are less toxic and less expensive.

In an editorial accompanying the two articles, Gerald Elfenbein, M.D., concluded that "high-dose chemotherapy should best be viewed as a launching pad from which to explore new methods of post-transplantation therapy to reduce the probability of relapse."

Chapter 56

Dose-Dense Chemotherapy

A new clinical trial has shown that reducing the interval between successive doses of a commonly used chemotherapy regimen improves survival in women whose breast cancer has spread to the lymph nodes. While previous research has evaluated the use of various forms of "dose-dense" chemotherapy, this is the first major controlled study to show a clear survival benefit for women with node-positive breast cancer. The study was conducted by Cancer and Leukemia Group B (CALGB) for the Breast Cancer Intergroup, a consortium of National Cancer Institute (NCI)-sponsored Cooperative Clinical Trials Groups, and was presented on December 12, 2002 at the 25th Annual San Antonio Breast Cancer Symposium.

"This study suggests that many women with breast cancer may benefit from chemotherapy administered on a condensed schedule," said Marc L. Citron, M.D., Albert Einstein College of Medicine, who is the lead investigator of the study. "With the availability of new drugs to control one of the most serious side effects of chemotherapy administration, we can further increase the chances of survival for women with breast cancer." The dose-dense regimen was made tolerable for patients because of the drug filgrastim, which helps prevent neutropenia, a serious complication of chemotherapy.

The researchers found that two dose-dense regimens provided significantly higher disease-free survival rates than two regimens

The information in this chapter is reprinted from "'Dose Dense' Chemotherapy Improves Survival in Breast Cancer Patients Compared to Conventional Chemotherapy," National Cancer Institute, December 12, 2002.

using conventional dosing, and that efficacy did not differ between the two dose-dense regimens. Among patients on the dose-dense regimens, disease-free survival was 82 percent after four years, compared to 75 percent for those who received conventional therapy. This difference corresponded to a 26 percent overall reduction in the risk of cancer recurrence. The findings confirm the predictions of a mathematical model developed in the 1980s that suggested the value of increased dose density, which was the impetus for the study.

"The improvement in outcome could well represent an important advance in our knowledge of the biology of breast cancer and how best to treat it," said Larry Norton, M.D., of Memorial Sloan-Kettering Cancer Center, senior investigator of the study and one of the developers of the original model. "If confirmed and extended by additional research, this finding could positively affect the care of thousands of patients throughout the world with breast cancer and perhaps, eventually, other diseases."

Study Design

Researchers tested both dose dense and conventional chemotherapy regimens in 1,973 women with node-positive primary breast cancer and no other metastases. Following surgical removal of their tumors, the women were assigned to one of four treatment regimens involving the standard chemotherapy drugs doxorubicin (A), paclitaxel (T), and cyclophosphamide (C):

- Sequential administration (A followed by T, followed by C) in three-week intervals (conventional)

- Sequential administration in two-week intervals, with filgrastim (dose dense)

- Concurrent administration (A and C together, followed by T) in three-week intervals

- Concurrent administration in two-week intervals, with filgrastim (dose dense)

Since frequent administration of chemotherapy can result in a condition called neutropenia, a decline in the number of a certain type of white blood cells, the researchers administered filgrastim to patients on the dose-dense regimens. Also known as the granulocyte-colony stimulating factor (G-CSF), filgrastim helps prevent neutropenia by stimulating the formation of white blood cells called neutrophils. Without it, chemotherapy dosing frequency is limited to longer intervals.

Study Results

"It is too soon to determine whether a dose-dense chemotherapy regimen with filgrastim should be the new standard of care," said Jeffrey Abrams, the oncologist in charge of breast cancer treatment trials at NCI. "However, the reduced risk of cancer recurrence and the low occurrence of side effects are encouraging, and further follow-up as well as other studies testing this approach will hopefully confirm the findings."

In addition to improved disease-free survival rates, the study indicated that dose-dense chemotherapy may also lead to higher overall survival rates. After three years, 92 percent of patients on the dose-dense therapy were alive, compared to 90 percent of those on the conventionally administered regimens. This difference corresponded to a 31 percent overall reduction in the risk of death. However, the study authors cautioned that additional follow-up is necessary to confirm this overall survival benefit.

Side effects were found to be no more severe among patients on the dose-dense regimens than among those on the conventional treatments, and patients on the dose-dense regimens suffered fewer cases of neutropenia. In addition, the study showed that sequential administration produced slightly fewer side effects than the concurrent regimens, with equal efficacy.

Future Directions for Study

Since the mathematical model that led to this study applies to most cancer types and many anti-cancer drugs, the researchers hypothesize that future clinical trials could examine the benefits of dose-dense chemotherapy using other drugs and in other types of cancer.

Chapter 57

Radiation Therapy for the Treatment of Breast Cancer

What Breast Cancer Patients Need to Know about Radiation Therapy

Radiation therapy (or radiotherapy) uses high-energy rays to stop cancer cells from growing and dividing. Radiation therapy is often used to destroy any remaining breast cancer cells in the breast, chest wall, or axilla (underarm) area after surgery. Occasionally, radiation therapy is used before surgery to shrink the size of a tumor. A common treatment for early stage breast cancer is breast-conserving therapy. Breast-conserving therapy (BCT) is the surgical removal of a breast lump (lumpectomy) and a surrounding margin of normal breast tissue. BCT is typically followed by at least six to seven weeks of radiation therapy. Treatment with radiation usually begins one month after surgery, allowing the breast tissue adequate time to heal. Radiation therapy may occasionally be recommended for women to destroy remaining cancer cells after mastectomy (surgical removal of the affected breast) or to shrink tumors in patients with advanced breast cancer.

External Beam Radiation

The most common type of radiation therapy used on women with breast cancer is called external beam radiation. External beam radiation is delivered from a source outside the body on the specific area of the body that has been affected by the cancer. Experts compare the experience of external beam radiation to having a diagnostic x-ray, except that radiation is usually administered for a longer period of time and at a higher dose.

Before radiation therapy begins, the physician will measure the correct angles for aiming the radiation beam at the specific area of the body and make ink marks on the patient's skin. As part of treatment after breast surgery, patients are typically treated with radiation five times per week for at least six weeks in an outpatient clinical setting. Each treatment generally lasts a few minutes; the entire radiation session after machine set-up typically lasts fifteen to thirty minutes. The procedure itself is pain-free. While the radiation is being administered, the technologist will leave the room and monitor the patient on a closed-circuit television. However, patients should be able to communicate with the technologist at any time over an intercom system.

Side effects of external beam therapy vary among patients. The most common side effect is fatigue. Fatigue (extreme tiredness) can be especially bothersome in the later weeks of treatment. Patients who experience fatigue after radiation sessions should get plenty of rest and try to maintain an active lifestyle. While many patients can still work and participate in normal activities during radiation therapy, some patients find it necessary to limit their work or activities until treatment has been completed.

Other common side effects of radiation therapy are neutropenia (sharp decrease in white blood cell count), swelling of the breast, a feeling of heaviness in the breast, a sunburn-type appearance of the breast skin, and loss of appetite. These side effects usually disappear after six to twelve months. Near the end of treatment with radiation, the breast skin may become moist. Patients should try to wear loose-fitting clothing and expose the skin to air as much as possible to help the skin heal quickly.

In most cases, the breast will look and feel the same after radiation therapy is completed, though it may be more firm. In rare cases, radiation therapy may cause changes in the breast size. Breasts may become larger due to fluid buildup (seroma) or smaller due to tissue changes. Some women may find that the breast skin is more sensitive after radiation, while others may find that it is less sensitive. Radiation therapy of the axillary (underarm) lymph nodes may cause lymphedema (chronic swelling of the arm) in some women. Women who have radiation to the lymph nodes will usually be instructed on arm exercises and other activities to help prevent lymphedema. Pregnant women are usually advised not to undergo radiation therapy because of possible harm to the fetus.

The following recommendations may help reduce pain from skin reactions to radiation therapy:

- Avoid any additional sun exposure to the area.

- Wear loose-fitting clothing, preferably cotton or other material that "breathes."

- Use warm or tepid water when bathing, rather than hot water.

- Avoid constricting bras (if a bra must be worn at all).

- Use cool compresses (not cold or ice packs, as that may cause additional skin damage).

- Lotions or powders on the treated area are generally not recommended.

- Specific creams should be approved by the radiation oncologist or his or her nurse. Often, there should not be any substance on the skin that could affect the radiation treatment or lead to a more serious burn injury (such as oil).

Patients should talk to their physicians about soothing oils or creams that may be allowed between (not during) treatment sessions.

Internal Radiation

Brachytherapy (also called internal radiation) is an experimental method currently being developed to use on breast cancer patients. Instead of using radiation beams from outside the body, radioactive substances are placed directly into the breast tissue next to the cancer. Brachytherapy involves the surgical placement of ten to twenty plastic catheters (tiny tubes called implants) into the breast tissue next to the tumor to help guide the radioactive materials to the correct area of the body. Technologists then insert pellets of radioactive substances (called Iridium-192) into the catheters. Nine or more times over the course of a week, the catheters are briefly connected to a high-dose-rate brachytherapy machine for internal radiation treatment. The treatments usually take about ten minutes each and are painless. The tubes are usually removed after a week.

Brachytherapy is not standard practice for breast cancer patients but is currently used on cancers in other areas of the body such as the mouth, cervix, or prostate.

Possible advantages of brachytherapy:

- The reduction of time a patient has to undergo radiation therapy from at least six weeks to one week.

- Less irritation of healthy breast tissues.

- Patients who must also undergo chemotherapy as part of their breast cancer treatment do not have to delay treatment for as much time.

- Fewer skin reactions, such as redness, rashes, or irritations.

Physicians are unsure whether brachytherapy is as effective in destroying breast cancer cells as external beam radiation therapy. Several clinical trials are currently being run to evaluate the safety and effectiveness of brachytherapy. Side effects of brachytherapy include risk of infection and breast swelling.

About Imaginis

Imaginis.com is an independent, award-winning, comprehensive resource for news and information on breast cancer prevention, screening, diagnosis, and treatment and related women's health topics such as hormone replacement therapy (HRT), multiple sclerosis, osteoporosis, and ovarian cancer. Imaginis.com also contains extensive information about medical procedures such as angiography, biopsy, CT, MR, nuclear medicine, ultrasound, x-ray imaging, and radiotherapy.

The goal of Imaginis.com is to provide women and their physicians with the most comprehensive and relevant information on breast health and related women's health issues. Imaginis content is created by an independent team of breast health specialists to ensure that it is up-to-date and accurate. Complicated medical terms are explained in everyday language to help individuals understand their options, make informed decisions, and achieve optimal health.

A Practical Guide for Radiation Therapy Patients

What Is Radiation Therapy?

Radiation therapy (sometimes called radiotherapy, x-ray therapy, or irradiation) is the treatment of disease using penetrating beams of high-energy waves or streams of particles called radiation.

Many years ago doctors learned how to use this energy to "see" inside the body and find disease. You've probably seen a chest x-ray or x-ray pictures of your teeth or your bones. At high doses (many times those used for x-ray exams) radiation is used to treat cancer and other illnesses.

The radiation used for cancer treatment comes from special machines or from radioactive substances. Radiation therapy equipment aims specific amounts of the radiation at tumors or areas of the body where there is disease.

How Does Radiation Therapy Work?

Radiation in high doses kills cells or keeps them from growing and dividing. Because cancer cells grow and divide more rapidly than most of the normal cells around them, radiation therapy can successfully treat many kinds of cancer. Normal cells are also affected by radiation but, unlike cancer cells, most of them recover from the effects of radiation.

To protect normal cells, doctors carefully limit the doses of radiation and spread the treatment out over time. They also shield as much normal tissue as possible while they aim the radiation at the site of the cancer.

The Goals and Benefits of Radiation Therapy

The goal of radiation therapy is to kill the cancer cells with as little risk as possible to normal cells. Radiation therapy can be used to treat many kinds of cancer in almost any part of the body. In fact, more than half of all people with cancer are treated with some form of radiation. For many cancer patients, radiation is the only kind of treatment they need. Thousands of people who have had radiation therapy alone or in combination with other types of cancer treatment are free of cancer.

Radiation treatment, like surgery, is a local treatment—it affects the cancer cells only in a specific area of the body. Sometimes doctors add radiation therapy to treatments that reach all parts of the body (systemic treatment) such as chemotherapy or biological therapy to improve treatment results. You may hear your doctor use the term *adjuvant therapy* for a treatment that is added to, and given after, the primary therapy.

Radiation therapy is often used with surgery to treat cancer. Doctors may use radiation before surgery to shrink a tumor. This makes it easier to remove the cancerous tissue and may allow the surgeon to perform less radical surgery.

Radiation therapy may be used after surgery to stop the growth of cancer cells that may remain. Your doctor may choose to use radiation therapy and surgery at the same time. This procedure, known as intraoperative radiation, is explained more fully in the "External Radiation Therapy" section.

In some cases, instead of surgery, doctors use radiation along with anticancer drugs (chemotherapy) to destroy the cancer. Radiation may be given before, during, or after chemotherapy. Doctors carefully tailor this combination treatment to each patient's needs depending on the type of cancer, its location, and its size. The purpose of radiation treatment before or during chemotherapy is to make the tumor smaller and thus improve the effectiveness of the anticancer drugs. Doctors sometimes recommend that a patient complete chemotherapy and then have radiation treatment to kill any cancer cells that might remain.

When curing the cancer is not possible, radiation therapy can be used to shrink tumors and reduce pressure, pain, and other symptoms of cancer. This is called palliative care or palliation. Many cancer patients find that they have a better quality of life when radiation is used for this purpose.

Risks of Radiation Therapy?

The brief high doses of radiation that damage or destroy cancer cells can also injure or kill normal cells. These effects of radiation on normal cells cause treatment side effects. Most side effects of radiation treatment are well known and, with the help of your doctor and nurse, easily treated.

Depending on the type and location of radiation therapy, there can be formation of scar tissue in the skin or organs. In some cases, this may cause problems years after treatment ends due to the scar tissue interfering with normal organ function. Most forms of radiation therapy also increase the risk of developing a second cancer in the area treated, unrelated to the first cancer.

Despite these problems, the risk of side effects is usually far less than the benefit of killing cancer cells. Your doctor will not advise you to have any treatment unless the benefits—control of disease and relief from symptoms—are greater than the known risks.

External Radiation Therapy: What to Expect

How does the doctor plan my treatment?

The high-energy rays used for radiation therapy can come from a variety of sources. Your doctor may choose to use x-rays, an electron beam, or cobalt-60 gamma rays. Some cancer treatment centers have special equipment that produces beams of protons or neutrons for radiation therapy. The type of radiation your doctor decides to use depends on what kind of cancer you have and how far into your body the radiation should go.

After a physical exam and a review of your medical history, the doctor plans your treatment. In a process called simulation, you will be asked to lie very still on an examining table while the radiation therapist uses a special x-ray machine to define your treatment port or field. This is the exact place on your body where the radiation will be aimed. Depending on the location of your cancer, you may have more than one treatment port.

Simulation may also involve CT scans or other imaging studies to plan how to direct the radiation. Depending on the type of treatment you will be receiving, body molds or other devices that keep you from moving during treatment (immobilization devices) may be made at this time. They will be used each time you have treatment to be sure that you are positioned correctly. Simulation may take from a half hour to about two hours.

The radiation therapist often will mark the treatment port on your skin with tattoos or tiny dots of colored, permanent ink. It's important that the radiation be targeted at the same area each time. If the dots appear to be fading, tell your radiation therapist who will darken them so that they can be seen easily.

Once simulation has been done, your doctor will meet with the radiation physicist and the dosimetrist. Based on the results of your medical history, lab tests, x-rays, other treatments you may have had, and the location and kind of cancer you have, they will decide how much radiation is needed, what kind of machine to use to deliver it, and how many treatments you should have.

After you have started the treatments, your doctor and the other members of your health care team will follow your progress by checking your response to treatment and how you are feeling at least once a week. When necessary, your doctor may revise the treatment plan by changing the radiation dose or the number and length of your remaining radiation sessions.

Your nurse will be available daily to discuss your concerns and answer any questions you may have. Be sure to tell your nurse if you are having any side effects or if you notice any unusual symptoms.

How long does the treatment take?

For most types of cancer, radiation therapy usually is given five days a week for six or seven weeks. (When radiation is used for palliative care, the course of treatment is shorter, usually two to three weeks.) The total dose of radiation and the number of treatments you need will depend on the size, location, and kind of cancer you have, your general health, and other medical treatments you may be receiving.

Using many small doses of daily radiation rather than a few large doses helps protect normal body tissues in the treatment area. Weekend rest breaks allow normal cells to recover.

It's very important that you have all of your scheduled treatments to get the most benefit from your therapy. Missing or delaying treatments can lessen the effectiveness of your radiation treatment.

What happens during the treatment visits?

Before each treatment, you may need to change into a hospital gown or robe. It's best to wear clothing that is easy to take off and put on again.

In the treatment room, the radiation therapist will use the marks on your skin to locate the treatment area and to position you correctly. You may sit in a special chair or lie down on a treatment table. For each external radiation therapy session, you will be in the treatment room about fifteen to thirty minutes, but you will be getting radiation for only about one to five minutes of that time. Receiving external radiation treatments is painless, just like having an x-ray taken. You will not hear, see, or smell the radiation.

The radiation therapist may put special shields (or blocks) between the machine and certain parts of your body to help protect normal tissues and organs. There might also be plastic or plaster forms that help you stay in exactly the right place. You need to remain very still during the treatment so that the radiation reaches only the area where it's needed and the same area is treated each time. You don't have to hold your breath—just breathe normally.

The radiation therapist will leave the treatment room before your treatment begins. The radiation machine is controlled from a nearby area. You will be watched on a television screen or through a window in the control room. Although you may feel alone, keep in mind that the therapist can see and hear you and even talk with you using an intercom in the treatment room. If you should feel ill or very uncomfortable during the treatment, tell your therapist at once. The machine can be stopped at any time.

The machines used for radiation treatments are very large, and they make noises as they move around your body to aim at the treatment area from different angles. Their size and motion may be frightening at first. Remember that the machines are being moved and controlled by your radiation therapist. They are checked constantly to be sure they're working right. If you have concerns about anything that happens in the treatment room, discuss these concerns with the radiation therapist.

What is hyperfractionated radiation therapy?

Radiation is usually given once daily in a dose that is based on the type and location of the tumor. In hyperfractionated radiation therapy, the daily dose is divided into smaller doses that are given more than once a day. The treatments usually are separated by four to six hours. Doctors are studying hyperfractionated therapy to learn if it is equal to, or perhaps more effective than, once-a-day therapy and whether there are fewer long-term side effects. Early results of treatment studies of some kinds of tumors are encouraging, and hyperfractionated therapy is becoming a more common way to give radiation treatments for some types of cancer.

What is intraoperative radiation?

Intraoperative radiation combines surgery and radiation therapy. The surgeon first removes as much of the tumor as possible. Before the surgery is completed, a large dose of radiation is given directly to the tumor bed (the area from which the tumor has been removed) and nearby areas where cancer cells might have spread. Sometimes intraoperative radiation is used in addition to external radiation therapy. This gives the cancer cells a larger amount of radiation than would be possible using external radiation alone.

What are the side effects of treatment?

External radiation therapy does not cause your body to become radioactive. The radiation does not remain in your body after treatment (exception: see internal radiation therapy, or brachytherapy) There is no need to avoid being with other people because you are undergoing treatment. Even hugging, kissing, or having sexual relations with others poses no risk of radiation exposure.

Most side effects of radiation therapy are related to the area that is being treated. Many patients have no side effects at all. Your doctor and nurse will tell you about the possible side effects you might expect and how you should deal with them. You should contact your doctor or nurse if you have any unusual symptoms during your treatment, such as coughing, sweating, fever, or pain.

The side effects of radiation therapy, although unpleasant, are usually not serious and can be controlled with medication or diet. They usually go away within a few weeks after treatment ends, although some side effects can last longer.

Throughout your treatment, your doctor will regularly check on the effects of the treatment. You may not be aware of changes in the cancer, but you probably will notice decreases in pain, bleeding, or other discomfort. You may continue to notice further improvement after your treatment is completed.

Your doctor may recommend periodic tests and physical exams to be sure that the radiation is causing as little damage to normal cells as possible. Depending on the area being treated, you may have routine blood tests to check the levels of red blood cells, white blood cells, and platelets, as radiation treatment can cause decreases in the levels of different blood cells.

What can I do to take care of myself during therapy?

Each patient's body responds to radiation therapy in its own way. That's why your doctor must plan, and sometimes adjust, your treatment. In addition, your doctor or nurse will give you suggestions for caring for yourself at home that are specific for your treatment and the possible side effects.

Nearly all cancer patients receiving radiation therapy need to take special care of themselves to protect their health and to help the treatment succeed.

- Before starting treatment, be sure your doctor knows about any medicines you are taking and if you have any allergies. Do not start taking any medicine (whether prescription or over-the-counter) during your radiation therapy without first telling your doctor or nurse.

- Fatigue is common during radiation therapy. Your body will use a lot of extra energy over the course of your treatment, and you may feel very tired. Be sure to get plenty of rest and sleep as often as you feel the need. It's common for fatigue to last for four to six weeks after your treatment has been completed.

- Good nutrition is very important. Try to eat a balanced diet that will prevent weight loss.

- Check with your doctor before taking vitamin supplements or herbal preparations during treatment.

- Avoid wearing tight clothes such as girdles or close-fitting collars over the treatment area.

- Be extra kind to your skin in the treatment area:

  - Ask your doctor or nurse if you may use soaps, lotions, deodorants, sun blocks, medicines, perfumes, cosmetics, talcum powder, or other substances in the treated area.

  - Wear loose, soft cotton clothing over the treated area.

  - Do not wear starched or stiff clothing over the treated area.

  - Do not scratch, rub, or scrub treated skin.

  - Do not use adhesive tape on treated skin. If bandaging is necessary, use paper tape and apply it outside of the treatment area. Your nurse can help you place dressings so that you can avoid irritating the treated area.

  - Do not apply heat or cold (heating pad, ice pack, etc.) to the treated area. Use only lukewarm water for bathing the area.

  - Use an electric shaver if you must shave the treated area but only after checking with your doctor or nurse. Do not use a preshave lotion or hair removal products on the treated area.

  - Protect the treatment area from the sun. Do not apply sunscreens just before a radiation treatment. If possible, cover treated skin (with light clothing) before going outside. Ask your doctor if you should use a sunscreen or a sun-blocking product. If so, select one with a protection factor of at least fifteen and reapply it often. Ask your doctor or nurse how long after your treatments are completed you should continue to protect the treated skin from sunlight.

- If you have questions, ask your doctor or nurse. They are the only ones who can properly advise you about your treatment, its side effects, home care, and any other medical concerns you may have.

Internal Radiation Therapy: What to Expect

When is internal radiation therapy used?

Your doctor may decide that a high dose of radiation given to a small area of your body is the best way to treat your cancer. Internal radiation therapy allows the doctor to give a higher total dose of radiation in a shorter time than is possible with external treatment.

Internal radiation therapy places the radiation source as close as possible to the cancer cells. Instead of using a large radiation machine, the radioactive material, sealed in a thin wire, catheter, or tube (implant), is placed directly into the affected tissue. This method of treatment concentrates the radiation on the cancer cells and lessens radiation damage to some of the normal tissue near the cancer. Some of the radioactive substances used for internal radiation treatment include cesium, iridium, iodine, phosphorus, and palladium.

In this chapter, "internal radiation treatment" refers to implant radiation. Health professionals prefer to use the term *brachytherapy* for implant radiation therapy. You may hear your doctor or nurse use the terms *interstitial radiation* or *intracavitary radiation;* each is a form of internal radiation therapy. Sometimes radioactive implants are called "capsules" or "seeds."

How is the implant placed in the body?

The type of implant and the method of placing it depend on the size and location of the cancer. Implants may be put right into the tumor (interstitial radiation), in special applicators inside a body cavity (intracavitary radiation) or passage (intraluminal radiation), on the surface of a tumor, or in the area from which the tumor has been removed. Implants may be removed after a short time or left in place permanently. If they are to be left in place, the radioactive substance used will lose radiation quickly and become nonradioactive in a short time.

When interstitial radiation is given, the radiation source is placed in the tumor in catheters, seeds, or capsules. When intracavitary radiation is used, a container or applicator of radioactive material is placed in a body cavity such as the uterus. In surface brachytherapy the radioactive source is sealed in a small holder and placed in or against the tumor. In intraluminal brachytherapy the radioactive source is placed in a body lumen or tube, such as the bronchus or esophagus.

Internal radiation also may be given by injecting a solution of radioactive substance into the bloodstream or a body cavity. This form of radiation therapy may be called unsealed internal radiation therapy.

For most types of implants, you will need to be in the hospital. You will be given general or local anesthesia so that you will not feel any pain when the doctor places the holder for the radioactive material in your body. In many hospitals, the radioactive material is placed in its holder or applicator after you return to your room so that other patients, staff, and visitors are not exposed to radiation.

How are other people protected from radiation while the implant is in place?

Sometimes the radiation source in your implant sends its high-energy rays outside your body. To protect others while you are having implant therapy, the hospital will have you stay in a private room. Although the nurses and other people caring for you will not be able to spend a long time in your room, they will give you all of the care you need. You should call for a nurse when you need one, but keep in mind that the nurse will work quickly and speak to you from the doorway more often than from your bedside. In most cases, your urine and stool will contain no radioactivity unless you are having unsealed internal radiation therapy.

There also will be limits on visitors while your implant is in place. Children younger than eighteen or pregnant women should not visit patients who are having internal radiation therapy. Be sure to tell your visitors to ask the hospital staff for any special instructions before they come into your room. Visitors should sit at least six feet from your bed, and the radiation oncology staff will determine how long your visitors may stay. The time can vary from thirty minutes to several hours per day. In some hospitals a rolling lead shield is placed beside the bed and kept between the patient and visitors or staff members.

What are the side effects of internal radiation therapy?

The side effects of implant therapy depend on the area being treated. You are not likely to have severe pain or feel ill during implant therapy. However, if an applicator is holding your implant in place, it may be somewhat uncomfortable. If you need it, the doctor will order medicine to help you relax or to relieve pain. If general anesthesia was used while your implant was put in place, you may feel drowsy, weak, or nauseated but these effects do not last long. If necessary, medications can be ordered to relieve nausea.

How long does the implant stay in place?

Your doctor will decide the amount of time that an implant is to be left in place. It depends on the dose (amount) of radioactivity needed for effective treatment. Your treatment schedule will depend on the type of cancer, where it is located, your general health, and other cancer treatments you have had. Depending on where the implant is placed, you may have to keep it from shifting by staying in bed and lying fairly still.

Temporary implants may be either low dose-rate (LDR) or high dose-rate (HDR). Low dose-rate implants are left in place for several days; high dose-rate implants are removed after a few minutes.

For some cancer sites, the implant is left in place permanently. If your implant is permanent, you may need to stay in your hospital room away from other people for a few days while the radiation is most active. The implant becomes less radioactive each day; by the time you are ready to go home, the radiation in your body will be much weaker. Your doctor will advise you if there are any special precautions you need to use at home.

What happens after the implant is removed?

Usually, an anesthetic is not needed when the doctor removes a temporary implant. Most can be taken out right in the patient's hospital room. Once the implant is removed, there is no radioactivity in your body. The hospital staff and your visitors will no longer have to limit the time they stay with you.

Your doctor will tell you if you need to limit your activities after you leave the hospital. Most patients are allowed to do as much as they feel like doing. You may need some extra sleep or rest breaks during your days at home, but you should feel stronger quickly.

The area that has been treated with an implant may be sore or sensitive for some time. If any particular activities, such as sports or sexual intercourse, cause irritation in the treatment area, your doctor may suggest that you limit these activities for a while.

Remote Brachytherapy

In remote brachytherapy, a computer sends the radioactive source through a tube to a catheter that has been placed near the tumor by the patient's doctor. The procedure is directed by the brachytherapy team, who watch the patient on closed-circuit television and communicate with the patient using an intercom. The radioactivity remains at the tumor for only a few minutes. In some cases, several remote treatments may be required and the catheter may stay in place between treatments.

Remote brachytherapy may be used for low dose-rate (LDR) treatments in an inpatient setting. High dose-rate (HDR) remote brachytherapy allows a person to have internal radiation therapy in an outpatient setting. High dose-rate treatments take only a few minutes. Because no radioactive material is left in the body, the patient can return home after the treatment. Remote brachytherapy has been used to treat cancers of the cervix, breast, lung, pancreas, prostate, and esophagus.

Managing Side Effects

Are side effects the same for everyone?

The side effects of radiation treatment vary from patient to patient. You may have no side effects or only a few mild ones through your course of treatment. Some people do experience serious side effects, however. The side effects that you have depend mostly on the radiation dose and the part of your body that is treated. Your general health also can affect how your body reacts to radiation therapy and whether you have side effects. Before beginning your treatment, your doctor and nurse will discuss the side effects you might experience, how long they might last, and how serious they might be.

Side effects may be acute or chronic. Acute side effects are sometimes referred to as "early side effects." They occur soon after the treatment begins and usually are gone within a few weeks of finishing therapy. Chronic side effects, sometimes called "late side effects," may take months or years to develop and usually are permanent.

The most common early side effects of radiation therapy are fatigue and skin changes. They can result from radiation to any treatment site. Other side effects are related to treatment of specific areas. For example, temporary or permanent hair loss may be a side effect of radiation treatment to the head. Appetite can be altered if treatment affects the mouth, stomach, or intestine.

Fortunately, most side effects will go away in time. In the mean-time, there are ways to reduce discomfort. If you have a side effect that is especially severe, the doctor may prescribe a break in your treatments or change your treatment in some way.

Be sure to tell your doctor, nurse, or radiation therapist about any side effects that you notice. They can help you treat the problems and tell you how to lessen the chances that the side effects will come back. The information discussed here can serve as a guide to handling some side effects, but it cannot take the place of talking with the members of your health care team.

Will side effects limit my activity?

Not necessarily. It will depend on which side effects you have and how severe they are. Many patients are able to work, prepare meals, and enjoy their usual leisure activities while they are having radia-tion therapy. Others find that they need more rest than usual and therefore cannot do as much. Try to continue doing the things you enjoy as long as you don't become too tired.

Your doctor may suggest that you limit activities that might irri-tate the area being treated. In most cases, you can have sexual rela-tions if you wish. You may find that your desire for physical intimacy is lower because radiation therapy may cause you to feel more tired than usual. For most patients, these feelings are temporary.

What causes fatigue?

Fatigue, feeling tired and lacking energy, is the most common symp-tom reported by cancer patients. The exact cause is not always known. It may be due to the disease itself or to treatment. It may also result from lowered blood counts, lack of sleep, pain, and poor appetite.

Most people begin to feel tired after a few weeks of radiation therapy. During radiation therapy, the body uses a lot of energy for healing. You also may be tired because of stress related to your ill-ness, daily trips for treatment, and the effects of radiation on normal cells. Feelings of weakness or weariness will go away gradually after your treatment has been completed.

You can help yourself during radiation therapy by not trying to do too much. If you do feel tired, limit your activities and use your lei-sure time in a restful way. Save your energy for doing the things that you feel are most important. Do not feel that you have to do every-thing you normally do. Try to get more sleep at night, and plan your day so that you have time to rest if you need it. Several short naps or breaks may be more helpful than a long rest period.

Sometimes, light exercise such as walking may combat fatigue. Talk with your doctor or nurse about how much exercise you may do while you are having therapy. Talking with other cancer patients in a support group may also help you learn how to deal with fatigue.

If you have a full-time job, you may want to try to continue to work your normal schedule. However, some patients prefer to take time off while they're receiving radiation therapy; others work a reduced number of hours. Speak frankly with your employer about your needs and wishes during this time. A part-time schedule may be possible or perhaps you can do some work at home. Ask your doctor's office or the radiation therapy department to help by trying to schedule treatments with your workday in mind.

Whether you're going to work or not, it's a good idea to ask family members or friends to help with daily chores, shopping, child care, housework, or driving. Neighbors may be able to help by picking up groceries for you when they do their own shopping. You also could ask someone to drive you to and from your treatment visits to help conserve your energy.

How are skin problems treated?

You may notice that your skin in the treatment area is red or irritated. It may look as if it is sunburned, or tanned. After a few weeks your skin may be very dry from the therapy. Ask your doctor or nurse for advice on how to relieve itching or discomfort.

With some kinds of radiation therapy, treated skin may develop a "moist reaction," especially in areas where there are skin folds. When this happens, the skin is wet and it may become very sore. It's important to notify your doctor or nurse if your skin develops a moist reaction. They can give you suggestions on how to care for these areas and prevent them from becoming infected.

During radiation therapy you will need to be very gentle with the skin in the treatment area. The following suggestions may be helpful:

- Avoid irritating treated skin.

- When you wash, use only lukewarm water and mild soap; pat dry.

- Do not wear tight clothing over the area.

- Do not rub, scrub, or scratch the skin in the treatment area.

- Avoid putting anything that is hot or cold, such as heating pads or ice packs, on your treated skin.

- Ask your doctor or nurse to recommend skin care products that will not cause skin irritation. Do not use any powders, creams, perfumes, deodorants, body oils, ointments, lotions, or home remedies in the treatment area while you're being treated and for several weeks afterward unless approved by your doctor or nurse.

- Do not apply any skin lotions within two hours of a treatment.

- Avoid exposing the radiated area to the sun during treatment. If you expect to be in the sun for more than a few minutes you will need to be very careful. Wear protective clothing (such as a hat with a broad brim and a shirt with long sleeves) and use a sunscreen. Ask your doctor or nurse about using sun-blocking lotions. After your treatment is over, ask your doctor or nurse how long you should continue to take extra precautions in the sun.

The majority of skin reactions to radiation therapy go away a few weeks after treatment is completed. In some cases, though, the treated skin will remain slightly darker than it was before and it may continue to be more sensitive to sun exposure. After some kinds of radiation therapy, particularly cobalt radiation, the exposed skin may develop a hard or woody texture over months or years. This is due to scarring within the skin from radiation injury, and is usually permanent.

How are side effects on the blood managed?

Radiation therapy can cause low levels of white blood cells and platelets. These blood cells normally help your body fight infection and prevent bleeding. If large areas of active bone marrow are treated, your red blood cell count may be low as well. If your blood tests show these side effects, your doctor may wait until your blood counts increase to continue treatments. Your doctor will check your blood counts regularly and change your treatment schedule if it is necessary.

Will eating be a problem?

Sometimes radiation treatment causes loss of appetite and interferes with eating, digesting, and absorbing food. Try to eat enough to help damaged tissues rebuild themselves. It is not unusual to lose one or two pounds a week during radiation therapy. You will be weighed weekly to monitor your weight.

It is very important to eat a balanced diet. You may find it helpful to eat small meals often and to try to eat a variety of different foods. Your doctor or nurse can tell you whether you should eat a special diet, and a dietitian will have some ideas that will help you maintain your weight.

Coping with short-term diet problems may be easier than you expect. There are a number of diet guides and recipe booklets for patients who need help with eating problems.

If it's painful to chew and swallow, your doctor may advise you to use a powdered or liquid diet supplement. Many of these products are available at drugstores and supermarkets and come in a variety of flavors. They are tasty when used alone or combined with other foods such as pureed fruit, or added to milkshakes. Some of the companies that make these diet supplements have recipe booklets to help you increase your nutrient intake. Ask your nurse, dietitian, or pharmacist for further information.

You may lose interest in food during your treatment. Fatigue from your treatments can cause loss of appetite. Some people just don't feel like eating because of stress from their illness and treatment or because the treatment changes the way food tastes. Even if you're not very hungry, it's important to keep your protein and calorie intake high. Doctors have found that patients who eat well can better cope with having cancer and with the side effects of treatment. Medications for appetite enhancement are now available; ask your doctor or nurse about them.

The following list suggests ways to perk up your appetite when it's poor and to make the most of it when you do feel like eating.

- Eat when you are hungry, even if it is not mealtime.

- Eat several small meals during the day rather than three large ones.

- Use soft lighting, quiet music, brightly colored table settings, or whatever helps you feel good while eating.

- Vary your diet and try new recipes. If you enjoy company while eating, try to have meals with family or friends. It may be helpful to have the radio or television on while you eat.

- Ask your doctor or nurse whether you can have a glass of wine or beer with your meal to increase your appetite. Keep in mind that, in some cases, alcohol may not be allowed because it could worsen the side effects of treatment.

- Keep simple meals in the freezer to use when you feel hungry.

- If other people offer to cook for you, let them. Don't be shy about telling them what you'd like to eat.

- Keep healthy snacks close by for nibbling when you get the urge.

- If you live alone, you might want to arrange for "Meals on Wheels" to bring food to you. Ask your doctor, nurse, social worker, or local social service agencies about "Meals on Wheels." This service is available in most large communities.

If you are able to eat only small amounts of food, you can increase the calories per serving by:

- Adding butter or margarine.

- Mixing canned cream soups with milk or half-and-half rather than water.

- Drinking eggnog, milkshakes, or prepared liquid supplements between meals.

- Adding cream sauce or melted cheese to your favorite vegetables.

Some people find they can drink large amounts of liquids even when they don't feel like eating solid foods. If this is the case for you, try to get the most from each glassful by making drinks enriched with powdered milk, yogurt, honey, or prepared liquid supplements.

Radiation Therapy and Emotional Effects

Nearly all patients being treated for cancer report feeling emotionally upset at different times during their therapy. It's not unusual to feel anxious, depressed, afraid, angry, frustrated, alone, or helpless. Radiation therapy may affect your emotions indirectly through fatigue or changes in hormone balance, but the treatment itself is not a direct cause of mental distress.

You may find that it's helpful to talk about your feelings with a close friend, family member, chaplain, nurse, social worker, or psychologist with whom you feel at ease. You may want to ask your doctor or nurse about meditation or relaxation exercises that might help you unwind and feel calmer.

Nationwide support programs can help cancer patients to meet others who share common problems and concerns. Some medical centers have formed peer support groups so that patients can meet to discuss their feelings and inspire each other.

Side Effects with Radiation Therapy for Breast Cancer

The most common side effects with radiation therapy for breast cancer are fatigue and skin changes. However there may be other side effects as well. If you notice that your shoulder feels stiff, ask your doctor or nurse about exercises to keep your arm moving freely. Other side effects include breast or nipple soreness, swelling from fluid buildup in the treated area, and skin reddening or tanning. Except for tanning, which may take up to six months to fade, these side effects will most likely disappear in four to six weeks.

If you are being treated for breast cancer and you are having radiation therapy after a lumpectomy or mastectomy, it's a good idea to go without your bra whenever possible or, if this makes you more uncomfortable, wear a soft cotton bra without underwires. This will help reduce skin irritation in the treatment area.

Radiation therapy after a lumpectomy may cause additional changes in the treated breast after therapy is complete. These long-term side effects may continue for a year or longer after treatment. The skin redness will fade, leaving your skin slightly darker, just as when a sunburn fades to a suntan. The pores in the skin of your breast may be enlarged and more noticeable. Some women report increased sensitivity of the skin on the breast; others have decreased feeling. The skin and the fatty tissue of the breast may feel thicker and firmer than it was before your radiation treatment. Sometimes the size of your breast changes—it may become larger because of fluid buildup or smaller because of the development of scar tissue. Many women have little or no change in size.

Your radiation therapy plan may include temporary implants of radioactive material in the area around your lumpectomy. A week or two after external treatment is completed, these implants are inserted during a short hospitalization. The implants may cause breast tenderness or a feeling of tightness. After they are removed, you are likely to notice some of the same effects that occur with external treatment. If so, let your doctor or nurse know about any problems that persist.

Most changes resulting from radiation therapy for breast cancer are seen within ten to twelve months after completing therapy. Occasionally small red areas called telangiectasias appear. These are areas of dilated blood vessels and the color may fade with time. If you see new changes in breast size, shape, appearance, or texture after this time, report them to your doctor at once.

Follow-up Care

What does "follow-up" mean?

Once you have completed your radiation treatments, it is important for your doctor to monitor the results of your therapy at regularly scheduled visits. These checkups are necessary to deal with radiation side effects and to detect any signs of recurrent disease. During these checkups your doctor will examine you and may order some lab tests and x-rays. The radiation oncologist also will want to see you for follow-up after your treatment ends and will coordinate follow-up care with your doctor.

Follow-up care might include more cancer treatment, rehabilitation, and counseling. Taking good care of yourself is also an important part of following through after radiation treatments.

Who provides care after therapy?

Most patients return to the radiation oncologist for regular follow-up visits. Others are referred to their original doctor, to a surgeon, or to a medical oncologist. Your follow-up care will depend on the kind of cancer that was treated and on other treatments that you had or may need.

What other care might be needed?

Just as every patient is different, follow-up care varies. Your doctor will prescribe and schedule the follow-up care that you need. Don't hesitate to ask about the tests or treatments that your doctor orders. Try to learn all the things you need to do to take good care of yourself.

Following are some questions that you may want to ask your doctor after you have finished your radiation therapy:

- How often do I need to return for checkups?

- Why do I need more x-rays, CT-scans, blood tests, and so on? What will these tests tell us?

- Will I need chemotherapy, surgery, or other treatments?

- How and when will you know if I'm cured of cancer?

- What are the chances that it will come back?

- How soon can I go back to my regular activities? Work? Sexual activity? Sports?

- Do I need to take any special precautions like staying out of the sun or avoiding people with infectious diseases?

- Do I need a special diet?

- Should I exercise?

- Can I wear a prosthesis?

- Can I have reconstructive surgery? How soon can I schedule it?

It's a good idea to write down the questions you want to ask your doctor and take them with you to your appointment. Some patients find that it's helpful to take a family member with them to help remember what the doctor says.

When Pain Is a Problem

Radiation therapy is not painful. However, some radiation side effects may cause discomfort. In addition, when radiation is used for palliation some discomfort or pain may remain. Sometimes patients need help to manage cancer pain. Over-the-counter pain medicine may be enough for mild pain. Remember that you should not use a heating pad or a warm compress to relieve pain in any area treated with radiation.

If your pain is severe, ask the doctor about prescription drugs or other methods of relief. Try to be specific about your pain (How severe is it on a scale of 0–10 where 0 is no pain and 10 is the worst pain you can imagine? Where is your pain? Is the pain throbbing, stabbing, or searing? Is it continuous or intermittent? What makes it better or worse?) when you tell the doctor about it so you can get the best pain management. If you are unable to get pain relief, you may want to ask your doctor for a referral to a pain specialist.

Because fear and worry can make pain worse, you may find that relaxation exercises are helpful. Other methods such as hypnosis, biofeedback, and acupuncture may be useful for some cancer pain. Be sure to discuss these complementary or alternative treatments with

413

your doctor or nurse. Sometimes complementary therapies can interfere with other treatment you are having. They can also be harmful when combined with other treatment.

Self-Care after Radiation Therapy

Patients who have had radiation therapy need to continue some of the special care they used during treatment, at least for a short while. For instance, you may have skin problems for several weeks after your treatments end. Continue to be gentle with skin in the treatment area until all signs of irritation are gone. Don't try to scrub off the marks in your treatment area. If tattoos were used to mark the treatment area, they are permanent and will not wash off. Your nurse can answer questions about skin care and help you with other concerns you may have after your treatment has been completed.

You may find that you still need extra rest after your therapy is over while your healthy tissues are recovering and rebuilding. Keep taking naps as needed and try to get more sleep at night. It may take some time to get your strength back, so resume your normal schedule of activities gradually. If you feel that you need emotional or social support, ask your doctor, nurse, or a social worker for information about support groups or other ways to express your feelings and concerns.

Returning to Work

Many people find that they can continue to work during radiation therapy because treatment appointments are short. If you have stopped working, you can return to your job as soon as you feel up to it. If your job requires lifting or heavy physical activity, you may need a change in your work responsibilities until you have regained your strength. Check with your employer to see if a "return to work" release from your doctor is required.

Chapter 58

Adjuvant Therapy for Breast Cancer: Questions and Answers

Researchers have been studying breast cancer for many years to learn how best to treat this disease. They have given special attention to ways to prevent breast cancer from recurring (returning) after primary treatment.

Scientists once thought that breast cancer metastasized (spread) first to nearby tissue and underarm lymph nodes before spreading to other parts of the body. They now believe that cancer cells may break away from the primary tumor in the breast and begin to metastasize even when the disease is in an early stage.

Adjuvant therapy is treatment given in addition to the primary therapy to kill any cancer cells that may have spread, even if the spread cannot be detected by radiologic or laboratory tests. Studies have shown that adjuvant therapy for breast cancer may increase the chance of long-term survival by preventing a recurrence.

What types of primary therapy are used for breast cancer?

Primary therapy for breast cancer generally involves lumpectomy and radiation therapy or modified radical mastectomy. A lumpectomy is the removal of the primary breast tumor and a small amount of surrounding tissue. Usually, most of the underarm lymph nodes are also removed. A lumpectomy is followed by radiation treatment to the breast. A modified radical mastectomy is the removal of the whole

---

Cancer Facts, National Cancer Institute, May 2002.

breast, most of the lymph nodes under the arm, and often the lining over the chest muscles. The smaller of the two chest muscles is sometimes taken out to help in removing the lymph nodes.

Doctors are evaluating a new procedure, called sentinel lymph node biopsy or sentinel node biopsy, in which only a single lymph node is removed and tested to determine if the breast cancer has spread to lymph nodes under the arm. Clinical trials (research studies with humans) are in progress to determine the role of this procedure in the treatment of breast cancer.

What types of adjuvant therapy are used for breast cancer?

Because the principal purpose of adjuvant therapy is to kill any cancer cells that may have spread, treatment is usually systemic (uses substances that travel through the bloodstream, reaching and affecting cancer cells all over the body). Adjuvant therapy for breast cancer involves chemotherapy or hormone therapy, either alone or in combination:

- Adjuvant chemotherapy is the use of drugs to kill cancer cells. Research has shown that using chemotherapy as adjuvant therapy for early stage breast cancer helps to prevent the original cancer from returning. Adjuvant chemotherapy is usually a combination of anticancer drugs, which has been shown to be more effective than a single anticancer drug.

- Adjuvant hormone therapy deprives cancer cells of the female hormone estrogen, which some breast cancer cells need to grow. Most often, adjuvant hormone therapy is treatment with the drug tamoxifen. Research has shown that when tamoxifen is used as adjuvant therapy for early stage breast cancer, it helps to prevent the original cancer from returning and also helps to prevent the development of new cancers in the other breast. The ovaries are the main source of estrogen prior to menopause. For premenopausal women with breast cancer, adjuvant hormone therapy may involve tamoxifen to deprive the cancer cells of estrogen. Drugs to suppress the production of estrogen by the ovaries are under investigation. Alternatively, surgery may be performed to remove the ovaries.

(Although this chapter focuses on systemic adjuvant therapy, radiation therapy is sometimes used as a local adjuvant treatment. Radiation therapy is considered adjuvant treatment when it is given

416

before or after a mastectomy. Such treatment is intended to destroy breast cancer cells that have spread to nearby parts of the body, such as the chest wall or lymph nodes. Radiation therapy is part of primary therapy, not adjuvant therapy, when it follows breast-sparing surgery.)

What are prognostic factors, and what do they have to do with adjuvant therapy?

Prognostic factors are characteristics of breast tumors that help predict whether the disease is likely to recur. Doctors consider these factors when they are deciding which patients might benefit from adjuvant therapy.

Several prognostic factors are commonly used to plan breast cancer treatment:

- **Tumor size.** Prognosis (probable outcome of the disease) is closely linked to tumor size. In general, patients with small tumors (2 centimeters [a little more than three-quarters of an inch] or less in diameter) have a better prognosis than do patients with larger tumors (especially those that are more than 5 centimeters [2 inches] in diameter).

- **Lymph node involvement.** Lymph nodes in the underarm are a common site of breast cancer spread. Doctors usually remove some of the underarm lymph nodes to determine whether they contain cancer cells. If cancer is found, the nodes are said to be "positive." If the lymph nodes are free of cancer, the nodes are said to be "negative." Breast cancer that is node-positive is more likely to recur than cancer that is node-negative, because if cancer cells have spread to the lymph nodes it is more likely that they have also spread elsewhere in the body.

- **Hormone receptor status.** Cells in the breast contain receptors for the female hormones estrogen and progesterone. These receptors allow the breast tissue to grow or change in response to changing hormone levels. Research has shown that about two-thirds of all breast cancers contain significant levels of estrogen receptors. These tumors are said to be estrogen-receptor-positive (ER+). About 40 percent to 50 percent of all breast cancers have progesterone receptors. These tumors are said to be progesterone-receptor-positive (PR+). ER+ tumors tend to grow less aggressively than ER- tumors. The result is a better prognosis for patients with ER+ tumors.

- **Histologic grade.** This term refers to how much the tumor cells resemble normal cells when viewed under the microscope. Tumors composed of cells that closely resemble normal breast cells and structures are called well differentiated. Tumors with cells that bear little or no resemblance to normal breast cells are called poorly differentiated. Tumors that have "in between" cells are called moderately differentiated. For most types of invasive breast cancer, patients who have tumors with cells that are well differentiated tend to have a better prognosis.

- **Proliferative capacity of a tumor.** This factor refers to the rate at which the cancer cells divide to form more cells. Cells that have a high proliferative capacity divide more often and are more aggressive (fast growing) than those with a low proliferative capacity. Patients who have tumors with cells that have a low proliferative capacity (i.e., divide less often and grow more slowly) tend to have a better prognosis. Scientists estimate the proliferative capacity of the tumor using such tests as flow cytometry, which includes the S-phase fraction measurement. The S-phase fraction is the percentage of tumor cells that are dividing. Tumors with a high S-phase fraction tend to have an increased risk of recurrence.

- **Oncogene activation.** The activation of an oncogene (a gene that causes or promotes unrestrained cell growth) can make normal cells become abnormal or convert a normal cell into a tumor cell. Patients whose tumor cells contain an oncogene called HER-2/neu, also called erb B2, may be more likely to have a recurrence. Some research studies suggest that HER-2/neu may be associated with resistance to certain anticancer drugs; however, more research is needed.

Who is given adjuvant therapy?

Although prognostic factors provide important information about the risk of recurrence, they do not enable doctors to predict exactly who will be cured by primary therapy and who may benefit from adjuvant therapy. Decisions about adjuvant therapy for breast cancer must be made on an individual basis, taking into account the prognostic factors described previously, the woman's menopausal status (whether she has gone through menopause), her general health, and her personal preference. This complicated decision-making process is best carried out by consulting an oncologist, a doctor who specializes in cancer treatment.

Clinical trials are in progress to learn how to identify women most likely to benefit from adjuvant therapy and those who do not require this treatment.

When is adjuvant therapy started?

Adjuvant therapy usually begins within six weeks after surgery, based on the results of clinical trials in which the therapy was started within that time period. Doctors do not know how effective adjuvant therapy is in reducing the chance of recurrence when treatment is started at a later time.

How is adjuvant therapy given, and how long does it last?

Chemotherapy is given by mouth or by injection into a blood vessel. Either way, the drugs enter the bloodstream and travel throughout the body. Chemotherapy is given in cycles: a treatment period followed by a recovery period, then another treatment period, and so on. Most patients receive treatment in an outpatient part of the hospital or at the doctor's office. Adjuvant chemotherapy usually lasts for three to six months.

In adjuvant hormone therapy, tamoxifen is taken orally. Tamoxifen enters the bloodstream and travels throughout the body. Most women take tamoxifen every day for five years. Studies have indicated that taking tamoxifen for longer than five years is not any more effective than taking it for five years. Premenopausal women may receive hormones by injection to suppress ovarian function. Alternatively, surgery can be performed to remove the ovaries.

What are some of the side effects of adjuvant therapy, and what can be done to help manage them?

The side effects of chemotherapy depend mainly on the drugs the patient receives. As with other types of treatment, side effects vary from person to person. In general, anticancer drugs affect rapidly dividing cells. These include blood cells, which fight infection, cause the blood to clot, and carry oxygen to all parts of the body. When blood cells are affected by anticancer drugs, patients are more likely to get infections, bruise or bleed easily, and may have less energy during treatment and for some time afterward. Cells in hair follicles and cells that line the digestive tract also divide rapidly. As a result of chemotherapy, patients may lose their hair and may have other side effects, such as loss of appetite, nausea, vomiting, diarrhea, or mouth sores.

Doctors can prescribe medications to help control nausea and vomiting caused by chemotherapy. They also monitor patients for any signs of other problems and may adjust the dose or schedule of treatment if problems arise. In addition, doctors advise women who have a lowered resistance to infection because of low blood cell counts to avoid crowds and people who are sick or have colds. The side effects of chemotherapy are generally short-term problems. They gradually go away during the recovery part of the chemotherapy cycle or after the treatment is over.

In general, the side effects of tamoxifen are similar to some of the symptoms of menopause. The most common side effects are hot flashes, vaginal discharge, and nausea. As is the case with menopause, not all women who take tamoxifen have these symptoms. Most of these side effects do not require medical attention.

Doctors carefully monitor women taking tamoxifen for any signs of more serious side effects. Women taking tamoxifen, particularly those who are receiving chemotherapy along with tamoxifen, have a greater risk of developing a blood clot. The risk of having a blood clot due to tamoxifen is similar to the risk of a blood clot when taking estrogen replacement therapy. Women taking tamoxifen also have an increased risk of stroke.

Among women who have not had a hysterectomy (surgery to remove the uterus), the risk of developing endometrial cancer (cancer of the lining of the uterus) and uterine sarcoma (cancer of the muscular wall of the uterus) is increased in those taking tamoxifen. Women who take tamoxifen should talk with their doctor about having regular pelvic exams, and should be examined promptly if they have pelvic pain or any abnormal vaginal bleeding.

Careful studies have shown that the risks of adjuvant therapy for breast cancer are outweighed by the benefit of the treatment—increasing the chance of survival. Still, it is important for women to share any concerns they may have about their treatment or side effects with their doctor or other health care provider.

More information and printed materials about the side effects of chemotherapy and tamoxifen can be obtained from the Cancer Information Service at 1-800-4-CANCER (1-800-422-6237).

How are doctors and scientists trying to answer questions about adjuvant therapy for breast cancer?

Doctors and scientists are conducting research studies called clinical trials to learn how to treat breast cancer more effectively. In these studies, researchers compare two or more groups of patients who receive different treatments. Such studies can show whether new treatments are more or less effective than standard ones and how the side effects compare. People who participate in clinical trials have the first opportunity to benefit from new treatments while helping to increase medical knowledge.

Women with breast cancer who are interested in taking part in a clinical trial should ask their doctor whether this would be appropriate for them. Information about current clinical trials can be obtained from the National Cancer Institute (NCI)-supported Cancer Information Service or the clinical trials page of the NCI's Web site at http://cancer.gov/clinical_trials/ on the internet.

Chapter 59

Herceptin (Trastuzumab): Questions and Answers

What is Herceptin? How does it work?

Herceptin® (trastuzumab) is a monoclonal antibody. It belongs to a group of drugs made in the laboratory that are designed to attack specific cancer cells. Herceptin is given intravenously (by injection into a blood vessel) to treat some breast cancers. Genentech, Inc., located in South San Francisco, manufactures Herceptin.

Herceptin targets cancer cells that "overexpress," or make too much of, a protein called HER-2 or erb B2, which is found on the surface of cancer cells. Herceptin slows or stops the growth of these cells. Herceptin is used only to treat cancers that overexpress the HER-2 protein.

Approximately 25 to 30 percent of breast cancers overexpress HER–2. These tumors tend to grow faster and are generally more likely to recur (come back) than tumors that do not overproduce HER-2.

The amount of HER-2 protein in the tumor is measured in the laboratory using a scale from 0 (negative) to 3+ (strongly positive). The result helps the doctor determine whether a patient might benefit from treatment with Herceptin. Patients whose tumors are strongly positive for HER-2 protein overexpression (a score of 3+ on the laboratory test) are more likely to benefit. There is no evidence of benefit in patients whose tumors do not overexpress HER-2 (a score of 0 or 1+ on the laboratory test).

Cancer Facts, National Cancer Institute, February 14, 2002.

How is Herceptin currently used in the treatment of cancer?

Herceptin is approved by the U.S. Food and Drug Administration (FDA) for the treatment of metastatic breast cancer (breast cancer that has spread to other parts of the body). Herceptin can be given by itself or along with chemotherapy.

Researchers continue to study Herceptin in clinical trials (research studies with people). These studies can show whether new treatments are more or less effective than standard ones and how the side effects compare.

What are some of the common side effects of Herceptin?

Side effects that most commonly occur during the first treatment with Herceptin include fever and chills. Other possible side effects include pain, weakness, nausea, vomiting, diarrhea, headaches, difficulty breathing, and rashes. These side effects generally become less severe after the first treatment with Herceptin.

Patients who receive Herceptin along with chemotherapy may experience side effects that are different from those of patients who take Herceptin by itself. Patients should discuss any concerns about the side effects of treatment with their doctor. The doctor may be able to make suggestions for managing side effects.

Can Herceptin cause any serious side effects?

Herceptin can cause damage to the heart muscle that can lead to heart failure. Symptoms of heart failure include shortness of breath, difficulty breathing, a fast or irregular heartbeat, increased cough, and swelling of the feet or lower legs.

Herceptin can also affect the lungs, causing severe or life-threatening breathing problems that require immediate medical attention.

Herceptin may also cause allergic reactions that can be severe or life-threatening. These reactions can involve a drop in blood pressure, shortness of breath, rashes, and wheezing. These reactions may be more common in patients who already have breathing difficulties or lung disease.

Because of these potentially life-threatening side effects, patients are evaluated carefully for any heart or lung problems before starting treatment and are monitored closely during treatment. Patients who develop any problems during or after treatment should call the doctor immediately or go to the nearest emergency care facility.

How did scientists study the effectiveness of Herceptin before it was approved by the FDA?

The safety and effectiveness of Herceptin were studied in two clinical trials with women whose metastatic breast cancers produced excess amounts of HER–2. In one clinical trial, women received either Herceptin and chemotherapy or chemotherapy alone. The women who received Herceptin and chemotherapy had slower tumor growth, greater reduction in tumor size, and longer survival than the women who received chemotherapy alone. In another trial, women received Herceptin by itself. In 14 percent of these women, the tumor got smaller or disappeared. Scientists continue to study the safety and effectiveness of Herceptin in clinical trials (see following).

Is Herceptin being studied to treat nonmetastatic breast cancer?

Yes. The National Cancer Institute (NCI) is sponsoring two large, multicenter phase III clinical trials of Herceptin as adjuvant therapy to treat node-positive breast cancer; this is breast cancer that has spread to the lymph nodes under the arm (regional lymph nodes), but not to other parts of the body. These trials will take place in hospitals and cancer centers around the country. Adjuvant therapy is treatment given in addition to the primary therapy to kill any cancer cells that may have spread, even if the spread cannot be detected by radiologic or laboratory tests.

- The National Surgical Adjuvant Breast and Bowel Project (NSABP) is comparing chemotherapy alone to chemotherapy plus Herceptin for patients with node-positive breast cancer. This trial will enroll 2,700 patients.

- The North Central Cancer Treatment Group (NCCTG) is leading an Intergroup study to compare three different treatments in patients with node-positive breast cancer. This trial will enroll 3,000 patients.

A third clinical trial comparing three different treatments in patients with node-positive breast cancer or patients with high-risk node-negative disease is being coordinated by the Jonsson Comprehensive Cancer Center at the University of California Los Angeles (UCLA) and the Breast Cancer International Research Group (BCIRG). High-risk node-negative patients include those who are under thirty-five years old or who have a tumor that is more than 2 centimeters (a little more than three-quarters of an inch) in diameter or a tumor that is estrogen- or progesterone-receptor negative (a tumor that does not depend on these hormones in order to grow). This trial will enroll 3,150 patients.

Patients who are interested in receiving Herceptin as adjuvant therapy for breast cancer should consider participating in a clinical trial. For more information about these and other clinical trials, patients and doctors may call the Cancer Information Service (CIS) at 1-800-4-CANCER (1-800-422-6237) or visit the NCI's website at http://cancer.gov on the internet.

Is Herceptin under study for cancers other than breast cancer?

Yes. Herceptin is also being studied in clinical trials for other types of cancer, including osteosarcoma (a type of bone cancer) and cancers of the lung, pancreas, salivary gland, colon, prostate, endometrium (lining of the uterus), and bladder. Some patients with these types of cancer have tumors that overexpress the HER-2 protein. These patients will be possible candidates for clinical trials with Herceptin.

Researchers are exploring the use of Herceptin by itself and in combination with anticancer drugs. They are also investigating the use of Herceptin with other types of cancer treatment.

Chapter 60

New Treatment Significantly Improves Long-Term Outlook for Breast Cancer Survivors

A Canadian-led international clinical trial has found that post-menopausal survivors of early-stage breast cancer who took the drug letrozole after completing an initial five years of tamoxifen therapy had a significantly reduced risk of cancer recurrence compared to women taking a placebo. The results of the study appear in the *New England Journal of Medicine.*

The clinical trial has been halted early because of the positive results, and researchers are notifying the 5,187 women worldwide who have participated in the study. Women on letrozole will continue taking the drug, and those on the placebo can begin taking letrozole, if they wish.

"This very important advance in breast cancer treatment will improve the outlook for many thousands of women," said Andrew von Eschenbach, M.D., director of the National Cancer Institute, which led the study in the United States. "This is one more example of the ability to interrupt the progression of a cancer using a drug that blocks a crucial metabolic pathway in the tumor cell."

Study researchers found that letrozole, when taken after five years of tamoxifen therapy, substantially increased the chance of remaining cancer free. In total, 132 women taking the placebo had their disease recur, compared to 75 on letrozole. Overall, letrozole reduced the risk of recurrence by 43 percent, so that after four years of participating in the

Reprinted from "New Treatment Significantly Improves Long-Term Outlook for Breast Cancer Survivors," National Cancer Institute, October 9, 2003.

trial, 13 percent of the women on the placebo, but only 7 percent of those on letrozole had recurred. Deaths from breast cancer were also reduced. Seventeen women taking the placebo died of breast cancer, compared to nine taking letrozole.

While tamoxifen is widely used to prevent breast cancer recurrence in postmenopausal women, it stops being effective after five years because, researchers believe, tumors become resistant to it.

"More than half of women who develop recurrent breast cancer do so more than five years after their original diagnosis," says Paul Goss, M.D., of Princess Margaret Hospital in Toronto. "For years, we have thought that we had reached the limit of what we could do to reduce the risk of recurrence with five years of tamoxifen. Our study ushers in a new era of hope by cutting these ongoing recurrences and deaths from breast cancer after tamoxifen by almost one half." Goss, a leading expert in novel hormone therapies for the treatment and prevention of breast cancer, conceived and chaired the international trial with letrozole.

A form of hormone therapy for the treatment of breast cancer, letrozole works by limiting the ability of an enzyme called aromatase to produce estrogen, a major growth stimulant in many breast cancers.

Mayo Clinic medical oncologist James Ingle, M.D., says, "Based on our findings, all postmenopausal women with hormone-receptor positive tumors completing about five years of tamoxifen should discuss taking letrozole with their doctors to reduce their risk of breast cancer recurrence." Ingle, from Rochester, Minnesota, led the research study in the United States.

With Canadian Cancer Society funding, the clinical trial was coordinated by the National Cancer Institute of Canada Clinical Trials Group at Queen's University, in partnership with the U.S. National Cancer Institute and its Clinical Trials Cooperative Groups. Novartis, which manufactures letrozole, also known as Femara®, provided the drug for the trial.

Women participated in the study for an average of 2.4 years and for as long as five years. The study found that women taking letrozole had a reduction in the number of recurrences of cancer in their previously affected breast, a reduction in the number of new cancers in their opposite breast, and a reduction in the spread of the cancer outside their breast.

The side effects of letrozole, a pill which is taken once a day, are very similar to those experienced by women undergoing menopause. They were generally mild in study participants. Women in the study will continue to be followed to more thoroughly assess any effects of long-term use of letrozole on bone strength or other organs. Until these are known, patients should be monitored closely.

"The Canadian Cancer Society is pleased to have made a key contribution to this study," says Barbara Whylie, M.D., director of Cancer Control Policy for the Canadian Cancer Society. "We estimate that more than twenty thousand Canadian women will be diagnosed with breast cancer this year and just over half of those are going to be eligible for this drug. That means these women will have a significantly improved hope for a future without cancer."

"This large trial only began in 1998 and we already have important results that will change clinical practice," says Jeffrey Abrams, M.D., coordinator of the U.S. National Cancer Institute's Cooperative Group breast cancer treatment trials. "This is a tribute to the patients and physicians who participated, since their efforts will now have a positive impact on so many lives."

Participants in the clinical trial were enrolled through hospitals, cancer centers, and institutes throughout Canada, the United States, England, Belgium, Ireland, Italy, Poland, Portugal, and Switzerland. The European Organization for Research and Treatment of Cancer and the International Breast Cancer Study Group coordinated the European component of the trial.

The Canadian Cancer Society is the largest charitable supporter of cancer research in Canada. It funds clinical trials research through its support of the National Cancer Institute of Canada Clinical Trials Group.

The National Cancer Institute is the primary U.S. agency for cancer research.

Additional Resources

For more information on the results of this clinical trial and what it might mean for you:

A Q&A on this finding can be found at: http://cancer.gov/newscenter/pressreleases/letrozoleQandA

More information on aromatase inhibitors can be found at: http://cancer.gov/clinicaltrials/developments/aromatase-inhibitors-digest

In Canada, call the Canadian Cancer Society at 1-888-939-3333, Monday to Friday, 9 A.M. to 6 P.M., or visit www.cancer.ca. Service is available in English and French.

In the United States, call the National Cancer Institute's Cancer Information Service at 1-800-422-6237, Monday to Friday, 9 A.M. to 4:30 P.M. or visit www.cancer.gov. Service is available in English and Spanish.

Chapter 61

Complementary Cancer Therapies

Introduction

Complementary therapies are treatments or health care practices that are not currently part of conventional medicine [2]. Use of such therapies in the United States is increasing, and this trend is reflected in the number of women with breast cancer who are seeking complementary therapy [3]. Moreover, a growing number of medical institutions now offer integrated approaches to cancer treatment, incorporating complementary therapies into standard treatment regimens.

Women living with breast cancer choose to supplement their conventional treatment with complementary therapies for a variety of reasons. Although conventional cancer treatments (such as surgery, radiation therapy, and chemotherapy) are constantly improving, many women want to feel they are doing something on a personal level to help fight the disease. These women may find that complementary therapies provide some sense of empowerment and control over their healing. For other women, using complementary therapies may offer hope for survival and improve their mental outlook. Still other women may wish to improve their quality of life by reducing the side effects of chemotherapy. Regardless of the reason, many women are increasingly turning to complementary therapies to cope with breast cancer. While these therapies cannot offer a cure for cancer, they can offer many potential physical, mental, and spiritual benefits when integrated with conventional treatment [4].

The Evidence for Complementary Therapies

Complementary therapies are considered unconventional because most of them have not yet undergone the rigorous testing of conventional therapies in terms of their safety and effectiveness. When considering the evidence around a particular complementary therapy, it is essential to understand what constitutes an adequate body of scientific research and to keep in mind a general hierarchy of evidence. Much of what we know about complementary therapies comes from anecdotal evidence—someone's personal report that a particular therapy is helpful in treating a particular disease or symptom. Although such anecdotal evidence may lead to the formal study of a particular therapy, it is not objective and is therefore not considered scientific evidence.

Conventional cancer treatments go through rigorous study before they become part of standard care. They are examined first in studies of cells and then in animals to determine their effectiveness and safety. Only the treatments that pass muster in both types of studies will be tested in humans. When a treatment finally reaches the human study phase (which can take many years), the first step is to rigorously assess its safety. Once this has been established, the treatment will be studied for its effectiveness. Treatments are accepted by the medical community only when they have undergone this extensive study and have been proven both safe and effective in humans.

Complementary therapies have not gone through this same rigorous evaluation and cannot be compared to conventional medical treatments in terms of safety or effectiveness in treating cancer. Although preliminary evidence from cellular and animal studies can highlight complementary therapies that hold future promise, this should not be misinterpreted as sufficient evidence that an intervention is safe or effective. At this time, all of the therapies listed in the following text are considered to be complementary and are not of proven clinical benefit.

The Role of Complementary Therapies in Cancer Care

Complementary therapies are used to supplement conventional treatment—not to replace it. It is vital to remember that no type of complementary therapy has ever been proven to cure cancer or to alter the progression of disease. Patients who choose to use any therapy in place of conventional cancer treatment may be putting themselves at great risk because ineffective treatments can lead to progression of the disease. On the other hand, some complementary therapies have been proven to enhance quality of life [4]. In general, most appear to be safe—given the limited data available—and may be a good option for breast cancer patients looking to alleviate stress, certain disease symptoms, and some side effects of surgery, chemotherapy, hormonal therapy, or radiation. Under the guidance of a physician, complementary therapies can offer women with breast cancer a number of mental and physical health benefits.

Because of this, it is important for women to be open with their physician about any complementary therapies they are taking— or considering taking—even if the physician does not directly ask about their use. Keeping physicians informed about all aspects of care can help ensure that therapeutic regimens are well integrated and can prevent harmful combinations. Unfortunately, there is much room for improvement in this area. A recent national survey found that over 60 percent of patients in the United States fail to inform their physician about complementary therapies they are using [5].

Complementary Therapy by Any Other Name

Many different terms have been used to describe unconventional therapy through the years: alternative therapy, complementary therapy, integrated therapy. And the way they are defined in the field of medicine continues to evolve as the views of unconventional therapy change. Today, the term "complementary therapy" is one of the most often used. However, "integrated therapy" is a term increasing in popularity, as many medical institutions have started to accept the value of some unconventional therapies and taken proactive, progressive steps to integrate them into their cancer treatment routines. For example, as part of the Dana Farber Cancer Institute in Boston, Massachusetts, the Zakim Center for Integrated Therapies offers patients massage therapy and acupuncture, among other services.

Types of Complementary Cancer Therapy

Although there are dozens of complementary therapies being used in cancer care, they can generally be grouped into five broad categories:

- Mind-body interventions
- Biological-based therapies
- Manipulative and body-based therapies
- Energy therapies
- Alternative medical systems

Based on theories from both ancient and modern cultures, these therapeutic practices encompass treatments for the mental, physical, and spiritual health of the patient. Most often, mind-body interventions tend to focus on improving the emotional well-being of the patient, while biological-based, manipulative, body-based, and energy therapies aim primarily to alleviate the physical side effects of cancer and chemotherapy. Alternative medical systems, on the other hand, are complete theories of health. As comprehensive therapy programs, they affect multiple lifestyle behaviors and often combine elements to improve all aspects of the patient's health.

Mind-Body Interventions

Mind-body interventions include prayer, meditation, guided imagery, music therapy, psychotherapy, and yoga. They are based on the belief that the mind has the capacity to influence health and healing. They can be very empowering because they facilitate the mind's capacity to affect bodily function and symptoms [6].

Mind-body interventions are considered safe and pose no risk to those who use them as part of a treatment plan.

Prayer, Meditation, and Guided Imagery

Prayer: Prayer is the most widely practiced mind-body intervention [7]. Because prayer is highly personalized, and the benefits highly subjective, it is difficult to accurately evaluate the benefits of prayer in a medical setting. However, many women report positive effects, both spiritually and physically, by including prayer as a part of their lives [7]. And there is even suggestive evidence that being prayed for by others (called intercessory prayer) could have some benefit for ill patients [8].

Meditation: Meditation is a relaxation technique that can enhance overall physical and mental health. Whether self-directed or guided by a professional, done with or without movement, meditation can help cancer patients to feel calm, focused, and relaxed [4]. The National Institutes of Health recommend it as a useful complementary therapy for the treatment of pain and anxiety [9]. Although meditation is not a cure or an effective treatment for cancer, it can improve the quality of life of cancer patients.

Guided Imagery: For centuries, people have used imagery as a relaxation and healing technique. This therapy involves visualizing images that promote feelings of tranquility or a sense of empowerment. A trained practitioner guides a patient through a series of calm-inducing images or may assist a patient in envisioning his or her body fighting cancer cells [4].

Scientific evidence has shown that guided imagery can be effective in reducing stress, anxiety, and depression in addition to alleviating pain and side effects of chemotherapy [4, 10–13]. Although guided imagery cannot cure cancer or alter the progression of the disease, it is completely safe and may offer many benefits to women with breast cancer.

Psychotherapy

Psychotherapy describes a group of counseling techniques that can be used to provide support, stress management, and coping skills to people undergoing the emotional stress of cancer diagnosis and treatment. Sessions may be conducted one-on-one with a therapist or in a group setting and may incorporate breathing exercises or other relaxation techniques.

There is no scientific evidence that any form of psychotherapy can treat cancer [4]. However, it has been shown to reduce stress and depression in breast cancer patients, which can greatly improve quality of life [14–17]. Although psychotherapy is generally considered safe, it may bring upsetting personal issues to the forefront and cause some emotional discomfort [4]. In general, however, forms of psychotherapy have a positive effect and increase optimism [15, 18].

Support Groups

Support groups are a popular form of psychotherapy that provide a place for people to share common feelings, concerns, and fears. By sharing these feelings with others, many people find their problems easier to handle. Support groups may address specific concerns through education, relaxation techniques, and group interaction. Some people may feel very comfortable sharing in a group setting, while others may be uncomfortable because confidentiality cannot be assured [4]. As with any form of psychosocial therapy, sessions may be upsetting due to the topics discussed. However, many women with breast cancer have found that support groups can reduce stress and depression and improve overall quality of life [4].

Some data suggest that support groups may have a positive impact on cancer survival, though the evidence is far from conclusive. In one well-known study, women with metastatic breast cancer who joined a support group as part of treatment lived an average of eighteen months longer than those who did not participate in a support group [19]. While these findings are quite intriguing because of the large benefit observed, more recent studies have failed to find a survival benefit linked with support group participation [20, 21].

Yoga and Music Therapy

Yoga: Yoga is a form of exercise that integrates the mind, body, and spirit. From the Sanskrit word meaning "union," yoga uses stretching, movement, breathing techniques, and meditation to induce a state of tranquility along with physical and mental well-being [4, 22].

Although yoga is not a treatment for cancer, it may enhance quality of life for patients by reducing stress and increasing feelings of relaxation [4, 23]. Since some of the postures included in the exercises may strain joints and muscles, women with breast cancer should consult with their physician before beginning yoga [4].

Music Therapy: Since the time of the ancient Greeks, music has been promoted as a healing technique for both emotional and physical well-being. Like other mind-body interventions, music therapy is used primarily to improve quality of life [24]. It involves passively listening to music or actively writing or performing music.

While there is no scientific evidence that music therapy can treat disease, it has been shown to reduce pain, stress, and depression in cancer patients [4, 10]. It has also been shown to relieve the nausea and vomiting associated with chemotherapy [10, 25].

Biological-Based Therapies

Biological-based therapies include herbal, vitamin, and mineral therapies, special diet regimens, and plant and animal derivatives.

Some of these therapies are based on remedies thousands of years old, while others are newly formulated. They come from cultures and science labs that span the globe and have formed the basis of one of the most widely used types of complementary cancer therapies.

While some biological-based therapies are supported by scientific evidence, others retain only their fabled uses. It is important to remember that many of these therapies, because they are natural products, are not regulated for safety and may not come in standardized potencies or doses. Some have severe side effects, especially for patients undergoing chemotherapy. And none of these therapies have been proven to halt or reverse the progression of disease. They should never be considered for use as a substitute for conventional treatment.

Melatonin

During the 1970s, scientists discovered that the hormone melatonin was connected with the sleep process. Since then, it has been used to aid sleep and to counter the effects of jet lag [4].

In the laboratory, studies of cells have shown that melatonin inhibits the growth of human breast cancer cells and greatly increases the effectiveness of the drug tamoxifen [26, 27]. However, human studies assessing melatonin as a cancer treatment have had conflicting results. Some have shown melatonin to be effective in increasing survival and improving quality of life, while others have shown it to have no effect on tumor growth [4].

In addition to its other properties, melatonin is a powerful antioxidant, which means it has the ability to neutralize highly active chemicals called free radicals that damage cells. The relationship between antioxidants and cancer is unclear. Free radicals have been linked to the development of cancer cells, and antioxidants—by limiting the cell damage caused by free radicals—may have some potential to suppress tumor growth [4]. Additionally, during chemotherapy, free radicals damage healthy tissues, and it is thought that antioxidants may help protect these tissues. On the other hand, some properties of antioxidants may actually interfere with the effectiveness of chemotherapy drugs [28]. At this time, antioxidant behavior is not well understood, but investigations are currently under way to establish their role in the treatment of cancer [29].

Because melatonin can stimulate the immune system, people with autoimmune disorders, such as rheumatoid arthritis, should avoid the supplement. Related to this and to melatonin's role in hormone regulation, people who take steroid medications should likely avoid melatonin as well [30]. People with depression should also avoid melatonin, as there is evidence that melatonin can make the condition worse [4]. Additionally, all women with breast cancer who are taking, or considering taking, melatonin as either a sleeping aid or as a complementary therapy should consult with their physician.

Coenzyme Q10

Coenzyme Q10 is both a coenzyme and an antioxidant [4, 31]. Coenzymes are substances that help enzymes function properly, and antioxidants are substances that protect cells from chemicals called free radicals [31].

Cellular and animal studies have found evidence that coenzyme Q10 stimulates the immune system and can increase resistance to illness [32–34]. Several studies have attempted to show that coenzyme Q10, when combined with conventional cancer treatment, enhances this treatment by boosting immune function in the body [35]. The few studies conducted in cancer patients, however, were greatly flawed in their design, and their reporting was incomplete [29, 31, 34, 35]. Therefore, although these studies suggest that coenzyme Q10 has the potential to increase survival and affect tumor growth, findings to date are inconclusive and unclear.

There are more promising results for the use of coenzyme Q10 to protect against heart damage related to chemotherapy. Many chemotherapy drugs can cause damage to the heart [4, 29, 31, 35], and initial animal studies found that coenzyme Q10 could reduce the adverse cardiac effects of these drugs [36–41]. These results have been repeated in cancer patients in several small studies and one clinical trial [34, 35].

While coenzyme Q10 appears to be safe, with no known serious side effects, it may adversely interact with certain prescription medications, such as blood-thinning drugs (anticoagulants) and the hormone insulin [34, 35]. For this reason, women should always alert their health care providers if they are using it.

Hydrazine Sulfate

Hydrazine sulfate is a compound found in tobacco plants, tobacco smoke, and some types of mushrooms [4, 42–44]. Its most common use as an unconventional therapy is to treat the severe weight loss and loss of appetite that may accompany advanced stages of cancer [4, 42, 43]. Although it is widely available in Europe, it is available in the United States only to those patients participating in research studies [4, 45].

The ability of hydrazine sulfate to improve quality of life among cancer patients—especially in terms of nutritional status—remains controversial, as does its effect on tumor growth [4, 42, 43, 46–55]. To date, no studies have specifically examined the effect of the compound in women with breast cancer.

Because of the chance of adverse interactions, hydrazine sulfate should not be taken with alcohol, tranquilizers, or barbiturates [4, 45, 55].

Calcium D-Glucarate

Calcium D-glucarate, also referred to as glucarate, is a plant compound found in fruits and vegetables, such as apples, grapefruit, and broccoli [4]. There is evidence from animal studies that glucarate may be useful in suppressing or reducing the growth of breast cancer tumors [56, 57]. However, human studies are needed to fully examine the potential role of glucarate in the treatment of breast cancer, and to date no solid data in humans exist [58].

Selenium

Selenium is a mineral found in seafood, liver, whole grains, cereals, and Brazil nuts [4]. Areas of the world with high levels of selenium in the soil—which gets taken up into food—tend to have lower rates of cancer death than areas with low levels of selenium [4, 59]. This evidence prompted scientists to examine the association between selenium and cancer, both as a preventive agent and in the treatment of the disease [60–63]. However, there is no evidence to date that selenium has any benefit in the prevention or treatment of breast cancer.

Notably, selenium is an essential nutrient that the body needs in small amounts. A healthy diet provides enough selenium for most people. Dietary supplements of selenium should be used with caution, as overdoses can be toxic, possibly harming the immune system [4, 59].

Shark Cartilage

The skeleton of a shark is composed mainly of cartilage. At one time, it was believed that sharks did not get cancer and the cartilage in their bodies was somehow responsible [64]. Although it is now known that sharks can get cancer, cartilage does appear to have physiological properties that may hold potential for treating cancer, and, as yet, no severe adverse effects have been linked to its use [4, 64–66].

A small number of studies in animals and cells have shown that cartilage inhibits the production of new blood vessels, which are vital for the growth of tumors [4, 59, 64]. However, studies in humans have shown no effect of shark cartilage on any type of cancer, including breast cancer [4, 64, 65, 66]. To further explore any potential cancer-related benefit, the National Cancer Institute is sponsoring a clinical trial to evaluate shark cartilage as a complementary therapy for lung cancer patients [4].

Special Diet Therapies

There are several special diet regimens, including macrobiotic and mega-vitamin diets, that proponents claim improve cancer survival and enhance quality of life. Although no diet has ever been found to cure cancer, a well-balanced diet can promote overall health. The primary concern with many special diets is that they may be nutritionally deficient [4]. Women with breast cancer who are investigating alternative diets should be wary of diets that are too restrictive.

Macrobiotic Diets: Macrobiotics is based on the principle of traditional Chinese medicine that an inner balance of energy maintains health. The balance in the diet comes from the complementary energies of yin, controlling the internal regions of the body, and yang, controlling the external regions of the body [67]. The warm energy of yang comes from sweet and pungent foods, while the cool energy of yin comes from sour, bitter, and salty foods [67]. In every aspect of the diet, from food selection to preparation to eating, these energies remain in balance. Modern day practitioners of macrobiotics combine these principles with the practice of avoiding foods they feel may contain toxins, such as dairy products, meats, and oily foods [4]. The macrobiotic diet consists mainly of organically grown whole grains, organically grown fruits and vegetables, fish, seaweed, and soy products.

If not taken to extremes, macrobiotics may offer some people health benefits. However, the original macrobiotics diet has been slowly simplified over time to include mainly brown rice and water. Such a restrictive diet led to severe nutritional deficiencies and even death in some followers. Though less extreme, other strict forms of macrobiotics—such as those that exclude all meat products—may also cause nutritional deficiencies and pose a dangerous threat to cancer patients struggling to maintain weight and nutrient levels [4]. Breast cancer patients considering macrobiotics should refrain from the more restrictive versions of the diet to avoid potential harm to their caloric and nutrient intake.

Mega-Vitamin Diet: Another dietary plan that proponents claim cures cancer is the mega-vitamin diet. In this regimen, high doses of vitamin C and other antioxidant vitamins are taken daily. This can involve taking hundreds of pills every day. There is no scientific evidence that high doses of any vitamin can cure cancer [68]. Furthermore, there is some concern that high doses of antioxidants may actually decrease the effectiveness of chemotherapy [4, 29]. Laboratory studies have found that tumor cells often contain large amounts of vitamin C, and some researchers speculate that this could actually enhance tumor growth or protect cancer cells from chemotherapy and possibly even radiation [69]. Studies of humans with cancer, though, are needed to back up these findings.

Of course, getting adequate vitamins and minerals is essential for good health. However, a healthy diet—possibly supplemented with a standard multivitamin tablet—is all most people need to meet their daily vitamin and mineral requirements.

Herbal Therapies

Herbal therapies encompass a wide range of natural and biological-based products. They are commonly used by cancer patients to relieve the mental stress and physical side effects associated with both cancer and cancer treatment [70]. A recent study reported that approximately 13 percent of women with breast cancer use herbal remedies [71]. Recent studies have found that anywhere from 14 percent to 49 percent of women with breast cancer use herbal remedies [71–73].

In 1993, the FDA relaxed restrictions on natural products, which led to an abundance of herbal remedies entering the marketplace. While severe side effects linked to these products appear rare—based on the current limited body of evidence—it is important to note that these products are not regulated or standardized for purity, consistency, or potency. Because many of these products are ingested, it is particularly important to be aware that the herbs might interfere with the action—and clearance—of hormonal therapy or chemotherapy drugs and could cause potential side effects that could be harmful, especially during treatment with chemotherapy.

Potential Dangers of Herbal Therapies in Patients Undergoing Surgery

Recent evidence has shown that several types of commonly used herbal therapies may be harmful to patients undergoing surgery [74].

Herbs can have a direct, adverse effect on the body, and people with certain medical conditions may be particularly sensitive. More importantly for cancer patients, herbal therapies can have dangerous interactions with certain medications and can also interfere with pharmaceutical drugs, rendering them useless. This can be extremely important when a patient is about to undergo surgery. Before any type of surgery, patients should be sure to tell their doctors if they have used any herbal supplements.

Table 61.1 highlights selected herbs and the potential problems that may result during surgery.

Table 61.1. Selected Herbs and Potential Problems during Surgery

Herb	Potential Problems During Surgery	When to Stop Before Surgery
Echinacea	• Hampered effectiveness of immunosuppression drugs • Allergic reaction to the herb	Unclear
Garlic	• Excessive bleeding	7 or more days
Ginkgo biloba	• Excessive bleeding	1½ or more days
Ginseng	• Low blood sugar • Excessive bleeding • Hampered effectiveness of the blood-thinning drug warfarin	7 or more days
Kava	• Increased sedation from anesthetics	1 or more day(s)
St. John's wort	• Interaction with numerous drugs, including steroids, warfarin, and calcium channel blockers	5 or more days
Valerian	• Increased sedation from anesthetics • Greater need for anesthetics (with long-term use)	Unclear

Adapted from Ang-Lee et al., 2001 [74]

Soy and Phytoestrogens

Countries with high soy intake, such as Japan, have low rates of breast cancer [4]. This pattern of disease prompted scientists to examine the relationship between soy products and breast cancer. Soybeans—as well as many other plants like flaxseed, certain grains, beans, fruits, vegetables, and the roots ginseng and black cohosh—contain chemicals called phytoestrogens, which mimic estrogen in the body. These estrogen-like qualities have created much controversy surrounding their role in the prevention and promotion of breast cancer [29].

In women without breast cancer, some studies have found that phytoestrogens may offer protection against developing the disease, while other studies have found no benefit [4, 75–80]. There is even some evidence from laboratory studies that soy can be harmful. Studies where estrogen-receptor-positive human breast cancer cells have been implanted in mice have found that soy diets can actually promote tumor growth [1, 81, 82].

At this time, unfortunately, no conclusions can be made about how soy affects the risk of breast cancer or the course of breast cancer in women who have the disease. More study is needed, and to help address this, the National Cancer Institute is currently conducting a clinical trial on the use of soy in breast cancer treatment. For more information on this trial, visit the National Cancer Institute's Clinical Trials website.

Outside of treatment, many women are also turning to soy products and other "natural hormones" (like black cohosh and wild yam cream) for the relief of hot flashes and other symptoms related to menopause. However, there is little evidence to date that such products offer any relief from menopausal symptoms.

Essiac

Essiac is an herbal tea that has purported healing properties. During the 1920s, a Canadian nurse named Rene Caisse met a patient who reported being cured of breast cancer by an herbal tea made by a Native American medicine man. Caisse got the recipe and became convinced of its healing power. She opened a clinic and began treating cancer patients with the remedy, which she called Essiac, her name spelled backward [4]. The tea was originally made from a mixture of burdock root, slippery elm inner bark, sheep sorrel, and Turkish rhubarb, and Caisse later added watercress, blessed thistle, red clover, and kelp [4, 29, 83].

While there are claims that Essiac can alleviate pain, enhance the immune system, improve appetite, and reduce the size of tumors, these claims remain unsubstantiated [83]. Leading medical institutions in both the United States and Canada have studied Essiac as a potential cancer treatment and found no conclusive evidence of any benefits [4].

Mistletoe (Iscador)

The European species of mistletoe, called iscador, has been noted since the time of the Druids for its purported healing qualities. This therapeutic species is neither grown nor commercially available in the United States, but it is a popular complementary therapy in Europe and Asia [4, 84, 85]. There, an extract from the plant's leaves and twigs is often injected directly into or near tumors [4, 84, 85]. At no time should part of the plant itself be eaten, as ingesting mistletoe can cause seizures and death [4, 84].

Cellular studies have established that iscador can activate immune system cells and can release chemicals that destroy cancer cells [86–88]. Additionally, several animal studies have had promising results for iscador as an anti-tumor agent [89, 90]. However, results from human studies have been inconclusive [4, 83, 85], and iscador should not be used as a substitute for conventional cancer treatment. Clinical trials are currently under way in Europe and will hopefully shed more light on the potential therapeutic use of this herb [83].

Green Tea

A traditional remedy in Asia, green tea is now gaining popularity in Western countries [4]. Black tea and green tea are both made from the dried leaves of the *Camellia sinesis* plant, but while black tea is made from fermented leaves, green tea is not [4, 91].

Green tea has been used as a medicinal stimulant and digestive remedy for five thousand years in China and Japan [91]. Herbalists claim that it relieves vomiting and diarrhea, but there are no studies of these effects in cancer patients [71]. Preliminary animal and cell studies have shown evidence that green tea may be beneficial in preventing and treating lung and breast cancer, but to date, no studies in humans have been conducted [91–94].

Ginger Root

Ginger has long been used as an herbal remedy for many ailments, including nausea, vomiting, and loss of appetite [4, 29]. Some research has shown that it can alleviate chemotherapy-induced nausea in cancer patients, and it is often used for this purpose [4, 29]. It comes in a variety of forms, including tea, powders, capsules, tablets, and candied slices [4, 29]. Ginger ale soft drinks may also contain small amounts of ginger, although many brands contain only ginger flavoring.

High doses of ginger may interfere with blood clotting in the body, and, therefore, patients with clotting problems or those planning to undergo surgery should refrain from using ginger [4, 29].

Milk Thistle

Milk thistle, a cousin of the daisy, has long been reported to have beneficial effects on the liver [71]. The seeds of the plant contain an antioxidant called silymarin, which has been suggested to protect the liver during chemotherapy treatment [29]. However, no formal studies have been done to evaluate this. Cellular studies have shown that silymarin can inhibit the growth of breast cancer cells, but these preliminary findings have not been repeated in animal or human studies [4]. Overall, there is no solid evidence that milk thistle has any cancer-related benefits.

Astragalus Root

Astragalus is a legume long used in traditional Chinese medicine to strengthen qi (the natural flow of energy in the body) and to protect against disease [4]. Western science has since become interested in it as a potential means of enhancing the immune system [4, 29]. Although there is preliminary evidence from cellular and animal studies to suggest that astragalus may enhance the effect of conventional cancer treatments, there have not yet been studies conducted in humans [4]. At this time, then, there does not appear to be any benefit of astragalus for women with breast cancer.

As with all complementary therapies, those who choose to take astragalus should consult with their physician beforehand. This is especially important for those who take drugs that suppress the immune response (such as steroids) or those who have diseases caused by an overactive immune system (such as lupus) [4].

St. John's Wort

Named for St. John the Baptist, St. John's wort has been used for centuries to treat everything from mental disorders and nerve pain to diarrhea and snakebites [4, 95]. Although many of these purported health benefits remain unproven, there is good evidence that the herb can effectively treat mild to moderate depression with fewer side effects than standard antidepressant drugs [4, 29, 96–98]. Its effectiveness in treating severe or clinical depression is much less clear and is currently being studied in a large-scale clinical trial [96, 99].

For cancer patients, one of the most important issues with St. John's wort is that it can interfere with a number of prescription drugs, including other antidepressants and certain types of chemotherapy [4, 95]. Additionally, St. John's wort can interfere with blood-clotting drugs that may be given to patients before and after surgery [74]. Thus, women with breast cancer who are considering taking St. John's wort should be sure to consult with their physicians beforehand and should discontinue use at least five days before surgery [4, 74].

Black Cohosh

Often called the "women's remedy," black cohosh is commonly used in Europe to relieve menstrual cramps and menopausal symptoms [4]. Unfortunately, at this time, there is not enough scientific evidence to conclude whether black cohosh is safe for cancer patients [4]. Several reviews of research have concluded that it may be effective in reducing many of the discomforts of menopause. However, a recent randomized trial found that breast cancer survivors who took black cohosh actually experienced the same number and intensity of hot flashes as those who did not take the herb [100]. Further complicating matters, the root of this plant appears to behave like estrogen in the human body, and some studies have shown that estrogen-like plant substances, or phytoestrogens, can stimulate the growth of breast tumors [29, 101]. Therefore, it is often advised that women with breast cancer avoid black cohosh.

Echinacea

Echinacea has been a common herbal remedy in the United States since the 1800s. Proponents of it as a cancer treatment claim that it can boost the immune system and stimulate the natural anticancer activity of white blood cells. However, there is no scientific evidence that echinacea can increase the body's natural defenses or protect it against cancer [4]. In addition, its safety remains uncertain, particularly among cancer patients. Using echinacea for more than eight weeks can not only cause liver damage but may also suppress the immune system. For patients undergoing surgery, these concerns are more serious and the use of echinacea should be avoided [74]. Moreover, it may interfere with several chemotherapy drugs [4].

Ginseng

The root of the ginseng plant has been used since ancient times to treat an array of health problems—from diabetes to lung disorders to severe wounds [4]. Ginseng is also thought to increase vitality and help fight disease [71]. In addition, researchers have speculated that it might inhibit tumor growth in cancer patients [71]. However, none of ginseng's purported health benefits, including those among cancer patients, have actually been supported by scientific evidence [4]. Thus, its beneficial effects remain largely unknown.

What is known about ginseng is that it has several serious side effects, including high blood pressure, and may interfere with medications that affect blood clotting, especially when these drugs are administered before or after surgery [71]. For women who are fasting before surgery, ginseng can also cause low blood sugar levels and should be discontinued at least seven days before surgery [74]. Moreover, some researchers have suggested that ginseng might be harmful to women with breast cancer since it behaves as a phytoestrogen in the body [71].

Chinese Herbal Medicine

Herbal therapy is an integral part of traditional Chinese medicine. Unlike Western medicine, traditional Chinese medicine seeks to restore a natural energy and balance to the body rather than to treat an underlying cause of disease [4, 102]. Approximately two thousand standardized herbal formulas are currently in use [67]. While some practitioners of traditional Chinese medicine claim that these herbal formulas can prevent and treat many forms of cancer, including breast cancer, there is no scientific evidence to support these reports [4]. However, it has been widely used among cancer patients—and shown to be effective in some studies—in relieving the side effects of conventional cancer therapy, alleviating pain, and improving quality of life [4]. In addition, some evidence suggests that Chinese herbal therapies, when combined with conventional therapy, may actually help increase survival and lower the risk of recurrence for some cancer patients [4, 102, 103].

Despite the possible benefits of Chinese herbal medicine, there are some drawbacks. First, it is difficult to know which particular herbs might be most beneficial, since the research studies done to date do not generally list the specific herbs being tested [4, 102]. Second, there are many potential side effects with herbal medicine, particularly because the formulas contain so many different types of herbs. Use of some herbal remedies can cause liver damage and may interfere with prescription drugs [4]. As a result, women who are interested in these therapies should consult with their physicians to ensure that the specific herbs they are considering will not interfere with their conventional therapy.

Manipulative and Body-Based Therapies

Manipulative and body-based treatment methods involve manual movement of the body, such as chiropractic treatment and massage therapy. Many of these therapies treat one part of the body in order to stimulate healing in another part [4]. While none of these treatments offer a cure for cancer or increase survival, they can provide relief from many of the side effects of the disease and its treatment. As with any treatment that involves joint or muscle manipulation, cancer patients should consult with their physician before undergoing any of these therapies [4].

Chiropractic Therapy

Chiropractic techniques manipulate the spine to improve quality of life through pain management and stress reduction [4, 104, 105]. Although chiropractic therapy is considered relatively safe, women with breast cancer should consult with their physician before undergoing treatment, as it manipulates joints and muscles [4].

Massage Therapy

For thousands of years, massage has been used to treat a variety of health conditions. It has been shown to promote relaxation and to reduce pain, anxiety, and stress through the rubbing, kneading, and manipulation of the body's muscles and soft tissues [4, 106–108]. Although the long-term effectiveness of massage in treating these symptoms is uncertain, it appears to be a safe way for cancer patients to manage pain and stress [4, 106–108]. As with other therapies that manipulate muscles, a patient should consult with her physician before undergoing this therapy [4].

Energy Therapies

Energy therapies encompass a variety of treatments that attempt to manipulate the body's internal energy to promote healing. According to traditional Chinese medical theory, internal energy flow, called qi, governs health. When this flow is out of balance, disease can develop.

To correct imbalance, energy therapies strive to realign the flow of energy through the body. These treatments may involve direct contact with the body, or they may concentrate only on the energy surrounding the body. Although no type of energy therapy has been shown to cure cancer or affect the progress of the disease, acupuncture, acupressure, and electrical nerve stimulation have been shown to have some positive benefits for breast cancer patients.

Acupuncture

Americans became interested in acupuncture during the 1970s when a *New York Times* reporter was treated with acupuncture for postoperative pain during a visit to China [109]. Since that time, it has become a popular complementary therapy among cancer patients. A 1999 study of breast cancer patients in the Midwest showed that 5 percent of women were interested in acupuncture as a complementary therapy [7], while a 2000 study of nearly three hundred breast cancer survivors found that 31 percent of women had tried acupuncture [110].

Acupuncture is based on the fundamental premise of Chinese medicine that the energy flow through the body, called qi, is responsible for a person's health. When this flow is disrupted, it is said that disease can occur [4, 111]. Acupuncture is the practice of inserting fine needles into points along the body where imbalances of energy flow, qi, can be corrected [112].

Although there is no evidence that acupuncture is a treatment for cancer itself, it can increase a woman's quality of life while she is undergoing conventional treatment [4]. Some research suggests that acupuncture influences neurotransmitters and endorphins, which are chemicals and hormones in the body that can reduce pain [111, 113, 114]. Acupuncture has been shown to alleviate the pain associated with breast cancer as well as to reduce some of the more common side effects of treatment, such as nausea, vomiting, hot flashes, and edema [4, 109, 115–121].

Acupuncture is one of the few complementary therapies for which government oversight and standards of use exist. The Food and Drug Administration (FDA) approved the use of acupuncture needles by licensed practitioners in 1996, and thirty-two states currently have standards for the training and licensing of practitioners [4]. This is particularly important since serious side effects (including infection, fainting, local internal bleeding, convulsions, hepatitis B, dermatitis, and nerve damage) can occur if a practitioner is not well trained [4].

449

When performed by a licensed practitioner, acupuncture is considered safe [4]. In fact, the incidence of adverse effects is much lower for acupuncture than it is for many pharmaceutical drugs used to treat the same conditions [112]. Nonetheless, side effects are possible and include mild discomfort and slight bruising at the points where the needles are inserted [122]. In addition, acupuncture is not advised for those with certain blood-clotting problems or those on blood-thinning drugs (anticoagulants), as it can cause bleeding in these patients [122].

Although Medicare does not cover the costs of acupuncture, many private health insurance plans and HMOs now cover these costs [4]. This suggests that acupuncture is being integrated into mainstream medicine.

Acupressure

Acupressure is based on the same underlying premise as acupuncture: that the internal energy flow through the body, called qi, is responsible for health. Rather than using tiny acupuncture needles, acupressure stimulates these energy points along the body using pressure from the fingertips. Although acupressure has not been well studied, it has been shown to reduce nausea in women with breast cancer and may offer other benefits, such as stress reduction [4, 123].

Electroacupuncture/Electrical Nerve Stimulation

Another variation of acupuncture is electrical nerve stimulation, or electroacupuncture. As the name suggests, this therapy involves the use of electrical impulses to stimulate points along the body targeted during a traditional acupuncture session [4]. The electrical impulses can be delivered through acupuncture needles, through metal probes placed near the skin, or through electrodes that are placed directly on the skin. Practitioners claim that this method enhances the therapeutic effect of acupuncture. Although it has not been studied as well as traditional acupuncture has, electroacupuncture can help reduce chemotherapy-induced nausea in some women with breast cancer [120]. Because this therapy is relatively new and little is known about the side effects, a woman should discuss it with her physician before undergoing treatment.

Alternative Medical Systems

Alternative medical systems are complete systems of health theory and practice that developed independently from conventional medicine [6]. Many of these systems of medicine are thousands of years old, much older than conventional practices, and are still often the preferred method of health treatment in many cultures. Examples include traditional Chinese medicine, Ayurveda, homeopathic medicine, and naturopathic medicine. Although many of these systems may help promote a healthy lifestyle, none of them offer an effective treatment for cancer [4]. When used as a complementary therapy, an alternative system may offer health benefits that can increase quality of life.

Traditional Chinese Medicine

Traditional Chinese medicine is based on the theory that the body's internal energy force, called qi, regulates health. This energy is kept in balance through a variety of means, including a macrobiotic diet, Chinese herbal medicine, acupuncture, massage, and meditation [4]. Some of these components may offer relief from cancer-related pain and the side effects of chemotherapy.

Ayurveda

Ayurveda is the traditional system of medicine in India. This ancient system focuses on harmony of the mind, body, and forces of nature. Like traditional Chinese medicine, ayurvedic theory suggests that disease is a result of an imbalance in these energies [4, 6]. Ayurveda incorporates diet, herbal therapies, yoga, meditation, massage, and imagery, which may be helpful in alleviating stress and the side effects of conventional cancer treatments [6]. There is no evidence that ayurveda can cure cancer or increase survival. Furthermore, several components of this therapy, including bloodletting and induced vomiting, can clearly be very dangerous and should be strictly avoided [4].

Conclusion

Complementary therapies have become an increasingly popular supplement to conventional cancer treatment. Unfortunately, it is too soon to predict whether any of these therapies will become effective cancer treatments. However, there is an ever-expanding body of evidence that many types of complementary therapies are effective in reducing the physical and mental effects of cancer diagnosis and treatment. By enhancing quality of life, complementary therapies offer hope for many women with breast cancer. As an increasing number of medical facilities are integrating these therapies into standard treatment regimens, more and more patients will have an opportunity to experience the potential benefits. By discussing complementary therapies with their physicians, women can help ensure that they receive safe and effective care.

The two major concerns about complementary therapies are the lack of FDA regulation (which means that the purity and potency of these products can be variable and potentially dangerous) and the lack of safety data for combining complementary therapies with traditional cancer therapies with proven effectiveness. For these reasons, many oncologists recommend that patients do not take complementary medicines together with chemotherapy or radiation therapy.

Questions for Your Provider

1. How do you feel about complementary therapies?

2. Have you ever referred a patient to a complementary practitioner?

3. Should I stop any complementary therapies that I am taking during chemotherapy and radiation therapy?

4. If I were to start a complementary therapy, what would you need to know about it from me?

Questions for Your Complementary Therapy Practitioner

1. Is the treatment you are suggesting potentially harmful in any way?

2. Is there any evidence that the treatment has been effective? Is the evidence scientific or anecdotal?

3. What are your credentials for practicing this therapy? Can you provide me with references?

4. What is the cost? Where do I have to go to get this treatment?

5. Is the treatment covered by my health insurance?

6. How can the purity and potency of the complementary products you are recommending be verified?

Adapted from Lerner 1994 [124].

References

1. Allred CD, Ju YH, Allred KF, et al. Dietary genistin stimulates growth of estrogen-dependent breast cancer tumors similar to that observed with genistein. *Carcinogenesis.* 22: 1667–73, 2001.

2. National Center for Complementary and Alternative Medicine. *About NCCAM.* 2001. http://nccam.nih.gov/about/aboutnccam/indcx.htm.

3. Eisenberg DM, Davis RB, Ettner SL, et al. Trends in alternative medicine use in the United States, 1990–1997: Results of a follow-up national survey. *JAMA.* 280: 1569–75, 1998.

4. American Cancer Society. *American Cancer Society's Guide to Complementary and Alternative Cancer Methods.* Atlanta, GA, American Cancer Society, 2000.

5. Eisenberg DM, Kessler RC, Van Rompay MI, et al. Perceptions about complementary therapies relative to conventional therapies among adults who use both: Results from a national survey. *Ann Intern Med.* 135: 344–51, 2001.

6. National Center for Complementary & Alternative Medicine. *What is complementary and alternative medicine (CAM)?* 2001. http://nccam.nih.gov/health/whatiscam/.

7. VandeCreek L, Rogers E and Lester J. Use of alternative therapies among breast cancer outpatients compared with the general population. *Altern Ther Health Med.* 5: 71–76, 1999.

8. Harris WS, Gowda M, Kolb JW, et al. A randomized, controlled trial of the effects of remote, intercessory prayer on outcomes in patients admitted to the coronary care unit. *Arch Intern Med.* 159: 2273–78, 1999.

9. National Institutes of Health. *Integration of Behavioral and Relaxation Approaches into the Treatment of Chronic Pain and Insomnia.* NIH Technology Statement Online. October 16–18, 1995. 1995. http://consensus.nih.gov/ta/017/017_intro.htm.

10. Frank JM. The effects of music therapy and guided visual imagery on chemotherapy induced nausea and vomiting. *Oncol Nurs Forum.* 12: 47–52, 1985.

11. Richardson MA. Coping, life attitudes, and immune response to imagery and group support after breast cancer treatment. *Alternative Therapies in Health and Medicine*. 3: 62–70, 1997.

12. Eller LS. Guided imagery interventions for symptom management. *Annu Rev Nurs Res*. 17: 57–84, 1999.

13. Rhodes VA and McDaniel RW. Nausea, vomiting, and retching: Complex problems in palliative care. *CA A Cancer Journal for Clinicians*. 51: 232–48, 2001.

14. Fukui S, Kugaya A, Okamura H, et al. A psychosocial group intervention for Japanese women with primary breast carcinoma. *Cancer*. 89: 1026–36, 2000.

15. Antoni MH, Lehman JM, Kilbourn KM, et al. Cognitive-behavioral stress management intervention decreases the prevalence of depression and enhances benefit finding among women under treatment for early-stage breast cancer. *Health Psychol*. 20: 20–32, 2001.

16. Classen C, Butler LD, Koopman C, et al. Supportive-expressive group therapy and distress in patients with metastatic breast cancer: A randomized clinical intervention trial. *Arch Gen Psychiatry*. 58: 494–501, 2001.

17. Rutledge DN and Raymon NJ. Changes in well-being of women cancer survivors following a survivor weekend experience. *Oncol Nurs Forum*. 28: 85–91, 2001.

18. Geiger AM, Mullen ES, Sloman PA, et al. Evaluation of a breast cancer patient information and support program. *Eff Clin Pract*. 3: 157–65, 2000.

19. Spiegel D, Bloom JR, Kraemer HC and Gottheil E. Effect of psychosocial treatment on survival of patients with metastatic breast cancer. *Lancet*. 2: 888–91, 1989.

20. Goodwin PJ, Leszcz M, Ennis M, et al. The effect of group psychosocial support on survival in metastatic breast cancer. *N Engl J Med*. 345: 1719–26, 2001.

21. Cunningham AJ, Edmonds CV, Jenkins GP, et al. A randomized controlled trial of the effects of group psychological therapy on survival in women with metastatic breast cancer. *Psychooncology*. 7: 508–17, 1998.

22. Leonard P. Zakim Center for Integrated Therapies. *Yoga.* 2001. http://www.dana-farber.org/pat/support/zakim_default.asp.

23. Coulter AH. Yoga and cancer: A move toward relaxation. *Alternative and Complementary Therapies.* 4: 150–55, 1998.

24. Leonard P. Zakim Center for Integrated Therapies. *Music Therapy.* 2001. http://www.dana-farber.org/pat/support/zakim_default.asp.

25. Ezzone S, Baker C, Rosselet R and Terepka E. Music as an adjunct to antiemetic therapy. *Oncol Nurs Forum.* 25: 1551–56, 1998.

26. Wilson ST, Blask DE and Lemus-Wilson AM. Melatonin augments the sensitivity of MCF-7 human breast cancer cells to tamoxifen in vitro. *J Clin Endocrinol Metab.* 75: 669–70, 1992.

27. Crespo D, Fernandez-Viadero C, Verduga R, et al. Interaction between melatonin and estradiol on morphological and morphometric features of MCF-7 human breast cancer cells. *J Pineal Res.* 16: 215–22, 1994.

28. Labriola D and Livingston R. Possible interactions between dietary antioxidants and chemotherapy. *Oncology (Huntingt).* 13: 1003–8; discussion 1008, 1011–12, 1999.

29. Dog TL, Riley D and Carter T. Traditional and alternative therapies for breast cancer. *Altern Ther Health Med.* 7: 36–42, 45–47; quiz 48, 149, 2001.

30. Braunwald E, Fauci AS and Isselbacher KJ. *Melatonin.* 2002. http://www.harrisonsonline.com/.

31. National Cancer Institute. *Coenzyme Q10.* 2001. http://www.nci.nih.gov/cancerinfo/pdq/cam/coenzymeQ10.

32. Bliznakov E, Casey A and Premuzic E. Coenzymes Q: Stimulants of the phagocytic activity in rats and immune response in mice. *Experientia.* 26: 953–54, 1970.

33. Hogenauer G, Mayer P and Drews J. The macrophage activating potential of ubiquinones., in K F. *Biomedical and Clinical Aspects of Coenzyme Q.* New York, NY, Elsevier Scientific Publishing Co., 1981.

34. National Center for Complementary and Alternative Medicine. *Cancer Facts: Complementary and Alternative Medicine: Questions and Answers about Coenzyme Q10*. 2001. http://cis.nci.nih.gov/fact/9_16.htm.

35. University of Texas-MD Anderson Cancer Center and Complementary/Integrative Medicine Education Resources. *Coenzyme Q10*. 1998. http://www.mdanderson.org/departments/CIMER/display.cfm?id=43EF7F77-0DAF-11D5-810D00508B603A14 &method=displayFull&pn=6EB86A59-EBD9-11D4-810100508B603A14.

36. Folkers K, Choe JY and Combs AB. *Rescue by coenzyme Q10 from the electrocardiographic abnormalities caused by the toxicity of adriamycin in the rat*. Washington, DC, National Academy of Sciences of the United States, 1976, 5178–80.

37. Combs AB, Choe JY, Truong DH and Folkers K. Reduction by coenzyme Q10 of the acute toxicity of adriamycin in mice. *Res Commun Chem Pathol Pharmacol*. 18: 565–68, 1977.

38. Choe JY, Combs AB and Folkers K. Prevention by coenzyme Q10 of the electrocardiographic changes induced by adriamycin in rats. *Res Commun Chem Pathol Pharmacol*. 23: 199–202, 1979.

39. Lubawy WC, Dallam RA and Hurley LH. Protection against anthramycin-induced toxicity in mice by coenzyme Q10. *J Natl Cancer Inst*. 64: 105–9, 1980.

40. Usui T, Ishikura H, Izumi Y, et al. Possible prevention from the progression of cardiotoxicity in adriamycin-treated rabbits by coenzyme Q10. *Toxicol Lett*. 12: 75–82, 1982.

41. Shinozawa S, Gomita Y and Araki Y. Protective effects of various drugs on adriamycin (doxorubicin)-induced toxicity and microsomal lipid peroxidation in mice and rats. *Biol Pharm Bull*. 16: 1114–17, 1993.

42. National Cancer Institute and CancerNet. *Hydrazine sulfate*. 2001. http://www.nci.nih.gov/cancerinfo/pdq/cam/hydrazinesulfate.

43. National Cancer Institute. *Paget's Disease of the Breast: Questions and Answers*. 2002. http://cis.nci.nih.gov/fact/6_39.htm.

44. National Cancer Institute. *Cancer Facts: National Cancer Institute Studies of Hydrazine Sulfate.* 2001. http://cis.nci.nih.gov/fact/9_18.htm.

45. Kaegi E. Unconventional therapies for cancer: 4. Hydrazine sulfate. Task Force on Alternative Therapies of the Canadian Breast Cancer Research Initiative. *CMAJ.* 158: 1327–30, 1998.

46. Toth B. Hydrazine, methylhydrazine and methylhydrazine sulfate carcinogenesis in Swiss mice: Failure of ammonium hydroxide to interfere in the development of tumors. *Int J Cancer.* 9: 109–18, 1972.

47. Gold J. Inhibition of gluconeogenesis at the phosphoenolpyruvate carboxykinase and pyruvate carboxylase reactions, as a means of cancer chemotherapy. *Oncology.* 29: 74–89, 1974.

48. Chlebowski RT, Bulcavage L, Grosvenor M, et al. Hydrazine sulfate influence on nutritional status and survival in non-small-cell lung cancer. *J Clin Oncol.* 8: 9–15, 1990.

49. Chlebowski RT, Heber D, Richardson B and Block JB. Influence of hydrazine sulfate on abnormal carbohydrate metabolism in cancer patients with weight loss. *Cancer Res.* 44: 857–61, 1984.

50. Nelson JA and Falk RE. The efficacy of phloridzin and phloretin on tumor cell growth. *Anticancer Res.* 13: 2287–92, 1993.

51. Kosty MP, Fleishman SB, Herndon JE, 2nd, et al. Cisplatin, vinblastine, and hydrazine sulfate in advanced, non-small-cell lung cancer: A randomized placebo-controlled, double-blind phase III study of the Cancer and Leukemia Group B. *J Clin Oncol.* 12: 1113–20, 1994.

52. Loprinzi CL, Goldberg RM, Su JQ, et al. Placebo-controlled trial of hydrazine sulfate in patients with newly diagnosed non-small-cell lung cancer. *J Clin Oncol.* 12: 1126–29, 1994.

53. Loprinzi CL, Kuross SA, O'Fallon JR, et al. Randomized placebo-controlled evaluation of hydrazine sulfate in patients with advanced colorectal cancer. *J Clin Oncol.* 12: 1121–25, 1994.

54. Filov VA, Gershanovich ML, Danova LA and Ivin BA. Experience of the treatment with Sehydrin (Hydrazine Sulfate, HS) in the advanced cancer patients. *Invest New Drugs.* 13: 89–97, 1995.

55. University of Texas-MD Anderson Cancer Center and Complementary/Integrative Medicine Education Resources. *Hydrazine Sulfate*. 1998. http://www.mdanderson.org/departments/ CIMER/display.cfm?id=35F66D07-F06A-11D4-810200508 B603A14&method=displayFull&pn=6EB86A59-EBD9-11D4-810100508B603A14.

56. Abou-Issa H, Moeschberger M, el-Masry W, et al. Relative efficacy of glucarate on the initiation and promotion phases of rat mammary carcinogenesis. *Anticancer Res*. 15: 805–10, 1995.

57. Abou-Issa H, Koolemans-Beynen A, Meredith TA and Webb TE. Antitumour synergism between non-toxic dietary combinations of isotretinoin and glucarate. *Eur J Cancer*. 784–88, 1992.

58. Heerdt AS, Young CW and Borgen PI. Calcium glucarate as a chemopreventive agent in breast cancer. *Isr J Med Sci*. 31: 101–5, 1995.

59. University of Texas-MD Anderson Cancer Center and Complementary/Integrative Medicine Education Resources. *Selenium*. 1998. http://www.mdanderson.org/departments/CIMER/ display.cfm?id=43EF7FE5-0DAF-11D5-810D00508B603A14 &method=displayFull&pn=6EB86A59-EBD9-11D4-810100508B603A14.

60. Clark LC. The epidemiology of selenium and cancer. *Fed Proc*. 44: 2584–89, 1985.

61. Combs GF, Jr. and Clark LC. Can dietary selenium modify cancer risk? *Nutr Rev*. 43: 325–31, 1985.

62. Ghadirian P, Maisonneuve P, Perret C, et al. A case-control study of toenail selenium and cancer of the breast, colon, and prostate. *Cancer Detect Prev*. 24: 305–13, 2000.

63. Mannisto S, Alfthan G, Virtanen M, et al. Toenail selenium and breast cancer—A case-control study in Finland. *Eur J Clin Nutr*. 54: 98–103, 2000.

64. National Cancer Institute. *Cartilage*. 2001. http://www.nci.nih .gov/cancerinfo/pdq/cam/cartilage.

65. Miller DR, Anderson GT, Stark JJ, et al. Phase I/II trial of the safety and efficacy of shark cartilage in the treatment of advanced cancer. *J Clin Oncol*. 16: 3649–55, 1998.

66. University of Texas-MD Anderson Cancer Center and Complementary/Integrative Medicine Education Resources. *Cartilage.* 1998. http://www.mdanderson.org/departments/CIMER/ display.cfm?id=43EF7F04-0DAF-11D5-810D00508B603A14 &method=displayFull&pn=6EB86A59-EBD9-11D4- 810100508B603A14.

67. Lu HC. *Chinese natural cures: Traditional methods for remedies and preventions.* New York, NY, Black Dog & Leventhal Publishers, Inc., 1994.

68. Cassileth B. Evaluating complementary and alternative therapies for cancer patients. *CA Cancer J Clin.* 49: 353–61, 1999.

69. Agus DB, Vera JC and Golde DW. Stromal cell oxidation: A mechanism by which tumors obtain vitamin C. *Cancer Res.* 59: 4555–58, 1999.

70. Tagliaferri M, Cohen I and Tripathy D. Complementary and alternative medicine in early-stage breast cancer. *Seminars in Oncology.* 28: 121–34, 2001.

71. Lee MM, Lin SS, Wrensch MR, et al. Alternative therapies used by women with breast cancer in four ethnic populations. *J Natl Cancer Inst.* 92: 42–47, 2000.

72. Ganz PA, Desmond KA, Leedham B, et al. Quality of life in long-term, disease-free survivors of breast cancer: A follow-up study. *J Natl Cancer Inst.* 94: 39–49, 2002.

73. DiGianni LM, Garber JE and Winer EP. Complementary and alternative medicine use among women with breast cancer. *J Clin Oncol.* 20: 34S–38S, 2002.

74. Ang-Lee MK, Moss J and Yuan CS. Herbal medicines and perioperative care. *JAMA.* 286: 208–16, 2001.

75. Barnes S, Grubbs C, Setchell KD and Carlson J. Soybeans inhibit mammary tumors in models of breast cancer. *Prog Clin Biol Res.* 347: 239–53, 1990.

76. Cassidy A, Bingham S and Setchell KD. Biological effects of a diet of soy protein rich in isoflavones on the menstrual cycle of premenopausal women. *Am J Clin Nutr.* 60: 333–40, 1994.

77. Fournier DB, Erdman JW, Jr. and Gordon GB. Soy, its components, and cancer prevention: A review of the in vitro, animal, and human data. *Cancer Epidemiol Biomarkers Prev*. 7: 1055–65, 1998.

78. Key TJ, Sharp GB, Appleby PN, et al. Soya foods and breast cancer risk: A prospective study in Hiroshima and Nagasaki, Japan. *Br J Cancer*. 81: 1248–56, 1999.

79. Messina M. Soy, soy phytoestrogens (isoflavones), and breast cancer. *Am J Clin Nutr*. 70: 574–75, 1999.

80. Messina M. Soyfoods and soybean phyto-oestrogens (isoflavones) as possible alternatives to hormone replacement therapy (HRT). *Eur J Cancer*. 36 Suppl 4: S71–72, 2000.

81. Hsieh CY, Santell RC, Haslam SZ and Helferich WG. Estrogenic effects of genistein on the growth of estrogen receptor-positive human breast cancer (MCF-7) cells in vitro and in vivo. *Cancer Res*. 58: 3833–38, 1998.

82. Allred CD, Allred KF, Ju YH, et al. Soy diets containing varying amounts of genistein stimulate growth of estrogen-dependent (MCF-7) tumors in a dose-dependent manner. *Cancer Res*. 61: 5045–50, 2001.

83. Kaegi E. Unconventional therapies for cancer: 1. Essiac. The Task Force on Alternative Therapies of the Canadian Breast Cancer Research Initiative. *CMAJ*. 158: 897–902, 1998.

84. Kaegi E. Unconventional therapies for cancer: 3. Iscador. Task Force on Alternative Therapies of the Canadian Breast Cancer Research Initiative. *CMAJ*. 158: 1157–59, 1998.

85. National Cancer Institute. *Mistletoe extracts*. 2001. http://www.nci.nih.gov/cancerinfo/pdq/cam/mistletoe.

86. Franz H. Mistletoe lectins and their A and B chains. *Oncology*. 43: 23–34, 1986.

87. Bocci V. Mistletoe (viscum album) lectins as cytokine inducers and immunoadjuvant in tumor therapy. A review. *J Biol Regul Homeost Agents*. 7: 1–6, 1993.

88. Samtleben R, Hajto T, Hostanska K, et al. Mistletoe lectins as immunostimulants (chemistry, pharmacology and clinic). in

Wagner H. *Immunomodulatory Agents from Plants.* Basel, Switzerland, Birkhauser Verlag, 1999.

89. Kuttan G, Vasudevan DM and Kuttan R. Isolation and identification of a tumour reducing component from mistletoe extract (Iscador). *Cancer Lett.* 41: 307–14, 1988.

90. Beuth J, Ko HL, Tunggal L, et al. Thymocyte proliferation and maturation in response to galactoside-specific mistletoe lectin-1. *In Vivo.* 7: 407–10, 1993.

91. Kaegi E. Unconventional therapies for cancer: 2. Green tea. The Task Force on Alternative Therapies of the Canadian Breast Cancer Research Initiative. *CMAJ.* 158: 1033–35, 1998.

92. Taniguchi S, Fujiki H, Kobayashi H, et al. Effect of (-)-epigallocatechin gallate, the main constituent of green tea, on lung metastasis with mouse B16 melanoma cell lines. *Cancer Lett.* 65: 51–54, 1992.

93. Sazuka M, Murakami S, Isemura M, et al. Inhibitory effects of green tea infusion on in vitro invasion and in vivo metastasis of mouse lung carcinoma cells. *Cancer Lett.* 98: 27–31, 1995.

94. Kavanagh KT, Hafer LJ, Kim DW, et al. Green tea extracts decrease carcinogen-induced mammary tumor burden in rats and rate of breast cancer cell proliferation in culture. *J Cell Biochem.* 82: 387–98, 2001.

95. National Center for Complementary and Alternative Medicine NIoH. *St. John's wort and the treatment of depression.* 2001. http://nccam.nih.gov/health/stjohnswort/index.htm.

96. Harrer G, Hubner WD and Podzuweit H. Effectiveness and tolerance of the hypericum extract LI 160 compared to maprotiline: A multicenter double-blind study. *J Geriatr Psychiatry Neurol.* 7 Suppl 1: S24–28, 1994.

97. Harrer G and Sommer H. Treatment of mild/moderate depressions with hypericum. *Phytomedicine.* 1: 3–8, 1994.

98. Linde K, Ramirez G, Mulrow CD, et al. St John's wort for depression—An overview and meta-analysis of randomised clinical trials. *BMJ.* 313: 253–58, 1996.

99. Shelton RC, Keller MB, Gelenberg A, et al. Effectiveness of St John's wort in major depression: a randomized controlled trial. *JAMA*. 285: 1978–86, 2001.

100. Jacobson JS, Troxel AB, Evans J, et al. Randomized trial of black cohosh for the treatment of hot flashes among women with a history of breast cancer. *J Clin Oncol*. 19: 2739–45, 2001.

101. McMichael-Phillips DF, Harding C, Morton M, et al. Effects of soy-protein supplementation on epithelial proliferation in the histologically normal human breast. *Am J Clin Nutr*. 68: 1431S–35S, 1998.

102. University of Texas-MD Anderson Cancer Center and Complementary/Integrative Medicine Education Resources. *Traditional Chinese Medicine*. 1998. http://www.mdanderson.org/departments/cimer/display.cfm?id=5A2F2735-F15F-11D4-810400508B603A14&method=displayFull&pn=6EB86A59-EBD9-11D4-810100508B603A14.

103. Adachi I and Watanabe T. Role of supporting therapy of Juzentaiho-to in advanced breast cancer patients. *Gan to Kagaku Ryoho* [Japanese journal of cancer & chemotherapy]. 16: 1538–43, 1989.

104. Schneider J and Gilford S. Integration of complementary disciplines into the oncology clinic. Part IV. The chiropractor's role in pain management for oncology patients. *Curr Probl Cancer*. 24: 231–41, 2000.

105. Schneider J and Gilford S. The chiropractor's role in pain management for oncology patients. *J Manipulative Physiol Ther*. 24: 52–57, 2001.

106. Ferrell-Torry AT and Glick OJ. The use of therapeutic massage as a nursing intervention to modify anxiety and the perception of cancer pain. *Cancer Nurs*. 16: 93–101, 1993.

107. Field TM. Massage therapy effects. *Am Psychol*. 53: 1270–81, 1998.

108. Grealish L, Lomasney A and Whiteman B. Foot massage. A nursing intervention to modify the distressing symptoms of pain and nausea in patients hospitalized with cancer. *Cancer Nurs*. 23: 237–43, 2000.

109. National Center for Complementary and Alternative Medicine. *Acupuncture.* 2001. http://nccam.nih.gov/health/acupuncture/index.htm.

110. Morris KT, Johnson N, Homer L and Walts D. A comparison of complementary therapy use between breast cancer patients and patients with other primary tumor sites. *Am J Surg.* 179: 407–11, 2000.

111. Vickers A and Zollman C. ABC of complementary therapy: Acupuncture. *BMJ.* 319: 973–76, 1999.

112. National Institutes of Health. *Acupuncture: National Institutes of Health Consensus Development Conference Statement.* Washington, DC, National Institutes of Health, 1997, 1–34.

113. Andersson S and Lundeberg T. Acupuncture—From empiricism to science: Functional background to acupuncture effects in pain and disease. *Med Hypotheses.* 45: 271–81, 1995.

114. Fu H. What is the material base of acupuncture? The nerves! *Med Hypotheses.* 54: 358–59, 2000.

115. Bardychev MS, Guseva LI and Zubova ND. Acupuncture in edema of the extremities following radiation or combination therapy of cancer of the breast and uterus. *Vopr Onkol.* 34: 319–22, 1988.

116. Dundee JW, Ghaly RG, Bill KM, et al. Effect of stimulation of the P6 antiemetic point on postoperative nausea and vomiting. *Br J Anaesth.* 63: 612–18, 1989.

117. Dundee JW, Ghaly RG, Fitzpatrick KT, et al. Acupuncture prophylaxis of cancer chemotherapy-induced sickness. *J R Soc Med.* 82: 268–71, 1989.

118. He JP, Friedrich M, Ertan AK, et al. Pain-relief and movement improvement by acupuncture after ablation and axillary lymphadenectomy in patients with mammary cancer. *Clin Exp Obstet Gynecol.* 26: 81–84, 1999.

119. Cumins SM and Brunt AM. Does acupuncture influence the vasomotor symptoms experienced by breast cancer patients taking tamoxifen? *Acupuncture in Medicine.* 18: 28, 2000.

120. Shen J, Wenger N, Glaspy J, et al. Electroacupuncture for control of myeloablative chemotherapy-induced emesis: A randomized controlled trial. *JAMA*. 284: 2755–61, 2000.

121. Tukmachi E. Treatment of hot flushes in breast cancer patients with acupuncture. *Acupuncture in Medicine*. 18: 22–27, 2000.

122. Leonard P. Zakim Center for Integrated Therapies. *Acupuncture*. 2001. http://www.dana-farber.org/pat/support/zakim_default.asp.

123. Dibble SL, Chapman J, Mack KA and Shih AS. Acupressure for nausea: Results of a pilot study. *Oncol Nurs Forum*. 27: 41–47, 2000.

124. Lerner, Michael. *Choices in Healing: Integrating the Best of Conventional and Complementary Approaches to Cancer*. Cambridge: MIT Press, 1994.

Chapter 62

Clinical Trials: An Overview

What Is a Clinical Trial?

Clinical trials are research studies in which people help doctors find ways to improve health and cancer care. Each study tries to answer scientific questions and to find better ways to prevent, diagnose, or treat cancer.

Why are there clinical trials?

A clinical trial is one of the final stages of a long and careful cancer research process. Studies are done with cancer patients to find out whether promising approaches to cancer prevention, diagnosis, and treatment are safe and effective.

What are the different types of clinical trials?

There are four types of clinical trials:

- Treatment trials test new treatments (like a new cancer drug, new approaches to surgery or radiation therapy, new

The information contained in this chapter is reprinted from the following sources: "What Is a Clinical Trial?" National Cancer Institute (NCI), reviewed December 2003; "Should I Take Part in a Clinical Trial?" NCI, reviewed December 2003; "How Do I Take Part in a Clinical Trial?" NCI, August 2001; "How Is a Clinical Trial Planned and Carried Out?" NCI, January 2003; and "Participating in a Trial: Questions to Ask Your Doctor," NCI, reviewed December 2003.

combinations of treatments, or new methods such as gene therapy).

- Prevention trials test new approaches, such as medicines, vitamins, minerals, or other supplements, that doctors believe may lower the risk of a certain type of cancer. These trials look for the best way to prevent cancer in people who have never had cancer or to prevent cancer from coming back or a new cancer occurring in people who have already had cancer.

- Screening trials test the best way to find cancer, especially in its early stages.

- Quality of Life trials (also called Supportive Care trials) explore ways to improve comfort and quality of life for cancer patients.

What are the phases of clinical trials?

Most clinical research that involves the testing of a new drug progresses in an orderly series of steps, called phases. This allows researchers to ask and answer questions in a way that results in reliable information about the drug and protects the patients. Clinical trials are usually classified into one of three phases:

- **Phase I trials:** These first studies in people evaluate how a new drug should be given (by mouth, injected into the blood, or injected into the muscle), how often, and what dose is safe. A phase I trial usually enrolls only a small number of patients, sometimes as few as a dozen.

- **Phase II trials:** A phase II trial continues to test the safety of the drug, and begins to evaluate how well the new drug works. Phase II studies usually focus on a particular type of cancer.

- **Phase III trials:** These studies test a new drug, a new combination of drugs, or a new surgical procedure in comparison to the current standard. A participant will usually be assigned to the standard group or the new group at random (called randomization). Phase III trials often enroll large numbers of people and may be conducted at many doctors' offices, clinics, and cancer centers nationwide.

Should I Take Part in a Clinical Trial?

Only you can make the decision about whether or not to partici-pate in a clinical trial. Before you make your decision, you should:

- Learn as much as possible about your disease and the trials that are available to you.

- Then, talk about this information and how you feel about it with your doctor or nurse, family members, and friends to help you determine what is right for you.

What are the potential risks and benefits of clinical trials?

Potential benefits include:

- Health care provided by leading physicians in the field of cancer research.

- Access to new drugs and interventions before they are widely available.

- Close monitoring of your health care and any side effects.

- A more active role in your own health care.

- Being among the first to benefit if the approach being studied is found to be helpful.

- An opportunity to make a valuable contribution to cancer re-search.

The potential risks include:

- New drugs and procedures may have side effects or risks un-known to the doctors.

- New drugs and procedures may be ineffective, or less effective, than current approaches.

- Even if a new approach has benefits, it may not work for you.

How are participants protected?

The government has a system designed to protect human research subjects. Before a government-funded clinical trial can begin, the trial plan (also called a protocol) must be approved. During the trial, review committees make sure that the plan is being followed and participants are being protected.

Regulations require the researchers performing studies to thoroughly inform patients about a study's treatments and tests and their possible benefits and risks before a patient decides whether to participate in any study. This process is called informed consent.

What is informed consent?

Informed consent is a process in which you learn the key facts about a clinical trial before you decide whether to participate. You will talk about these facts with the research doctor or nurse, and they will also be included in a written consent form that you can take home to read and discuss. The consent form will include details about:

- the study approach
- the intervention given in the trial
- the possible risks and benefits
- the tests you may have

Don't hesitate to ask questions until you have all the information you need. While informed consent begins before you agree to participate in a trial, you should feel free to ask the health-care team any questions you have at any point. Informed consent continues as long as you are in the study. You can change your mind and leave the study whenever you want—before the study starts or at any time during the study or follow-up period.

Could I receive a placebo?

In treatment trials involving people who have cancer, placebos ("dummy" pills that contain no active ingredient) are very rarely used. Many treatment trials are designed to compare a new treatment with a standard treatment, which is the best treatment currently known for a cancer based on results of past research. In these studies, patients are randomly assigned to one group or another. When no standard treatment exists for a cancer, a study may compare a new treatment with a placebo. However, you will be told about this possibility during informed consent, before you decide whether or not to take part in the study.

What happens during a trial?

If you decide to participate in a clinical trial, you will work with a research team. Team members may include doctors, nurses, social workers, dietitians, and other health care professionals. They will provide your care, monitor your health carefully, and give you specific instructions about the study.

Participating in a trial may mean that you will have more tests and doctor visits than you would if you weren't in the study. Team members also may continue to stay in contact with you after the trial ends. To make the trial results as reliable as possible, it is important for participants to follow the research team's instructions. That means having all doctor visits and tests, taking medicines on time, and completing logs or answering questionnaires.

How Do I Take Part in a Clinical Trial?

Once you've decided that participating in a clinical trial could prove beneficial to you, there are other factors to consider that might affect your participation.

Who is eligible to participate in a clinical trial?

Each study has its own guidelines for who can participate, called eligibility criteria. Generally, participants in a study are alike in key ways, such as the type and stage of cancer, age, gender, or previous treatments. The eligibility criteria are included in the study plan. To find out if you are eligible for a particular study, talk to your doctor or the doctor or nurse in charge of enrolling patients in the study.

Where are trials conducted?

If you were to participate in a clinical trial, you might receive your treatment at a large cancer center, a university hospital, or your local medical center or physician's office.

Depending on the type of trial and on the intervention it's designed to study, the trial may include participants at one or two highly specialized centers or it may involve hundreds of locations at the same time. You would participate in the trial under the guidance of a team including your physician and other health professionals, who would report your experience with the treatment back to the center responsible for the trial's overall coordination. Experts then use the information from all the participants to evaluate the intervention that the trial is testing.

Who pays for the patient care costs on a clinical trial?

Even if you have health insurance, your coverage may not include some or all of the costs associated with a clinical trial. This is because some health plans define clinical trials as "experimental" or "investigational" procedures. Because lack of coverage for these costs can keep people from enrolling in trials, the National Cancer Institute is working with major health plans and managed care groups to find solutions.

How Is a Clinical Trial Planned and Carried Out?

In order to make a decision about whether to participate in a clinical trial, it helps to understand more about how trials are conceived and run. You will also want to know what happens when a trial is over.

Where do the ideas for trials come from?

The ideas for clinical trials often originate in the laboratory. Researchers develop a clinical trial protocol (the plan for a trial) after laboratory studies indicate the promise of a new drug or procedure. The first trials of a particular drug or procedure are focused on safety, and following trials focus on whether the drug or procedure works.

What is a protocol?

Every trial has a person in charge, usually a doctor, who is called the principal investigator. The principal investigator prepares a plan for the study, called a protocol. The protocol explains what the study will do, how it will be carried out, and why each part of the study is necessary. The protocol usually includes:

- The reason for doing the study
- How many people will be in the study
- Who is eligible to participate in the study
- What study drugs participants will take
- What medical tests they will have and how often
- What information will be gathered

Every doctor or research center that takes part in the trial uses the same protocol. This ensures that patients are treated identically no matter where they are receiving treatment, and that information from all the participating centers can be combined and compared.

Who sponsors clinical trials?

Clinical trials are sponsored by organizations or individuals who are seeking better treatments for cancer or better ways to prevent or detect cancer.

Individual physicians at cancer centers and other medical institutions can sponsor clinical trials themselves.

The National Cancer Institute (NCI) sponsors a large number of clinical trials. The NCI has a number of programs designed to make clinical trials widely available in the United States. Thousands of investigators at over a thousand sites participate in various aspects of NCI's clinical trials programs. These include the following:

- **Cancer Centers Program:** About sixty research-oriented institutions have been designated as NCI Comprehensive or Clinical Cancer Centers for their scientific excellence. The centers are key partners in the NCI's efforts to bring the benefits of clinical research directly to you. Located throughout the country, they play an important role in cancer research, delivery of the highest quality cancer care, and outreach and education for the public and professionals.

- **Cooperative Clinical Trials Program:** This program brings together groups of researchers, cancer centers, and community physicians into a national NCI-supported network. The network consists of a number of Cooperative Groups that seek to define the key unanswered questions in cancer and then conduct high-quality clinical trials at many sites around the country to answer these questions. The Cooperative Groups enroll about twenty thousand new patients in treatment trials each year. Important phase III trials run by the Cooperative Groups help establish the state of the art for cancer therapy. Additionally, the Groups perform large cancer prevention trials.

- **Guide to Cooperative Group Web Sites:** the Cooperative Group sites provide a wide variety of information and resources for non-member visitors, along with password-protected members-only areas. All clinical trials conducted by the Cooperative Groups are listed in NCI's clinical trials database, PDQ (see the User's Guide for information on how to search the database.) To search for trials sponsored by one or more of the groups, use the Lead Organization or Cooperative Group field at the bottom of PDQ's advanced search form to either type in the name of a group or use a browse list to look up group names alphabetically.

- **The Community Clinical Oncology Program (CCOP):** This program makes clinical trials available in a large number of local communities in the United States by linking community physicians with researchers in cancer centers. Local hospitals throughout the country affiliate with a cancer center or a cooperative group. This enables doctors to offer people participation in clinical trials more easily, without having to travel long distances or leave their usual caregivers. Several of these programs focus on encouraging minority populations to participate in trials.

Drug companies or companies that make diagnostic equipment (like x-ray machines) sponsor trials of their products, hoping to demonstrate that their products are safe and effective. The U.S. Food and Drug Administration (FDA) will permit companies to sell a product only after it has been proven safe and effective in clinical trials.

What happens when a clinical trial is over?

After a phase I or II trial is completed, the researchers look carefully at the data collected during the trial and decide whether to:

- Move on to the next phase trial with the treatment, or
- Stop testing the treatment because it is not safe or effective

When a phase III trial comes to an end, the researchers must look at the data and decide if the results have medical importance. When the analysis is complete, the researchers will inform the medical community and the public of the study results.

In most cases, the results of trials are published in scientific or medical journals. To find out if the results of a study you participated in was published:

- Ask the doctor or nurse in charge of your treatment.
- Find out the official name of your study and search for the study in the PubMed database of medical publications. If you have trouble locating the study or searching for it, the research librarian at a university or medical library may be able to help.

Most medical and scientific journals have in place a process of peer review, in which experts critique the report before it is published, to make sure that the analysis and conclusions are sound. Particularly important results are likely to be featured by the print or electronic media, and widely discussed at scientific meetings and by patient advocacy groups. Once an intervention is proven safe and effective in a clinical trial, it may become the new standard of practice. In this way the development of better interventions for prevention, for treatment, or for detection and diagnosis is an ongoing, continuous process that builds progressively on itself to improve the quality of cancer care and prevention available to us all.

Participating in a Trial: Questions to Ask Your Doctor

Anyone considering a clinical trial should feel free to ask any questions or bring up any issues concerning the trial at any time. The following suggestions may give you some ideas as you think about your own questions.

The Study

1. What is the purpose of the study?

2. Why do researchers think the approach may be effective?

3. Who will sponsor the study?

4. Who has reviewed and approved the study?

5. How are study results and safety of participants being checked?

6. How long will the study last?

7. What will my responsibilities be if I participate?

Possible Risks and Benefits

1. What are my possible short-term benefits?

2. What are my possible long-term benefits?

3. What are my short-term risks, such as side effects?

4. What are my possible long-term risks?

5. What other options do people with my risk of cancer or type of cancer have?

6. How do the possible risks and benefits of this trial compare with those options?

Participation and Care

1. What kinds of therapies, procedures, or tests will I have during the trial?

2. Will they hurt, and if so, for how long?

3. How do the tests in the study compare with those I would have outside of the trial?

4. Will I be able to take my regular medications while in the clinical trial?

5. Where will I have my medical care?

6. Who will be in charge of my care?

Personal Issues

1. How could being in this study affect my daily life?

2. Can I talk to other people in the study?

Cost Issues

1. Will I have to pay for any part of the trial such as tests or the study drug?

2. If so, what will the charges likely be?

3. What is my health insurance likely to cover?

4. Who can help answer any questions from my insurance company or health plan?

5. Will there be any travel or child care costs that I need to consider while I am in the trial?

Tips for Asking Your Doctor about Trials

When you talk with your doctor or members of the research team:

1. Consider taking a family member or friend along, for support and for help in asking questions or recording answers.

2. Plan ahead what to ask—but don't hesitate to ask any new questions you think of while you're there.

3. Write down your questions in advance, to make sure you remember to ask them all.

4. Write down the answers, so that you can review them whenever you want.

5. Consider bringing a tape recorder to make a taped record of what's said (even if you write down answers).

Chapter 63

Clinical Trials and Insurance Coverage: A Resource Guide

As you consider enrolling in a clinical trial, you will face the critical issue of how to cover the costs of care. Even if you have health insurance, your coverage may not include some or all of the patient care costs associated with a clinical trial. This is because some health plans define clinical trials as "experimental" or "investigational" procedures.

A growing number of states have passed legislation or instituted special agreements requiring health plans to pay the cost of routine medical care you receive as a participant in a clinical trial.

Because lack of coverage for these costs can keep people from enrolling in trials, the National Cancer Institute is working with major health plans and managed care groups to find solutions. In the meantime, there are strategies that may help you deal with cost and coverage barriers. This chapter answers frequently asked questions about insurance coverage for clinical trial participation.

The material here is mainly concerned with treatment clinical trials, since other types of trials (prevention, screening, etc.) are newer and generally not covered by health insurance at all. However, the information provided here may become more relevant for prevention and other types of trials as these trials grow more common.

In 2000, Medicare began covering beneficiaries' patient care costs in clinical trials. Up-to-date information about what Medicare will

Reprinted from "Clinical Trials and Insurance Coverage: A Resource Guide," National Cancer Institute, January 2002.

cover can be found on the website (http://cms.hhs.gov) of the Centers for Medicare and Medicaid (formerly the Health Care Financing Administration). A summary of Medicare coverage as of January 2001 is included in this chapter.

If you do not have any health insurance, you may find this chapter helpful for understanding some of the costs that trials involve.

Basics

What costs do trials involve, and who is usually responsible for paying them?

There are two types of costs associated with a clinical trial: patient care costs and research costs.

Patient care costs fall into two categories:

- Usual care costs, such as doctor visits, hospital stays, clinical laboratory tests, x-rays, and so on, which occur whether you are participating in a trial or receiving standard treatment. These costs have usually been covered by a third-party health plan, such as Medicare or private insurance.

- Extra care costs associated with clinical trial participation, such as the additional tests that may or may not be fully covered by the clinical trial sponsor or research institution. The sponsor and the participant's health plan need to resolve coverage of these costs for particular trials.

Research costs are those associated with conducting the trial, such as data collection and management, research physician and nurse time, analysis of results, and tests purely performed for research purposes. Such costs are usually covered by the sponsoring organization, such as the National Cancer Institute (NCI) or a pharmaceutical company.

What criteria do health plans use to make decisions about reimbursement for trials?

Health insurance companies and managed care companies decide which health care services they will pay for by developing a coverage policy regarding the specific services. In general, the most important factor determining whether something is covered is a health plan's judgment as to whether the service is established or investigational. Health plans usually designate a service as established if there is a certain amount of scientific data to show that it is safe and effective. If the health plan does not think that such data exist in sufficient quantity, the plan may label the service as investigational.

Health care services delivered within the setting of a clinical trial are very often categorized as investigational and not covered. This is because the health plan thinks that the major reason to perform the clinical trial is that there is not enough data to establish the safety and effectiveness of the service being studied. Thus, for some health plans, any mention of the fact that the patient is involved in a clinical trial results in a denial of payment.

Your health plan may define specific criteria that a trial must meet before extending coverage, such as:

- **Sponsorship:** Some plans may cover costs only of trials sponsored by organizations whose review and oversight of the trial is careful and scientifically rigorous, according to standards set by the health plan.

- **Trial phase and type:** Some plans may cover patient care costs only for the clinical trials they judge to be "medically necessary" on a case-by-case basis. Trial phase may also affect coverage; for example, while a plan may be willing to cover costs associated with phase III trials, which include treatments that have already been successful with a certain number of people, the plan may require some documentation of effectiveness before covering a phase I or phase II trial.

  While health plans are interested in efforts to improve prevention and screening, they currently seem less likely to have a review process in place for these trials. Therefore, it may be more difficult to get coverage for the care costs associated with them.

- **Cost "neutrality":** Some health plans may limit coverage to trials they consider cost-neutral (i.e., not significantly more expensive than the treatments considered standard).

- **Lack of standard therapy:** Some plans limit coverage of trials to situations in which no standard therapy is available.

- **Facility and personnel qualifications:** A health plan may require that the facility and medical staff meet specific qualifications to conduct a trial involving unique services, especially intensive therapy such as high-dose chemotherapy with bone marrow or stem cell transplantation.

Some plans, especially smaller ones, will not cover any costs associated with a clinical trial. Policies vary widely, but in most cases your best bet is to have your doctor start discussions with the health plan.

Medicare Coverage

For up-to-date information about Medicare coverage of clinical trials, go to the website (http://cms.hhs.gov) for the Centers for Medicaid and Medicare (formerly the Health Care Financing Administration). As of January 2001, the following information was accurate:

If I'm in a clinical trial, what will Medicare pay?

- Anything normally covered is still covered when it is part of a clinical trial. This includes tests, procedures, and doctor visits that are ordinarily covered.

- Anything normally covered even if it is a service or item associated with the experimental treatment. For example, Medicare will pay for the intravenous administration of a new chemotherapy drug being tested in a trial, including any therapy to prevent side effects from the new drug.

- Anything normally covered even if it resulted from your being in the clinical trial. For example, a test or hospitalization resulting from a side effect of the new treatment that Medicare would ordinarily cover.

What costs are not covered?

- Investigational items or services being tested in a trial. Sponsors of clinical trials often provide the new drug free, but make sure you ask your doctor before you begin.

- Items or services used solely for the data collection needs of the trial.

- Anything being provided free by the sponsor of the trial.

What kinds of clinical trials are covered?

In general, cancer treatment and diagnosis trials are covered if:

- They are funded by the National Cancer Institute (NCI), NCI-designated cancer centers, NCI-sponsored Clinical Trials

Cooperative Groups, and all other federal agencies that fund cancer research. Other trials may be eligible for coverage and doctors can ask Medicare to pay the patients' costs. Ask your doctor about this before you begin.

- They are designed to treat or diagnose your cancer.

- The purpose or subject of the trial is within a Medicare benefit category. For example, cancer diagnosis and treatment are Medicare benefits, so these trials are covered. Cancer prevention trials are not currently covered.

Strategies

What can I do to increase the likelihood of coverage?

There are several steps you can follow to deal with coverage issues up front when deciding to enter a clinical trial. Along the way, enlist the help of family members and your doctor or other health professionals. You may find the following checklist useful:

- **Understand the costs associated with the trial.** Ask your doctor or the trial's contact person about the costs that must be covered by you or your health plan. Are these costs significantly higher than those associated with standard therapy? Also, inquire about the experience of other patients in the trial. Have their plans paid for their care? Have there been any persistent problems with coverage? How often have the trial's administrators been successful in getting plans to cover patient care costs?

- **Understand your health plan.** Be sure you know what's in your policy; request and carefully review the actual contract language. If there's a specific exclusion for "experimental treatment," look closely at the policy to see how the plan defines such treatment and under what conditions it might be covered. If it is not clearly defined, call the plan's customer service line, consult their website, or write to them. Ask for specific information about clinical trials coverage.

- **Work closely with your doctor.** Talk with your doctor about the paperwork he or she submits to your health plan. If there have been problems with coverage in the past, you might ask your doctor or the hospital to send an information package to the plan that includes studies supporting the procedure's safety, benefits, and medical appropriateness. This package might include: publications from peer-reviewed literature about the proposed therapy that demonstrate patient benefits; a letter that uses the insurance contract's own language to explain why the treatment, screening method, or preventive measure should be covered; letters from researchers that explain the clinical trial; and support letters from patient advocacy groups. Be sure to keep your own copy of any materials that the doctor sends to your health plan for future reference.

- **Work closely with your company's benefits manager.** This person may be helpful in enlisting the support of your employer to request coverage by the health plan.

- **Give your health plan a deadline.** Ask the hospital or cancer center to set a target date for the therapy. This will help to ensure that coverage decisions are made promptly.

- **Take advantage of all information resources available to you.**

What if my claim is denied after I begin participating in a trial?

If a claim is denied, read your policy to find out what steps you can follow to make an appeal. The National Coalition for Cancer Survivorship suggests that you and your doctor demonstrate to the health plan that:

- the therapy is not just a research study, but also a valid procedure that benefits patients;

- your situation is similar to that of other patients who are participating in clinical trials as part of a covered benefit;

- possible complications have been anticipated and can be handled effectively.

You also may wish to contact your state insurance counseling hotline or insurance department for more help, or write your state insurance commissioner describing the problem.

Where else can I turn for assistance?

It's never easy to deal with financial issues when you or a loved one faces cancer. Unfortunately, costs can present a significant barrier to clinical trials participation.

The range of insurance issues and health plan contracts makes it impossible to deal with all of them here. You may wish to consult this partial list of publications, organizations, and websites for more information:

Publications

What Cancer Survivors Need to Know about Health Insurance
National Coalition for Cancer Survivorship
1010 Wayne Avenue, Suite 770
Silver Spring, MD 20910
Toll-Free: 877-622-7937
Phone: 301-650-9127
Fax: 301-565-9670
Website: http://www.canceradvocacy.org
E-mail: info@canceradvocacy.org

Cancer Treatments Your Insurance Should Cover
Association of Community Cancer Centers
11600 Nebel Street, Suite 201
Rockville, MD 20852
Phone: 301-984-9496
Fax: 301-770-1949
Website: http://www.accc-cancer.org/main2001.shtml

Managed Care Answer Guide
Patient Advocate Foundation
700 Thimble Shoals Boulevard, Suite 200
Newport News, VA 23606
Toll-Free: 800-532-5274
Phone: 757-873-8999
Website: http://www.patientadvocate.org/pdf/pubs/mc_answer-guide.pdf
E-mail: help@patientadvocate.org

Medicare

Helpline: 800-444-4606
Website: http://www.medicare.gov

481

Assistance Programs

Candlelighters Childhood Cancer Foundation
PO Box 498
Kensington, MD 20895
Toll-free: 800-366-2223
Phone: 301-962-3520
Fax: 301-962-3521
Website: http://www.candlelighters.org
E-mail: staff@candlelighters.org

The Ombudsman Program helps families of children with cancer and survivors of childhood cancer resolve a range of problems, including insurance coverage difficulties. Local groups appoint a parent advocate who works with the treatment center on behalf of families.

Medical Care Management Corporation
5272 River Road, Suite 650
Bethesda, MD 20816-1405
Phone: 301-652-1818
Fax: 617-375-7777
Website: http://www.mcman.com
E-mail: mcman@mcman.com

Working for a range of clients, including health plans, employers, and patients, MCMC conducts independent, objective reviews of high-technology medical care cases to assist in decision making. While it does charge for its services, MCMC also offers a volunteer program for those who cannot afford to pay.

More Information Resources

OncoLink, a service of the University of Pennsylvania Cancer Center
3400 Spruce Street, 2 Donner
Philadelphia, PA 19104-4283
Fax: 215-349-5445
Website: http://www.oncolink.com

In addition to general cancer information, this website features a section on financial information for patients (http://www.oncolink.com/

resources/resources.cfm?c=6). Among the topics: viatical settlements, life insurance, a glossary of financial and medical terms, and news about billing and insurance.

American's Health Insurance Plans
601 Pennsylvania Ave., NW
South Bldg., Suite 500
Washington, DC 20004
Phone: 202-778-3200
Fax: 202-331-7487
Website: http://www.ahip.net
E-mail: webmaster@ahip.net

The website section "For Consumers" includes a fact sheet on clinical research that describes various health plans' efforts to support research initiatives and collaborate with academic health centers and universities.

Initiatives to Expand Coverage

The good news is that there has been a recent nationwide effort to assure clinical trials coverage, with the National Cancer Institute (NCI) involved in several new initiatives.

NCI's Department of Defense Agreement

An innovative 1996 agreement between NCI and the Department of Defense (DoD) has given thousands of DoD cancer patients more options for care and greater access to state-of-the-art treatments. Patients who are beneficiaries of TRICARE/CHAMPUS, the DoD's health program, are covered for NCI-sponsored phase II and phase III clinical treatment trials. NCI and DoD are refining a system that allows physicians and patients to determine quickly what current trials meet their needs and where they are taking place.

NCI's Department of Veterans Affairs Agreement

A 1997 agreement with the Department of Veterans Affairs provides coverage for eligible veterans of the armed services to participate in NCI-sponsored prevention, diagnosis, and treatment studies nationwide.

Other Developments

- **Midwest Health Plans Agreement**: Some NCI Cooperative Groups have reached agreements with several insurers in Wisconsin and Minnesota to provide more than 200,000 people there with coverage for patient care costs if they participate in a cooperative group-sponsored trial.

- **Pediatric Cancer Care Network:** This network, a cooperative agreement among the Children's Cancer Group, the Pediatric Oncology Group, and the Blue Cross Blue Shield System Association (BCBS) nationwide, will ensure that children of BCBS subscribers receive care at designated centers of cancer care excellence and may promote the enrollment of children in Cooperative Group clinical trials.

Part Seven

Post-Treatment Concerns

Chapter 64

Breast Cancer Recurrence

Occasionally breast cancer can return after primary treatment. There are three types of recurrent breast cancer:

- **Local recurrence:** Cancerous tumor cells remain in the original site, and over time, grow back. Most physicians do not consider local breast cancer recurrence to be the spread of breast cancer, but rather, failure of the primary treatment. Even after mastectomy (surgical removal of the affected breast), portions of the breast skin and fat remain and local recurrence is possible (however, it is uncommon).

- **Regional recurrence:** A regional recurrence of breast cancer is more serious than local recurrence because it usually indicates that the cancer has spread past the breast and the axillary (underarm) lymph nodes. Regional breast cancer recurrences can occur in the pectoral (chest) muscles, in the internal mammary lymph nodes under the breastbone and between the ribs, in the supraclavicular nodes (above the collarbone), and in the nodes surrounding the neck.

- **Distant recurrence:** A distant breast cancer recurrence, also known as a metastasis (spread), is the most dangerous type of recurrence. Once out of the breast, cancer usually spreads first to the axillary (underarm) lymph nodes. In 25 percent of distant recurrences, breast cancer spreads from the lymph nodes to bone. Other sites breast cancer may spread to include the bone marrow, lungs, liver, brain, or other organs.

Often, a diagnosis of recurrent cancer is more devastating or psychologically difficult for a woman than her initial breast cancer diagnosis. Women who have recurrent breast cancer are encouraged to discuss their feelings with a counselor or therapist and consider joining a support group.

Local and Regional Recurrence

Breast cancer most commonly recurs in the same area as the original cancer had occurred. Women with ductal carcinoma in situ (DCIS) who are treated with breast-conserving therapy (lumpectomy and radiation) are at a slightly higher risk of experiencing a recurrence than those women who are treated with mastectomy (removal of the affected breast). However, several studies have shown that women treated with breast-conserving therapy who have local recurrence of DCIS are not at any significantly greater risk of dying from the disease than women treated with mastectomy. DCIS is a common type of cancer that is confined to the milk ducts of the breast.

A recurrence of noninvasive breast cancer is less serious than a recurrence of invasive cancer. In general, invasive local recurrences are more aggressive since they have a second chance of spreading (metastasizing) to other areas of the body.

Once recurrent breast cancer has been detected, physicians will order additional tests to determine to what extent the cancer has spread. These tests may include: bone scan, chest x-ray, CAT scan, MRI scan, and liver blood tests. Treatment of a local recurrence often depends on how the initial treatment was performed. If lumpectomy was performed, recurrent breast cancer will usually be treated with mastectomy. A local recurrence after mastectomy will usually present itself as a small lump in the mastectomy scar or under the skin. This type of recurrence often goes undetected for some time because it may be mistaken for a leftover stitch or scar tissue from the mastectomy operation. Once the lump grows, breast biopsy is performed to determine whether it is cancerous.

Breast reconstruction rarely hides recurrent breast cancer. Local recurrences with implants are most often in front of the implant, and recurrences with TRAM flap procedures are along the edge of the breast skin (not in the flap).

Women whose initial breast cancer was aggressive are more likely to have recurrences than other women. Inflammatory breast cancer with cancer cells in the lymphatics of the skin or breast often recurs. (Lymphatics are key components of the body's immune system). Also, women with large tumors or several cancerous lymph nodes may experience recurrent breast cancer. Often, these types of recurrent cancers are treated with mastectomy (if it was not performed during primary treatment) followed by radiation therapy to the chest wall.

Regional breast cancer recurrences are rare, occurring in approximately 2 percent of all breast cancer cases. Most often, regional recurrence appears as a cancerous axillary (underarm) lymph node that was not removed during primary treatment. Treatment involves simply removing the cancerous node. Regional recurrence in the lymph nodes of the neck or above the collarbone usually indicates more aggressive cancers.

Besides local and regional recurrences, a new cancer may occasionally occur years after the initial cancer. Usually, the new cancer is in a different area of the breast and does not have the same pathology. For example, the original cancer is ductal carcinoma in situ (DCIS) and the second cancer appears as invasive lobular carcinoma. Second cancers are treated as new cancers, independent of the first cancer.

Distant Recurrence

A distant recurrence of breast cancer is called metastatic disease. Metastatic breast cancer (Stage IV) is serious and the survival rate is considerably lower than for women whose cancer is confined to the breast or axillary (underarm) lymph nodes. Breast cancer has the potential to spread to almost any region of the body. The most common region is bone, followed by the lungs and liver.

Symptoms of metastatic breast cancer may include:

- Bone pain (possible indication of bone metastases)

- Shortness of breath (possible indication of lung metastases)

- Lack of appetite (possible indication of liver metastases)

- Weight loss (possible indication of liver metastases)

- Neurological pain or weakness, headaches (possible indication of neurological metastases)

These symptoms are sometimes but not always associated with metastatic breast cancer. Additionally, having one or more of these symptoms does not necessarily mean a woman has metastatic breast cancer. Any changes in health should be reported to a physician for further examination. Metastatic breast cancer is usually diagnosed by bone scan, CAT scan, MRI scan, or liver blood tests.

Surgery is rarely an option for metastatic breast cancer because the cancer is not usually confined to one specific spot on the given organ. Instead, treatment options include one or more of the following: chemotherapy, radiation therapy, or hormonal (drug) therapies. Patients with advanced breast cancer may wish to consider entering into a clinical trial designed to evaluate the effectiveness of newly developed treatments.

About Imaginis

Imaginis.com is an independent, award-winning, comprehensive resource for news and information on breast cancer prevention, screening, diagnosis, and treatment and related women's health topics such as hormone replacement therapy (HRT), multiple sclerosis, osteoporosis, and ovarian cancer. Imaginis.com also contains extensive information about medical procedures such as angiography, biopsy, CT, MR, nuclear medicine, ultrasound, x-ray imaging, and radiotherapy.

The goal of Imaginis.com is to provide women and their physicians with the most comprehensive and relevant information on breast health and related women's health issues. Imaginis content is created by an independent team of breast health specialists to ensure that it is up-to-date and accurate. Complicated medical terms are explained in everyday language to help individuals understand their options, make informed decisions, and achieve optimal health.

Chapter 65

Breast Reconstruction

General Description of Breast Implant Surgery

Breast implant procedures can be performed on an outpatient (not hospitalized) basis or at a hospital. Breast implant surgery can be done under local anesthesia (only breast area numbed) or under general anesthesia (put to sleep). Breast implant surgery can last from one to several hours depending on whether the implant is inserted behind (submuscular) or in front of (subglandular) the chest muscle and whether surgery is performed on one or both breasts. If the surgery is done in a hospital, the length of the hospital stay will vary according to the type of surgery, the development of any postoperative complications, and your general health. It may also depend on the type of coverage your insurance provides. Before surgery, your doctor should discuss with you the extent of surgery, the estimated time it will take, and the choice of drugs for pain and nausea.

Your Expectations

Your consideration of breast implants should be based on realistic expectations of the outcome. You may also want to talk with women who have had this surgery at least a year ago by the same surgeon. Keep in mind, however, that there is no guarantee that your results will match those of other women.

Reprinted from "Breast Implants: An Informational Update," U.S. Food and Drug Administration, Center for Devices and Radiological Health, August 2000.

491

Your results will depend on many individual factors, such as:

- your overall health
- chest structure and body shape
- healing capabilities (which may be hindered by radiation and chemotherapy, smoking, alcohol, and various medications)
- bleeding tendencies/likelihood
- prior breast surgery(ies)
- possibility of infection
- the skill and experience of the surgical team
- the type of surgical procedure
- the type and size of implant

You will be given general or local anesthesia, and in most cases, antibiotics. The surgery may last several hours.

Scarring is a natural outcome of surgery, and your doctor can describe the location, size, and appearance of the scars you can expect to have. For most women, scars will fade over time to thin lines, although the darker your skin, the more prominent the scars are likely to be. You should ask your doctor about the types of surgical procedures, where your scar will be, and what to expect after surgery.

Postoperative Care

Your doctor should describe the usual postoperative (after surgery) recovery process, the possible complications that can arise, and the expected recovery period. Following the operation, as with any surgery, some pain, swelling, bruising, and tenderness can be expected. These complications may last for a month or longer, but they should disappear with time.

Medications for pain and nausea can be prescribed. Some women may experience bleeding and some may experience fever, warmth, or redness of the breast, or other symptoms of infection. These symptoms should be reported immediately to your doctor. You should be told about wound healing and how to care for your wound. Drains may be used for a few days.

Postoperative care may involve the use of a postoperative bra, compression bandage, or jog bra for extra support and positioning while you heal. At your doctor's recommendation, you will most likely be able to return to work within a few days, although you should avoid any strenuous activities that could raise your pulse and blood pressure for at least a couple of weeks. Your doctor may also recommend breast massage exercises.

Ask your doctor about a schedule of follow-up examinations, limits on your activities, precautions you should take, and when you can return to your normal routine. (If you are enrolled in a clinical study, your doctor should give you a schedule for follow-up examinations set by the study plan.)

Special Surgical Concerns for Women with Breast Cancer

The following issues should be considered for women with breast cancer:

- The physical and cosmetic results with breast implants may be affected by chemotherapy, radiation therapy, or any other factor that significantly alters the healing process.

- Skin necrosis (cell death) may occur because circulation to the remaining tissue has been changed by a mastectomy (breast removal). Also, skin necrosis may be increased as a result of radiation treatment.

- It usually takes more than one operation to achieve the desired cosmetic outcome, especially if this procedure includes building a new nipple.

Choices in Reconstructive Procedures

The type of breast reconstruction procedure available to you depends on your medical situation, breast shape and size, general health, lifestyle, and goals. Women with small or medium-sized breasts are the best candidates for breast reconstruction.

Breast reconstruction can be accomplished by the use of a breast implant, your own tissues (a tissue flap), or a combination of the two. A tissue flap is a section of skin, fat, or muscle that is moved from your stomach, back, or other area of your body to the chest area and shaped into a new breast.

Whether you have reconstruction with or without breast implants, you will probably undergo additional surgeries to improve symmetry

493

and appearance. For example, after your breast has healed from the original implant surgery, you may want to build a new nipple and darken the areola (skin around the nipple). This procedure can usually be performed on an outpatient basis. Ask your doctor to explain the various ways this can be done, such as using a skin graft from the opposite breast or tattooing the area.

Ask your doctor about the pros and cons of each implant technique. If you decide to have reconstruction for one breast, you may need to think about surgery on the other breast to achieve a similar appearance.

Breast Reconstruction with Breast Implants

Your surgeon will decide whether your health and medical condition makes you an appropriate candidate for breast implant reconstruction. Women with larger breasts may require reconstruction with a combination of a tissue flap and an implant. Your surgeon may recommend breast implantation of the opposite, uninvolved breast in order to make them more alike (maximize symmetry) or he or she may suggest breast reduction (reduction mammoplasty) or a breast lift (mastopexy) to improve symmetry. Mastopexy involves removing a strip of skin from under the breast or around the nipple and using it to lift and tighten the skin over the breast. Reduction mammoplasty involves removal of breast tissue and skin. If it is important to you not to alter the unaffected breast, you should discuss this with your surgeon, as it may affect the breast reconstruction methods considered for your case.

Timing of Breast Implant Reconstruction

The following description applies to reconstruction following mastectomy, but similar considerations apply to reconstruction following breast trauma or for reconstruction for congenital defects. The breast reconstruction process may begin at the time of your mastectomy (immediate reconstruction) or weeks to years afterward (delayed reconstruction). Immediate reconstruction may involve placement of a breast implant, but typically involves placement of a tissue expander, which will eventually be replaced with a breast implant. It is important to know that any type of surgical breast reconstruction may take several steps to complete.

Two potential advantages to immediate reconstruction are that your breast reconstruction starts at the time of your mastectomy and that there may be cost savings in combining the mastectomy procedure with the first stage of the reconstruction. However, there may be a higher risk of complications such as deflation with immediate reconstruction, and your initial operative time and recuperative time may be longer.

A potential advantage to delayed reconstruction is that you can delay your reconstruction decision and surgery until other treatments, such as radiation therapy and chemotherapy, are completed. Delayed reconstruction may be advisable if your surgeon anticipates healing problems with your mastectomy, or if you just need more time to consider your options.

There are medical, financial, and emotional considerations to choosing immediate versus delayed reconstruction. You should discuss with your surgeon, plastic surgeon, and oncologist the pros and cons with the options available in your individual case.

Surgical Considerations to Discuss

Discuss the advantages and disadvantages of the following options with your surgeon and your oncologist:

Immediate Reconstruction

- One-stage immediate reconstruction with a breast implant (implant only).

- Two-stage immediate reconstruction with a tissue expander followed by delayed reconstruction several months later with a breast implant.

Delayed Reconstruction

- Two-stage delayed reconstruction with a tissue expander followed several months later by replacement with a breast implant.

Breast Implant Reconstruction Procedures

One-Stage Immediate Breast Implant Reconstruction

Immediate one-stage breast reconstruction may be done at the time of your mastectomy. After the general surgeon removes your breast tissue, the plastic surgeon will then implant a breast implant that completes the one-stage reconstruction.

Two-Stage (Immediate or Delayed) Breast Implant Reconstruction

Breast reconstruction usually occurs as a two-stage procedure, starting with the placement of a breast tissue expander, which is replaced several months later with a breast implant. The tissue expander placement may be done immediately, at the time of your mastectomy, or be delayed until months or years later.

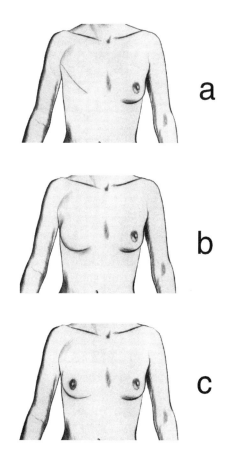

Figure 65.1. Breast reconstruction with an implant: (a) post-mastectomy; (b) stage 1: tissue expander; (c) stage 2: breast implant and nipple/areola reconstruction. (Source: NCI Visuals Online, National Cancer Institute.)

Tissue Expansion

During a mastectomy, the general surgeon often removes skin as well as breast tissue, leaving the chest tissues flat and tight. To create a breast shaped space for the breast implant, a tissue expander is placed under the remaining chest tissues.

The tissue expander is a balloon-like device made from elastic silicone rubber. It is inserted unfilled, and over time, sterile saline fluid is added by inserting a small needle through the skin to the filling port of the device. As the tissue expander fills, the tissues over the expander begin to stretch, similar to the gradual expansion of a woman's abdomen during pregnancy. The tissue expander creates a new breast-shaped pocket for a breast implant.

Tissue expander placement usually occurs under general anesthesia in an operating room. Operative time is generally one to two hours. The procedure may require a brief hospital stay, or be done on an outpatient basis. Typically, you can resume normal daily activity after two to three weeks.

Because the chest skin is usually numb from the mastectomy surgery, it is possible that you may not experience pain from the placement of the tissue expander. However, you may experience feelings of pressure or discomfort after each filling of the expander, which subsides as the tissue expands. Tissue expansion typically lasts four to six months.

Placing the Breast Implant

After the tissue expander is removed, the breast implant is placed in the pocket. The surgery to replace the tissue expander with a breast implant (implant exchange) is usually done under general anesthesia in an operating room. It may require a brief hospital stay or be done on an outpatient basis.

Breast Reconstruction without Implants: Tissue Flap Procedures

The breast can be reconstructed by surgically moving a section of skin, fat, and muscle from one area of your body to another. The section of tissue may be taken from such areas as your abdomen, upper back, upper hip, or buttocks.

The tissue flap may be left attached to the blood supply and moved to the breast area through a tunnel under the skin (a pedicled flap), or it may be removed completely and reattached to the breast area by microsurgical techniques (a free flap). Operating time is generally longer with free flaps, because of the microsurgical requirements.

Flap surgery requires a hospital stay of several days and generally a longer recovery time than implant reconstruction. Flap surgery also creates scars at the site where the flap was taken and possibly on the reconstructed breast. However, flap surgery has the advantage of being able to replace tissue in the chest area. This may be useful when the chest tissues have been damaged and are not suitable for tissue expansion. Another advantage of flap procedures over implantation is that alteration of the unaffected breast is generally not needed to improve symmetry.

The most common types of tissue flaps are the TRAM (transverse rectus abdominus musculocutaneous) flap, which uses tissue from the abdomen, and the Latissimus dorsi flap, which uses tissue from the upper back.

It is important for you to be aware that flap surgery, particularly the TRAM flap, is a major operation and more extensive than your mastectomy operation. It requires good general health and strong emotional motivation. If you are very overweight, smoke cigarettes, have had previous surgery at the flap site, or have any circulatory problems, you may not be a good candidate for a tissue flap procedure. Also, if you are very thin, you may not have enough tissue in your abdomen or back to create a breast mound with this method.

The TRAM Flap (Pedicle or Free)

During a TRAM flap procedure, the surgeon removes a section of tissue from your abdomen and moves it to your chest to reconstruct the breast. The TRAM flap is sometimes referred to as a "tummy tuck" reconstruction because it may leave the stomach area flatter.

A pedicle TRAM flap procedure typically takes three to six hours of surgery under general anesthesia; a free TRAM flap procedure generally takes longer. The TRAM procedure may require a blood transfusion. Typically, the hospital stay is two to five days. You can resume normal daily activity after six to eight weeks. Some women, however, report that it takes up to one year to resume a normal lifestyle. You may have temporary or permanent muscle weakness in the abdominal area. If you are considering pregnancy after your reconstruction, you should discuss this with your surgeon. You will have a large scar on your abdomen and may also have additional scars on your reconstructed breast.

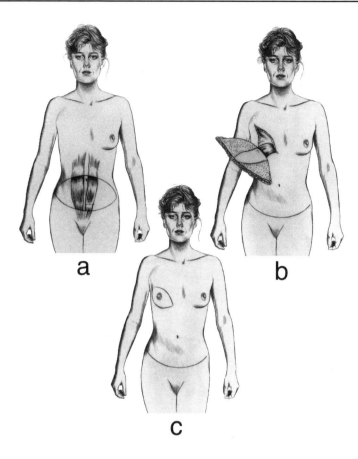

Figure 65.2. TRAM flap: (a) post-mastectomy; (b) TRAM flap; (c) final result with nipple/areola reconstruction. (Source: NCI Visuals Online, National Cancer Institute.)

The Latissimus Dorsi Flap with or without Breast Implants

During a Latissimus Dorsi flap procedure, the surgeon moves a section of tissue from your back to your chest to reconstruct the breast. Because the Latissimus Dorsi flap is usually thinner and smaller than the TRAM flap, this procedure may be more appropriate for reconstructing a smaller breast.

The Latissimus Dorsi flap procedure typically takes two to four hours of surgery under general anesthesia. Typically, the hospital stay

499

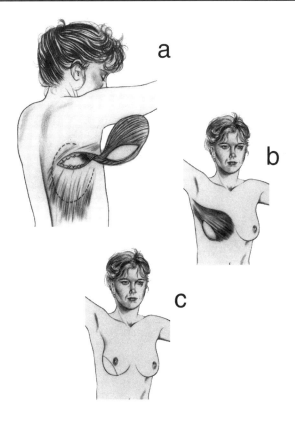

Figure 65.3. *Latissimus Dorsi flap: (a) back view; (b) front view; (c) final result with nipple/areola reconstruction. (Source: NCI Visuals Online, National Cancer Institute.)*

is two to three days. You can resume daily activity after two to three weeks. You may have some temporary or permanent muscle weakness and difficulty with movement in your back and shoulder. You will have a scar on your back, which can usually be hidden in the bra line. You may also have additional scars on your reconstructed breast.

Chapter 66

Lymphedema: A Brief Overview and Steps to Prevention

Lymphedema: A Brief Overview

What Is Lymphedema?

Lymphedema is an accumulation of lymphatic fluid in the interstitial tissue that causes swelling, most often in the arm(s) or leg(s), and occasionally in other parts of the body. Lymphedema can develop when lymphatic vessels are missing or impaired (primary), or when lymph vessels are damaged or lymph nodes removed (secondary).

When the impairment becomes so great that the lymphatic fluid exceeds the lymphatic transport capacity, an abnormal amount of protein-rich fluid collects in the tissues of the affected area. Left untreated, this stagnant, protein-rich fluid not only causes tissue channels to increase in size and number, but also reduces oxygen availability in the transport system, interferes with wound healing, and provides a culture medium for bacteria that can result in lymphangitis (infection).

Lymphedema should not be confused with edema resulting from venous insufficiency, which is not lymph-edema. However, untreated venous insufficiency can progress into a combined venous/lymphatic disorder that is treated in the same way as lymphedema.

What Causes Lymphedema?

Primary lymphedema, which can affect from one to as many as four limbs or other parts of the body, can be present at birth, develop at the onset of puberty (praecox), or develop in adulthood (tarda), all from unknown causes, or associated with vascular anomalies such as hemangioma, lymphangioma, Port Wine Stain, and Klippel-Trenaunay syndrome.

Secondary lymphedema, or acquired lymphedema, can develop as a result of surgery, radiation, infection, or trauma. Specific surgeries, such as surgery for melanoma or breast, gynecological, head and neck, prostate or testicular, bladder, or colon cancer, all of which currently require removal of lymph nodes, put patients at risk of developing secondary lymphedema. If lymph nodes are removed, there is always a risk of developing lymphedema.

Secondary lymphedema can develop immediately postoperatively, or weeks, months, or even years later. It can also develop when chemotherapy is unwisely administered to the already affected area (the side on which the surgery was performed) or after repeated aspirations of a seroma (a pocket of fluid that occurs commonly postoperatively) in the axilla, around the breast incision, or in the groin area. This often causes infection and, subsequently, lymphedema.

Aircraft flight has also been linked to the onset of lymphedema in patients post–cancer surgery (likely due to the decreased cabin pressure). Always be sure to wear a compression garment (sleeve, stocking) when you fly, even if you do not have lymphedema.

Another cause of lower extremity lymphedema is that resulting from the use of Tamoxifen. This medication can cause blood clots and subsequent DVT (deep venous thrombosis).

Radiation therapy, used in the treatment of various cancers and some AIDS-related diseases (such as Kaposi-Sarcoma), can damage otherwise healthy lymph nodes and vessels, causing scar tissue to form that interrupts the normal flow of the lymphatic fluid. Radiation can also cause skin dermatitis or a burn similar to sunburn. It is important to closely monitor the radiated area for any skin changes, such as increased temperature, discoloration (erythema) or blistering, which can lead into the development of lymphedema. Be sure to keep the area soft with lotion recommended by your radiation oncologist.

Lymphedema can develop secondary to lymphangitis (an infection), which interrupts normal lymphatic pathway function. A severe traumatic injury in which the lymphatic system is interrupted or damaged in any way may also trigger the onset of lymphedema. Although extremely rare in developed countries, there is a form of lymphedema called Filariasis that affects as many as two hundred million people worldwide (primarily in the endemic areas of southeast Asia, India, and Africa). When the filarial larvae from a mosquito bite enters the lymphatic system, these larvae mature into adult worms in the peripheral lymphatic channels, causing severe lymphedema in the arms, legs, and genitalia (also known as Elephantiasis).

Symptoms of Lymphedema

Lymphedema can develop in any part of the body or limb(s). Signs or symptoms of lymphedema to watch out for include: a full sensation in the limb(s); skin feeling tight; decreased flexibility in the hand, wrist, or ankle; difficulty fitting into clothing in one specific area; or ring, wristwatch, or bracelet tightness. If you notice persistent swelling, it is very important that you seek immediate medical advice (and get at least one second opinion), as early diagnosis and treatment improve both the prognosis and the condition.

Lymphedema develops in a number of stages, from mild to severe (referred to as Stage 1, 2 and 3).

Stage 1 (Spontaneously Reversible)

Tissue is still at the "pitting" stage, which means that when pressed by fingertips, the area indents and holds the indentation. Usually, upon waking in the morning, the limb or affected area is normal or almost normal size.

Stage 2 (Spontaneously Irreversible)

The tissue now has a spongy consistency and is "non-pitting," meaning that when pressed by fingertips, the tissue bounces back without any indentation forming). Fibrosis found in Stage 2 lymphedema marks the beginning of the hardening of the limbs and increasing size.

Stage 3 (Lymphostatic Elephantiasis)

At this stage the swelling is irreversible and usually the limb is very large. The tissue is hard (fibrotic) and unresponsive; some patients consider undergoing reconstructive surgery called "debulking" at this stage.

When lymphedema remains untreated, protein-rich fluid continues to accumulate, leading to an increase of swelling and a hardening or fibrosis of the tissue. In this state, the swollen limb becomes a perfect culture medium for bacteria and subsequent recurrent lymphangitis (infections). Moreover, untreated lymphedema can lead into a decrease or loss of functioning of the limb, skin breakdown, chronic infections, and, sometimes, irreversible complications. In the most severe cases, untreated lymphedema can develop into a rare form of lymphatic cancer called lymphangiosarcoma (most often in secondary lymphedema).

Lymphangitis (Infection)

Signs and symptoms of lymphangitis (infection) may include some or all of the following: rash, red blotchy skin, itching of the affected area, discoloration, increase of swelling or temperature of the skin, heavy sensation in the limb (more so than usual), pain, and in many cases a sudden onset of high fever and chills.

Treatment for infections: immediately discontinue all current lymphedema treatment modalities (including manual lymphatic drainage, bandaging, pumps, and wearing of compression garments) and contact your physician as soon as possible. The antibiotics of choice for these types of lymphatic infections are those in the penicillin family (note: people who develop side effects, such as yeast infections or gastric upset, can take Bicillin injections for two weeks), if no allergies are present. **Note: Always carry antibiotics or a prescription with you when you travel.**

Treatments for Lymphedema

Planning the treatment program depends on the cause of the lymphedema. For example, if the initial signs and symptoms of swelling are caused by infection (redness, rash, heat, blister, or pain may indicate an infection), antibiotics will first need to be prescribed. Treating an infection often reduces some of the swelling and discoloration.

If the lymphedema is not caused by infection, and depending on the severity of the lymphedema, the recommended treatment plan should be determined using an approach based on the Complex Decongestive Therapy (CDT) methods, which consist of: (a) manual lymphatic drainage; (b) bandaging; (c) proper skin care and diet; (d) compression garments (sleeves, stockings, devices such as Reid Sleeve, CircAid leggings, Legacy Sleeve, as well as other alternative approaches); (e) remedial exercises; (f) self-manual lymphatic drainage and bandaging, if instruction is available; and (g) continuing to follow prophylactic methods at all times.

Contraindications

1. Post–cancer surgery lymphedema patients who experience a sudden marked increase of swelling should immediately cease treatment and be checked by their physician for possible recurrent tumor or disease. Tumor growth can block the lymphatic flow, causing a worsening of the condition. Although not yet proven in a controlled clinical study, many lymphedema specialists believe that patients with recurrent or metastatic disease should not undergo complete decongestive therapy (CDT) in order not to promote the spreading of the cancer. Be sure to discuss this treatment with your doctor.

2. Patients with a sudden onset of lymphangitis (infection) should immediately discontinue treatment until the infection is cleared. Patients with histories of vascular disease and who are taking anticoagulants should have a Doppler and ultrasound to rule out deep-venous thrombosis before being treated. During treatment, these patients should be followed closely and regular laboratory tests should be performed.

3. Patients who have congestive heart failure must be monitored closely to avoid moving too much fluid too quickly, for which the heart may not be able to compensate.

4. If pain is present, discontinue all treatment until the pain subsides or the underlying cause has been determined.

Eighteen Steps to Prevention: Upper Extremities

Who Is at Risk?

At risk is anyone who has had either a simple mastectomy, a lumpectomy, or a modified radical mastectomy in combination with axillary node dissection or radiation therapy. Lymphedema can occur immediately postoperatively, within a few months, after a couple of years, or twenty years or more after cancer therapy. With proper education and care, lymphedema can be avoided, or, if it develops, kept well under control.

The following instructions should be reviewed carefully preoperatively and discussed with your physician or therapist.

1. Absolutely do not ignore any slight increase of swelling in the arm, hand, fingers, or chest wall. Consult with your doctor immediately.

2. Never allow an injection or a blood drawing in the affected arm(s). Wear a lymphedema alert bracelet.

3. Have blood pressure checked on the unaffected arm, or on the leg (thigh), if bilateral lymphedema/at-risk arms.

4. Keep the edemic or at-risk arm(s) spotlessly clean. Use lotion (Eucerin, Lymphoderm, Curel, or whatever works best for you) after bathing. When drying, be gentle, but thorough. Make sure the affected arm is dry in any creases and between the fingers.

5. Avoid vigorous, repetitive movements against resistance with the affected arm (scrubbing, pushing, pulling).

6. Avoid heavy lifting with the affected arm. Never carry heavy handbags or bags with over-the-shoulder straps on your affected side.

7. Do not wear tight jewelry or elastic bands around affected fingers or arm(s).

8. Avoid extreme temperature changes when bathing or washing dishes, and it is recommended that saunas and hot tubs be avoided (at least keep affected arm out of the hot tub). Protect the arm from the sun at all times.

9. Try to avoid any type of trauma (bruising, cuts, sunburn or other burns, sports injuries, insect bites, cat scratches) to the arm(s). Watch for subsequent signs of infection.

10. Wear gloves while doing housework, gardening, or any type of work that could result in even a minor injury.

11. When manicuring your nails, avoid cutting your cuticles (inform your manicurist).

12. Exercise is important, but consult with your therapist. Do not overtire an arm at risk: if it starts to ache, lie down and elevate it. Recommended exercises: walking, swimming, light aerobics, bike riding, and specially designed ballet or yoga. (Do not lift more than fifteen pounds.)

13. When traveling by air, patients with lymphedema (or who are at risk) must wear a well-fitted compression sleeve. Additional bandages may be required on a long flight. Increase fluid intake while in the air.

14. Patients with large breasts should wear light breast prostheses (heavy prostheses may put too much pressure on the lymph nodes above the collar bone). Soft padded shoulder straps may have to be worn. Wear a well-fitted bra: not too tight, ideally with no underwire.

15. Use an electric razor to remove hair from axilla. Maintain electric razor properly, replacing heads as needed.

16. Patients with lymphedema should wear a well-fitted compression sleeve during all waking hours. At least every four to six months, see your therapist for follow-up. If the sleeve is too loose, most likely the arm circumference has reduced or the sleeve is worn.

17. Warning: If you notice a rash, itching, redness, pain, increase of temperature, or fever, see your physician immediately. An inflammation (or infection) in the affected arm could be the beginning or worsening of lymphedema.

18. Maintain your ideal weight through a well-balanced, low sodium, high-fiber diet. Avoid smoking and alcohol. Lymphedema is a high-protein edema, but eating too little protein will not reduce the protein element in the lymph fluid; rather, this may weaken the connective tissue and worsen the condition. The diet should contain easily digested protein (chicken, fish, tofu).

Unfortunately, prevention is not a cure. But, as a cancer or lymphedema patient, you are in control of your ongoing cancer checkups and the continued maintenance of your lymphedema.

Chapter 67

What Breast Cancer Survivors Need to Know about Osteoporosis

The Impact of Breast Cancer

The National Cancer Institute reports that one in eight women in the United States (approximately 13.3 percent) will develop breast cancer in her lifetime. In fact, next to skin cancer, breast cancer is the most common type of cancer among U.S. women.

While the exact cause of breast cancer is not known, the risk of developing it increases with age. Most breast cancers occur in women in their fifties, and the risk is particularly high in women over the age of sixty. Because of their age, these women are already at increased risk for osteoporosis. Given the rising incidence of breast cancer and the improvement of long-term survival rates, bone health and fracture prevention have become important health issues among breast cancer survivors.

Facts about Osteoporosis

Osteoporosis is a condition in which the bones become less dense and more likely to fracture. Fractures from osteoporosis can result in significant pain and disability. It is a major health threat for an estimated forty-four million Americans, 68 percent of whom are women.

Risk factors for developing osteoporosis include: thinness or small frame; family history of the disease; being postmenopausal or having

Fact Sheet, National Institutes of Health Osteoporosis and Related Bone Diseases—National Resource Center, August 2003.

had early menopause; abnormal absence of menstrual periods; prolonged use of certain medications, such as glucocorticoids; low calcium intake; physical inactivity; smoking; and excessive alcohol intake.

Osteoporosis is a silent disease that can often be prevented. However, if undetected, it can progress for many years without symptoms until a fracture occurs. It has been called "a pediatric disease with geriatric consequences," because building healthy bones in one's youth is important to help prevent osteoporosis and fractures later in life.

The Breast Cancer-Osteoporosis Link

Women who have had breast cancer treatment may be at increased risk for osteoporosis for several reasons. First, estrogen has a protective effect on bone, and reduced levels of the hormone trigger bone loss. Because of chemotherapy or surgery, many breast cancer survivors experience a loss of ovarian function and, consequently, a drop in estrogen levels. Women who were premenopausal prior to their cancer treatment tend to go through menopause earlier than those who have not had the disease.

Studies also suggest that chemotherapy may have a direct negative effect on bone. In addition, the breast cancer itself may actually stimulate the production of osteoclasts, the cells that break down bone.

Osteoporosis Management Strategies

Several strategies can reduce one's risk for osteoporosis or lessen the effects of the disease in women who have already been diagnosed.

Nutrition

Some studies have found a link between diet and breast cancer. However, it is not yet clear which foods or supplements may play a role in reducing breast cancer risk. As far as bone health is concerned, a well-balanced diet rich in calcium and vitamin D is important. Good sources of calcium include low-fat dairy products, dark green, leafy vegetables, and calcium-fortified foods and beverages. Also, supplements can help ensure that the calcium requirement is met each day. The Institute of Medicine recommends a daily calcium intake of 1,000 mg in men and women between the ages of nineteen and fifty, increasing to 1,200 mg in those over fifty.

Vitamin D plays an important role in calcium absorption and bone health. It is synthesized in the skin through exposure to sunlight.

Some individuals may require vitamin D supplements in order to achieve the recommended intake of 400–800 International Units (IU) each day.

Exercise

Like muscle, bone is living tissue that responds to exercise by becoming stronger. The best exercise for bones is weight-bearing exercise that forces you to work against gravity. Some examples include walking, stair-climbing, and dancing. Regular exercise such as walking may help prevent bone loss and provide many other health benefits. Recent research suggests that exercise may also reduce breast cancer risk in younger women.

Healthy Lifestyle

Smoking is bad for bones, as well as the heart and lungs. In addition, smokers may absorb less calcium from their diets. While some studies have found a slightly higher risk of breast cancer in women who drink alcohol, evidence also suggests that alcohol can negatively affect bone health. Those who drink heavily are more prone to bone loss and fracture, because of poor nutrition as well as an increased risk of falling.

Bone Density Test

Specialized tests known as bone mineral density (BMD) tests measure bone density in various sites of the body. These tests can detect osteoporosis before a fracture occurs and predict one's chances of fracturing in the future. A woman recovering from breast cancer should ask her physician whether she might be a candidate for a bone density test.

Medication

There is no cure for osteoporosis. However, medications are available for the prevention and treatment of the disease in postmenopausal women, men, and those taking glucocorticoid medications.

Although there is a lack of studies that specifically address the use of these medications in women with breast cancer, bisphosphonates, a class of the osteoporosis treatment medications, are being studied for and have demonstrated some success in their ability to treat breast cancers that have metastasized to bone.

In addition, another osteoporosis treatment medication, raloxifene, is currently being evaluated for its ability to decrease breast cancer risk. Raloxifene, a selective estrogen receptor modulator (SERM), has been shown to reduce the risk of breast cancer in women with osteoporosis. The National Institutes of Health is currently sponsoring STAR (Study of Tamoxifen and Raloxifene) to compare the effectiveness of raloxifene with that of tamoxifen in preventing breast cancer in postmenopausal women at high risk of developing the disease.

Chapter 68

Questions and Answers about Sexuality for Women with Breast Cancer

As a woman who is receiving chemotherapy or radiation therapy for breast cancer or who has had breast surgery, you may have questions and worries about the effect of these treatments on your sexuality and your ability to have children. This chapter contains answers to some common questions asked by women who have been treated for breast cancer. If you find that you have additional questions as you read this information, please discuss them with your doctor or nurse.

Is my disease catching? Can my partner get cancer from me if we have sex?

No, cancer is not catching. You cannot give cancer to your partner by kissing, hugging, or having intercourse.

If I am receiving radiation therapy as part of my treatment, am I radioactive? Can I transmit radiation to my partner during intimacy or sex?

No, you are not radioactive. You cannot give radiation to your partner by any form of touching, including intercourse.

513

Sometimes I am very tired or don't feel well enough to have intercourse. When this happens, how can I let my partner know that my feelings about him have not changed?

Chemotherapy, radiation therapy, or cancer itself, as well as many of the concerns you have right now, may make you feel tired or not physically up to par for periods of time. When this happens, you may want to be intimate with your sexual partner in ways other than intercourse: body touching, hugging, kissing, stroking, massage, or gentle, loving words or gestures. These are but a few ways to express tenderness and love. There are many other ways that you and your partner can discuss and experiment with to make each other feel special and loved.

Sometimes during a time of illness and recovery, partners are hesitant to talk to each other about physical, emotional, or sexual needs. Your partner is probably concerned about your physical stamina and might feel protective of you. You might start a conversation about what you feel comfortable doing, or show your partner through actions. You might also want to ask your partner what you can do to please him as well as discuss what might be pleasing to the two of you.

My vagina is dry, which makes intercourse painful. Is there anything I can do?

A dry vagina is a fairly common side effect of chemotherapy. Vaginal lubricating jellies can make your vagina less dry during intercourse. We recommend that you use a non-water-based vaginal lubricating jelly. These jellies can be purchased in drugstores without a prescription, or ask your doctor to recommend one.

Will chemotherapy affect menstruation?

Usually. If you were having regular menstrual periods before beginning chemotherapy, you might stop ovulating after taking some of the drugs, and you will probably stop menstruating during the course of your chemotherapy. Ask your doctor or nurse how your particular treatments will affect your menstrual and ovulation cycles.

Will I begin menstruating again after I discontinue the chemotherapy?

This answer depends on the type of chemotherapy used, and the age of the patient. Not all chemotherapy permanently stops menstrual cycles. One of the most effective drugs for the treatment of breast cancer is cyclophosphamide (Cytoxan®) or the related alkylating agents. Almost all of these drugs cause ovulation and menstruation to stop during treatment. All standard adjuvant chemotherapy combinations for breast cancer contain cyclophosphamide or a related drug. ("Adjuvant" describes the "preventive" chemotherapy given after a mastectomy or lumpectomy when all the tests show no evidence of remaining tumor).

Most patients who are more than forty years old will stop their menstrual periods during the time they take chemotherapy, and only 5 percent to 25 percent of these women will resume regular menstrual periods. But only about 40 percent of women who are younger than forty will stop having menstrual periods, and about half of the women whose periods stop will resume having them. They will probably go through menopause earlier than if they had not taken chemotherapy.

Will I need to use birth control while I am on chemotherapy?

Yes. If you have not gone through menopause, it is very important not to become pregnant while you are receiving chemotherapy. You must use some form of birth control, but not birth control pills. If you have an Intrauterine Device (IUD), let your doctor know.

If you have questions about which methods of birth control you can use, ask your doctor. Your doctor can help you choose an effective means of birth control, such as a diaphragm, condoms, or a barrier cream or gel.

Will it be possible for me to become pregnant after chemotherapy?

The ability to become pregnant depends on the normal functioning of the ovaries. The ovaries of younger women are more resistant to chemotherapy. If a woman's ovaries stay normal during chemotherapy or return to normal function after she stops chemotherapy, she can become pregnant. A woman will have regular menstrual cycles if the ovaries are functioning normally. However, many women who do not have regular periods can still become pregnant. Occasionally a woman who thinks she has gone through "the change" (menopause) because she has stopped having menstrual periods does get pregnant. A special blood test of the hormone levels can determine fairly accurately whether a patient has gone through menopause.

515

Is it safe for me to become pregnant after I have completed my chemotherapy?

Many doctors have reported that, in their experience, pregnancy has no adverse effects on women who have recovered from breast cancer. The general recommendation is that a woman wait at least two to three years after breast cancer is diagnosed before becoming pregnant. This allows enough time to determine whether the tumor is likely to recur (come back).

We do not recommend that patients become pregnant if their tumors have ever recurred. However, if a patient has not had a tumor recurrence after her mastectomy (or lumpectomy and radiation) and if she did not have an aggressive type of tumor, it is probably safe for her to become pregnant two to three years after diagnosis. If you have any questions about becoming pregnant after your treatment, ask your doctor.

Will I have hot flashes if I stop menstruating because I'm on chemotherapy? If so, is there anything I can do to alleviate them?

Hot flashes are a sign that the ovaries are no longer producing enough estrogen (a female hormone). The amount of estrogen necessary to prevent hot flashes is less than the amount necessary to have normal menstrual periods. Therefore, many women will stop having menstrual periods, but will not have hot flashes. The closer the patient is to age forty, however, the more likely it is that she will have hot flashes and also experience menopause.

Hot flashes are not a medically serious problem, but they can be very annoying. Often just knowing that these are hot flashes and are not serious is enough to reduce the anxiety associated with them.

Treatment generally starts with mild tranquilizing agents, such as alprazolam (Xanax®) during the day or triazolam (Halcion®) during the night. If this is not enough, another medication, Bellergal-S®, is often helpful. This tablet is a combination of three drugs. The side effects of Bellergal-S® may include constipation, slight difficulty starting the urine stream, dryness of the mouth, and occasionally blurred vision. The usual dose is one tablet twice a day. Because of the side effects, some patients prefer taking Bellergal-S® only at night. This drug is worth trying as long as the patient is aware of the possible side effects.

A third treatment is a drug called clonidine (Catapres®) that is commonly used to treat high blood pressure. It is usually taken once or twice a day. Blood pressure should be checked regularly to make sure it does not decrease too much as a result of the medication.

In some patients, the hot flashes are unbearable and there is no alternative except to use some sort of hormone. It is not safe for patients who have breast cancer to take estrogen, because estrogen therapy could cause tumors to recur. When hormone treatment is necessary, progesterone or testosterone (the male hormone) is used. This treatment is given as a last resort and after the patient and her doctor have frankly discussed the risks of the therapy versus the quality of life improvements it will bring.

What other side effects might I have because ovulation and menstrual cycles have changed? What can I do to relieve them?

Usually, the most disturbing side effects (besides the hot flashes) occur in the vagina. Two things happen: the tissue lining the wall of the vagina gets thin, and there is less lubrication in the vagina during sexual intercourse.

The tissues of the vagina and also in the urethra (the opening from the bladder to the outside) need estrogen to keep them soft and yet thick enough to resist normal wear and tear. When ovulation and the menstrual cycle stop, less estrogen is produced. Without enough estrogen, these tissues become thin and tend to bleed easily during sexual intercourse.

Sometimes, vitamin A and D ointment can help thicken the vaginal lining and reduce bleeding during intercourse. The ointment is available in drugstores without a prescription. Apply the cream to the vagina and the area around it one to three times a day. If this does not work, ask your doctor about other alternatives.

There may also be less lubrication in the vagina, which may make intercourse painful. Vaginal lubricating jellies can be used during intercourse to increase lubrication. Non-water-based lubricants are recommended, and are available in drugstores without a prescription.

Can I have intercourse while I am wearing my infusion pump? If so, is there a safe and comfortable way to do so?

If you feel well enough for sexual activity, it is all right to have intercourse as long as the infusion pump is protected. It is important not to pull on the tubing that connects the pump to you and to your catheter. Perhaps tucking the pump under an armpit will be comfortable if you are lying on your back. If you generally make love very vigorously, you may have to do it less actively while you are wearing your pump.

Depending on your chemotherapy, you may not feel physically well enough for sex. If the chemotherapy causes nausea, you may receive antinausea medications. These medications cause drowsiness and may also decrease vaginal lubrication.

If you are not feeling well or if you are not comfortable wearing your pump during intercourse, you may want to be intimate with your partner in other ways. Touching, massaging, and stroking may be a mutually acceptable substitute for sexual intercourse when you are wearing your pump.

Two books may be helpful in finding and discussing alternate ways to sexual expression. One is Maggie Scarf's book, *Intimate Partners: Patterns in Love and Marriage,* which discusses normal sexual functioning and describes exercises to teach couples how to please each other by touch. The second book, by Dagmar O'Connor (the director of the Sexual Therapy Program at St. Luke's Roosevelt Hospital Center in New York City), discusses alternative ways to make sexual interaction pleasurable for couples who have committed and long-term relationships. Her book is titled *How to Make Love to the Same Person for the Rest of Your Life and Still Love It.* Both of these books suggest that it is healthy to try new solutions when the situation changes. Some of these solutions may simply involve a different way of looking at the situation. If you are too overwhelmed by your illness to think about reading at this time, you may want to ask your partner to read these books or, even better, read them aloud to you!

I am self-conscious about my body since my breast surgery and wonder if I will be a "turn-off" to my partner.

Your perception of your body may not be at all how your partner sees you. If you experienced love and affection for one another before your surgery, there is every reason to think these same feelings are present now. You may have lost a breast, but you have not lost the ability to love and be loved.

I have always had large breasts and feel very "one-sided" and "unbalanced" when I wear a nightgown or pajamas since I've had a mastectomy.

After a mastectomy many women are more comfortable wearing a leisure or lightweight bra with a lightweight prosthesis when they go to bed. Also, some nightgowns are made so that ruffles can be added to the front, giving a fuller appearance to the side of the mastectomy. For an added touch of femininity, you might want to dab on your favorite cologne before going to bed.

Information on obtaining a prosthesis is available through the Reach to Recovery program sponsored by the American Cancer Society. Volunteers provide shopping information and samples of breast prostheses for women after their mastectomies. To schedule a visit, ask your nurse or doctor for information on this program.

Many patients may be good candidates for breast reconstruction at the mastectomy site. For women who do consider it, reconstruction is a more permanent alternative to wearing a prosthesis. Ask your doctor for more information about breast reconstruction and if it would be a good option for you.

I have had a prosthetic implant. Will massaging, squeezing, or caressing a breast dislodge or damage the implant?

Massaging, squeezing, or caressing a breast with a prosthetic implant usually will not cause any harm. In fact, many plastic surgeons recommend that the breast be massaged regularly to prevent scarring from occurring around the prosthesis.

Severe or blunt blows to the breast might damage the implant. If you suspect that the implant has been damaged, contact your doctor.

It seems to me that some of my friends, co-workers, relatives, and others are very awkward when they are around me, and they don't know how to handle the fact that I've had breast cancer.

Remember, other people will take their cue from you. If you are comfortable using words like "breast," "cancer," "breast surgery," "mastectomy," and "chemotherapy," others may pick up on this attitude, and they too will be able to add these words to their vocabularies.

Occasionally, an awkward situation may occur, such as a prosthesis slipping out of place, a person staring at your chest, or even someone repeating a joke about breasts. If you should be in a situation similar to this, please try to have a sense of humor—humor is wonderful and can help you through a tough and trying time. What has happened to you is certainly not funny, but humor often diffuses an awkward situation.

Every time I get an ache or pain now, I think that perhaps I have a new cancer.

This anxiety is very common and will subside as time goes on. Be sure you follow your doctor's instructions for follow-up appointments and proper care of your body. If you feel you have a medical problem, discuss it with your doctor as soon as possible.

I seem to be having a difficult time accepting what has happened to me.

As with so many things in life, adjustments of any type take time. Do not be too hard on yourself. Soon you will probably be doing everything you did before your treatment or surgery, and maybe even more because of an added determination!

Sometimes it helps to talk to someone who has had the same type of surgery as you had. If you do not know anyone, call the local office of the American Cancer Society. Their Reach to Recovery program can put you in touch with someone who has had the same type of surgery. Again, having a sense of humor and using it to relieve anxiety and enjoy the good things in life often helps to reduce a stressful situation. Sharing your sense of humor with your partner, your family, and your friends may ease stress and brighten your lives.

You may find that some of these questions or answers may not seem appropriate for you or your situation, and that's okay. If you have any special concerns or questions that are not discussed in this chapter, please discuss them with your doctor or nurse.

Chapter 69

How to Talk to Your Children, Family, and Friends about Breast Cancer

How to Talk to Your Children

Parents find it very difficult to tell their children about cancer. There are a couple of basic guidelines that can help parents discuss their cancer diagnosis with their children. However, the type of discussion you have with your children will depend on their ages. Children of any age can sense when something is wrong, and they usually imagine the worst possible problem. Telling them what is going on can actually alleviate some anxiety and fear that they may be feeling. It is important to answer only the questions your children ask and nothing more. Children, especially between the ages of six and ten, can handle only little bits of information at a time. As they ask for more detail you can provide it to them, but try to focus on what their concerns are for the moment. Answer your children's questions as honestly as possible. An environment of honesty and openness can help children deal with the crisis that results when a parent is diagnosed with cancer.

Up to Two Years Old

For small children, their biggest concern comes from the disruption of their daily routine. They do not understand the concept of cancer, but will be disturbed if their parent is away for several days, or is too tired to play. Establish a new routine as soon as possible, one that can accommodate your recovery and treatment needs. Ask for help from friends and family to give them extra attention and love.

Ages Two to Seven Years

For younger children, it is very common that they assume they might be responsible for you getting cancer. For instance, they may think that because they got in trouble at school you got cancer. Use simple terms to explain your illness, like "good" and "bad" cells. Remind your children often that cancer is not something you catch and that they did not do anything to cause your cancer.

Try to explain the treatments and procedures that you will have in terms of how it will affect them and their routine. For instance, "I will be having chemotherapy next week, and it will make me very tired. I won't be able to drive you to school then, but Susie's mother will come to our house to pick you up at your regular time." Or, "When I have the medicine that will remove my cancer cells, my hair will fall out and you will see me without any hair. Sometimes I will wear a hat or a wig to keep me warm and comfortable. My hair will grow back."

Ages Seven to Twelve Years

School-aged children will understand more about the causes and effects of a serious illness, but you should still keep your explanations simple. They may hesitate to bring up a concern or a fear they have because they are afraid of burdening the parent who is facing cancer. It is good to ask them once a week how things are going and how they are feeling. By encouraging them to verbalize their concerns, you are teaching them how to handle crisis in a positive way, and you will also have a sense of how your child is coping. Be sure to watch for changes in school performance, as well as eating and sleeping patterns. Any changes may be an indicator that your child is worried and unable to verbalize his or her feelings.

Ages Twelve and Older

Children at this age can understand most aspects of breast cancer causes and treatments. You should spend time listening to their concerns and trying to help them get the best information to answer their questions. Older teenagers may want to know detailed information about breast cancer and may want to do their own research about the illness. Others may want to rely only on what you tell them.

Each child may respond differently to his or her parent's illness. Some may get angry and distant. Others may feel insecure and scared. If they are having a hard time talking to you, encourage them to talk with other members of the family, or to a teacher or friend.

Just like you, children will have to react to the wide range of emotions that occur when cancer invades a family. Fear, sadness, insecurity, anger, and curiosity are just some of the feelings they will have. Keep talking to and with them. Try to plan activities for the whole family on a regular basis. Most importantly, try to give them extra love and attention—it will benefit everyone.

Talking with Family and Friends

Telling people who are mature and sensitive enough to handle a disclosure of cancer will relieve you of the burden of inventing explanations, or being on guard against discovery of your illness. You may find unexpected sources of support and understanding from others, including people who have struggled with a life-threatening illness.

Here are ten suggestions on communicating with your friends and family:

- Be honest and direct. Give clear guidelines about what others can do to help you.

- Don't assume people know what you need, or what the "right" thing to do is.

- If you don't feel like company, say that you appreciate their concern but would much rather they visit you at another time, when you feel better.

- Some people are better at coping with a crisis than others. Most people truly care, but don't know what to say or do. Accept their limitations.

- If you just need to be with someone or want them to just listen to you, tell them so. Explain to them that you don't expect answers or solutions; you just want them to listen to your concerns.

- Coping with breast cancer may reveal long-standing problems in a relationship, like poor communication or lack of trust— problems clearly not caused by cancer. Recognizing this may allow you to let go of old behaviors and patterns while identifying ongoing stressful relationships.

- Even thoughtful family and friends may be impatient for you to "get over" your experience. You have survived an ordeal—do not let their expectations pressure you to ignore your feelings.

- Give yourself permission to explore ways to enhance your health and self-esteem. Focus on building a stronger sense of self and purpose to survive your treatments.

- You can become preoccupied with the cancer so much that certain feelings linger and you may become stuck in the process of emotional healing. Get assistance from a support group or therapist to help you move forward.

- While it is not your responsibility to take care of others' feelings, understand that they, too, are trying to cope.

Part Eight

Additional Help and Information

Chapter 70

Glossary of Breast Cancer–Related Terms

abnormal: Not normal. May be cancerous or premalignant.

abscess: A pocket of pus that forms as the body's defenses attempt to wall off infection-causing germs.

adjuvant therapy: Treatment given after the primary treatment to increase the chances of a cure. Adjuvant therapy may include chemotherapy, radiation therapy, hormone therapy, or biological therapy.

aggressive: A quickly growing cancer.

alopecia: The lack or loss of hair from areas of the body where hair is usually found. Alopecia can be a side effect of some cancer treatments.

alteration, altered: Change; different from original.

anesthesia: Drugs or gases given before and during surgery so the patient won't feel pain. The patient may be awake or asleep.

anesthesiologist: A doctor who gives drugs or gases that keep you comfortable during surgery.

areola: The colored tissue that encircles the nipple.

The terms in this glossary were excerpted from several documents produced by the National Cancer Institute (NCI), including "Understanding Breast Cancer Treatment" (1998); "Understanding Breast Changes" (1998); "Clinical Trials and Insurance Coverage" (2002); and the NCI online dictionary available at www.cancer.gov/dictionary, accessed April 2004.

aromatase inhibitor: A drug that prevents the formation of estradiol, a female hormone, by interfering with an aromatase enzyme. Aromatase inhibitors are used as a type of hormone therapy for postmenopausal women who have hormone-dependent breast cancer.

aspiration: Removal of fluid from a cyst or cells from a lump, using a needle and syringe.

atypical hyperplasia: Cells that are both abnormal (atypical) and increased in number. Benign microscopic breast changes known as atypical hyperplasia moderately increase a woman's risk of developing breast cancer.

average risk (for breast cancer): A measure of the chances of getting breast cancer without the presence of any specific factors known to be associated with the disease.

axillary dissection: Surgery to remove lymph nodes found in the armpit region. Also called axillary lymph node dissection.

axillary lymph node: A lymph node in the armpit region that drains lymph channels from the breast.

benign: Not cancerous; cannot invade neighboring tissues or spread to other parts of the body.

benign breast changes: Noncancerous changes in the breast. Benign breast conditions can cause pain, lumpiness, nipple discharge, and other problems.

biological therapy: Treatment that uses the body's immune system to fight cancer or to lessen the side effects that may be caused by some cancer treatments. Also known as immunotherapy.

biopsy: Removal of a sample of tissue that is then examined under a microscope to check for cancer cells.

bone marrow: The soft material inside bones. Blood cells are produced in the bone marrow.

bone marrow transplantation: A procedure to replace bone marrow that has been destroyed by treatment with high doses of anticancer drugs or radiation. Transplantation may be autologous (an individual's own marrow saved before treatment), allogeneic (marrow donated by someone else), or syngeneic (marrow donated by an identical twin).

brachytherapy: A procedure in which radioactive material sealed in needles, seeds, wires, or catheters is placed directly into or near a tumor. Also called internal radiation, implant radiation, or interstitial radiation therapy.

BRCA1 and BRCA2 genes: The principal genes that, when altered, indicate an inherited susceptibility to breast cancer. These gene alterations are present in 80 to 90 percent of hereditary cases of breast cancer.

breast cancer in situ: Very early or noninvasive abnormal cells that are confined to the ducts or lobules in the breast. Also known as DCIS or LCIS.

breast-conserving surgery: An operation to remove the breast cancer but not the breast itself. Also called breast-sparing surgery.

breast density: Glandular tissue in the breast common in younger women, making it difficult for mammography to detect breast cancer.

breast implants: Silicone rubber sacs, which are filled with silicone gel or sterile saline, used for breast reconstruction after mastectomy.

breast reconstruction: Surgery to rebuild the shape of the breast after a mastectomy.

breast self-exam: An exam by a woman of her breasts to check for lumps or other changes.

calcifications: Small deposits of calcium in tissue, which can be seen on mammograms.

cancer: A general name for more than one hundred diseases in which abnormal cells grow out of control. Cancer cells can invade and destroy healthy tissues, and they can spread through the bloodstream and the lymphatic system to other parts of the body.

carcinoma: Cancer that begins in tissues lining or covering the surfaces (epithelial tissues) of organs, glands, or other body structures. Most cancers are carcinomas.

carcinoma in situ: Cancer that is confined to the cells where it began, and has not spread into surrounding tissues.

cell: The smallest unit of tissue that makes up any living thing. Cells have very specialized structure and function and are able to reproduce when needed.

chemoprevention: The use of drugs or vitamins to prevent cancer in people who have precancerous conditions or a high risk of cancer, or to prevent the recurrence of cancer in people who have already been treated for it.

chemotherapy: Treatment with drugs to kill or slow the growth of cancer cells; also used to shrink tumors before surgery.

chromosomes: Structures located in the nucleus of a cell, containing genes.

clavicle: Collarbone.

clear margins: An area of normal tissue that surrounds cancerous tissue, as seen during examination under a microscope.

clinical breast exam: A physical examination by a doctor or nurse of the breast, underarm, and collarbone area, first on one side, then on the other.

clinical trial: A type of research study that uses volunteers to test new methods of screening, prevention, diagnosis, or treatment of a disease. The trial may be carried out in a clinic or other medical facility. Also called a clinical study.

computed tomography (CT) scanning: An imaging technique that uses a computer to organize the information from multiple x-ray views and construct a cross-sectional image of areas inside the body.

computer-aided diagnosis (CAD): the use of special computer programs to scan mammographic images and flag areas that look suspicious.

core needle biopsy: The use of a small cutting needle to remove a core of tissue for microscopic examination.

cyclic breast changes: Normal tissue changes that occur in response to the changing levels of female hormones during the menstrual cycle. Cyclic breast changes can produce swelling, tenderness, and pain.

cyst: Fluid-filled sac. Breast cysts are benign.

diagnosis: The process of identifying a disease by the signs and symptoms.

diagnostic mammogram: The use of a breast x-ray to evaluate the breasts of a woman who has symptoms of disease such as a lump, or whose screening mammogram shows an abnormality.

digital mammography: A technique for recording x-ray images in computer code, which allows the information to enhance subtle, but potentially significant, changes.

duct: A small channel in the breast through which milk passes from the lobes to the nipple.

ductal carcinoma in situ (DCIS): Cancer that is confined to the ducts of the breast tissue.

ductal lavage: A method used to collect cells from milk ducts in the breast. Ductal lavage may be used in addition to clinical breast examination and mammography to detect breast cancer.

estrogen: A female hormone; one of the hormones that can help some breast cancer tumors grow.

estrogen receptor test: Lab test to determine if breast cancer depends on estrogen for growth.

excisional biopsy: The surgical removal (excision) of an abnormal area of tissue, usually along with a margin of healthy tissue, for microscopic examination. Excisional biopsies remove the entire lump from the breast.

external radiation: Radiation therapy that uses a machine to aim high-energy rays at the cancer. Also called external-beam radiation.

false negative (mammograms): Breast x-rays that miss cancer when it is present.

false positive (mammograms): Breast x-rays that indicate breast cancer is present when the disease is truly absent.

fat necrosis: Lumps of fatty material that form in response to a bruise or blow to the breast.

fibroadenoma: Benign breast tumor made up of both structural (fibro) and glandular (adenoma) tissues.

fine needle aspiration: The use of a slender needle to remove fluid from a cyst or clusters of cells from a solid lump.

frozen section: A sliver of frozen biopsy tissue. A frozen section provides a quick preliminary diagnosis but is not 100 percent reliable.

gene: The basic unit of heredity found in all cells of the body.

generalized breast lumpiness: Breast irregularities and lumpiness, commonplace and noncancerous. Sometimes called "fibrocystic disease" or "benign breast disease."

genetic change: An alteration in a segment of DNA, which can disturb a gene's behavior and sometimes leads to disease.

glands: Lymph nodes.

gynecologist: A doctor who specializes in the care and treatment of women's reproductive systems.

hormonal therapy: The use of hormones to treat cancer patients by removing, blocking, or adding to the effects of a hormone on an organ or part of the body.

hormone receptor tests: Lab tests that determine if a breast cancer depends on female hormones (estrogen and progesterone) for growth.

hormone replacement therapy: Hormone-containing medications taken to offset the symptoms and other effects of the hormone loss that accompanies menopause.

hormones: Chemicals produced by various glands in the body, which produce specific effects on specific target organs and tissues.

hyperfractionation: A way of giving radiation therapy in smaller-than-usual doses two or three times a day instead of once a day.

hyperplasia: Excessive growth of cells. Several types of benign breast conditions involve hyperplasia.

immune system: The body's own natural defense system against infection or disease.

implant: A silicone gel-filled or saline-filled sac inserted under the chest muscle to restore breast shape.

incisional biopsy: The surgical removal of a portion of an abnormal area of tissue, by cutting into (incising) it, for microscopic examination.

infection: Invasion of body tissues by microorganisms such as bacteria and viruses.

infiltrating cancer: Cancer that has spread to nearby tissue, lymph nodes under the arm, or other parts of the body. (Same as invasive cancer.)

inflammation: The body's protective response to injury (including infection). Inflammation is marked by heat, redness, swelling, pain, and loss of function.

intraductal carcinoma: Abnormal cells that are contained within the milk duct and have not spread outside the duct. Also known as DCIS (ductal carcinoma in situ).

intraductal papilloma: A small wartlike growth that projects into a breast duct.

invasive cancer: Cancer that has spread to nearby tissue, lymph nodes under the arm, or other parts of the body. (Same as infiltrating cancer.)

laser beam scanning: a technology being studied in research for breast cancer detection that shines a laser beam through the breast and records the image produced, using a special camera.

leukocytes: White blood cells that defend the body against infections and other diseases.

lobes, lobules: Milk-producing tissues of the breast. Each of the breast's fifteen to twenty lobes branches into smaller lobules, and each lobule ends in scores of tiny bulbs. Milk originates in the bulbs and is carried by ducts to the nipple.

lobular carcinoma in situ, LCIS: Abnormal cells in the lobules of the breast; a sign that a woman is at increased risk of developing breast cancer.

localization biopsy: The use of mammography to locate tissue containing an abnormality that can be detected only on mammograms, so it can be removed for microscopic examination.

lumpectomy: Surgery to remove only the cancerous breast lump; usually followed by radiation therapy.

lymph nodes: Small bean-shaped organs (sometimes called lymph glands); part of the lymphatic system. Lymph nodes under the arm drain fluid from the chest and arm. During surgery, some underarm lymph nodes are removed to help determine the stage of breast cancer.

lymphatic system: The tissues and organs that produce, store, and transport cells that fight infection and disease.

lymphedema: Swelling in the arm caused by fluid that can build up when underarm lymph nodes are removed during breast cancer surgery or damaged by radiation.

macrocalcifications: Coarse calcium deposits. They are most likely due to aging, old injuries, or inflammations and usually are associated with benign conditions.

magnetic resonance imaging (MRI): A technique that uses a powerful magnet linked to a computer to create detailed pictures of areas inside the body.

malignant: Cancerous; capable of invading, spreading, and destroying tissue.

mammary duct ectasia: A benign breast condition in which ducts beneath the nipple become dilated and sometimes inflamed, and which can cause pain and nipple discharge.

mammogram: An x-ray of the breast.

mammography: The examination of breast tissue using x-rays.

mastectomy: Surgery to remove the breast (or as much of the breast as possible).

mastitis: Infection of the breast. Mastitis is most often seen in nursing mothers.

menopause: The time when a woman's monthly menstrual periods cease. Menopause is sometimes called the "change of life."

menstrual cycle: The monthly cycle of discharge, during a woman's reproductive years, of blood and tissues from the uterus.

metastasis or metastatic: Spread of cancer from the original part of the body to another. Cells that have metastasized are like those in the original (primary) tumor.

microcalcifications: Tiny deposits of calcium that can be detected by mammography. A cluster of small specks of calcium may indicate that cancer is present.

mutation: A change in the number, arrangement, or molecular sequence of a gene.

needle biopsy: Use of a needle to extract cells or bits of tissue for microscopic examination.

negative: A lab test result that is normal; failing to show a positive result for the specific disease or condition for which the test is being done.

nipple discharge: Fluid coming from the nipple.

nonpalpable cancer: Cancer in breast tissue that can be seen on mammograms but that cannot be felt.

oncologist, medical oncologist, or cancer specialist: A doctor who uses chemotherapy or hormonal therapy to treat cancer.

oncology nurse: A nurse with special training in caring for cancer patients.

oncology pharmacy specialist: A person who prepares anticancer drugs in consultation with an oncologist.

one-step procedure: Biopsy and surgical treatment combined into a single operation.

osteoporosis: A condition of mineral loss that causes a decrease in bone density and an enlargement of bone spaces, producing bone fragility.

ovaries: The pair of female reproductive organs that produce eggs and hormones.

palpation: Use of the fingers to press body surfaces, so as to feel tissues and organs underneath. Palpating the breast for lumps is a crucial part of a physical breast examination.

pathologist: A doctor who diagnoses disease by studying cells and tissues under a microscope.

pathology report: Diagnosis made by a pathologist based on microscopic evidence.

patient advocate: A person who helps a patient work with others who have an effect on the patient's health, including doctors, insurance companies, employers, case managers, and lawyers. A patient advocate helps resolve issues about health care, medical bills, and job discrimination related to a patient's medical condition.

permanent section: Biopsy tissue specially prepared and mounted on slides so that it can be examined under a microscope by a pathologist.

phase I trial: The first step in testing a new treatment in humans. These studies test the best way to give a new treatment and the best dose. Because little is known about the possible risks and benefits of the treatments being tested, phase I trials usually include only a small number of patients who have not been helped by other treatments.

phase II trial: A study to test whether a new treatment has an anti-cancer effect (for example, whether it shrinks a tumor or improves blood test results) and whether it works against a certain type of cancer.

phase III trial: A study to compare the results of people taking a new treatment with the results of people taking the standard treatment. In most cases, studies move into phase III only after a treatment seems to work in phases I and II. Phase III trials may include hundreds of people.

physical therapist: A health professional who teaches exercises that help restore arm and shoulder movement and build back strength after breast cancer surgery.

phytochemicals: Naturally occurring chemicals found in plants that may be important nutrients for reducing a person's cancer risk.

plastic surgeon or reconstructive surgeon: A doctor who can surgically rebuild (reconstruct) a woman's breast.

platelets: The part of a blood cell that helps prevent bleeding by causing blood clots to form at the site of an injury.

positive: A lab test result that reveals the presence of a specific disease or condition for which the test is being done.

positron emission tomography (PET scanning): A technique that uses signals emitted by radioactive tracers to construct images of the distribution of the tracers in the human body.

primary care doctor: A doctor who usually manages your health care and can discuss cancer treatment choices with you.

progesterone: A female hormone; one of the hormones that can help some breast cancers grow.

progesterone receptor test: Lab test to determine if a breast cancer depends on progesterone for growth.

prophylactic mastectomy: Surgery to remove a breast that is not known to contain breast cancer, for the purpose of reducing an individual's cancer risk.

prosthesis: An artificial replacement of a part of the body. A breast prosthesis is a breast form that may be worn under clothing. Also, a technical name for an implant that is placed under the chest muscle in breast reconstruction.

psychologist: A specialist who can talk with you and your family about emotional and personal matters, and can help you make decisions.

rad: A unit of measure for radiation. It stands for radiation absorbed dose.

radiation: Energy carried by waves or by streams of particles. Various forms of radiation can be used in low doses to diagnose disease and in high doses to treat disease.

radiation therapy: Treatment with high-energy x-rays to kill cancer cells. Radiation can be used in low doses to diagnose breast cancer and in high doses to treat breast cancer.

radical mastectomy: Surgery for breast cancer in which the breast, chest muscles, and all of the lymph nodes under the arm are removed.

radiologist: A doctor with special training in the use of x-rays (and related technologies such as ultrasound) to image body tissues and to treat disease.

raloxifene: A drug that belongs to the family of drugs called selective estrogen receptor modulators (SERMs) and is used in the prevention of osteoporosis in postmenopausal women. Raloxifene is also being studied as a cancer prevention drug.

recurrence: The return of cancer, at the same site as the original (primary) tumor or in another location, after the tumor had disappeared.

risk factor: A condition that increases a person's chances of getting a disease. Risk factors do not necessarily cause a disease; rather, they are indicators, statistically associated with an increase in likelihood.

sclerosing adenosis: A benign breast disease that involves the excessive growth of tissues in the breast's lobules.

screening: Checking for disease when there are no symptoms.

screening mammogram: Breast x-ray used to look for signs of disease such as cancer in people who are symptom-free.

selective estrogen receptor modulator (SERM): A drug that acts like estrogen on some tissues but blocks the effect of estrogen on other tissues. Tamoxifen and raloxifene are SERMs.

sentinel lymph node: The first lymph node(s) to which cancer cells spread after leaving the area of the primary tumor. Presence of cancer cells in this node alerts the doctor that the tumor has spread to the lymphatic system.

side effect: A problem that occurs when treatment affects tissues or organs other than the ones being treated. Some common side effects of cancer treatment are fatigue, pain, nausea, vomiting, decreased blood cell counts, hair loss, and mouth sores.

silicone: A synthetic gel that is used as an outer coating on breast implants and to make up the inside filling of some implants.

sonogram: The image produced by ultrasound.

specimen x-ray: An x-ray of tissue that has been surgically removed (surgical specimen).

stage, or staging: Classification of breast cancer according to its size and extent of spread.

standard therapy: In medicine, treatment that experts agree is appropriate, accepted, and widely used. Health care providers are obligated to provide patients with standard therapy. Also called standard of care or best practice.

stem cell: The immature cells in blood and bone marrow from which all mature blood cells develop.

stem cell transplantation: A method of replacing immature blood-forming cells that were destroyed by cancer treatment. The stem cells are given to the person after treatment to help the bone marrow recover and continue producing healthy blood cells.

stereotactic localization biopsy: A technique that employs three-dimensional x-ray to pinpoint a specific target area. It is used in conjunction with needle biopsy of nonpalpable breast abnormalities.

surgeon or surgical oncologist: A doctor who performs biopsies and other surgical procedures such as removing a lump or a breast.

surgical biopsy: The surgical removal of tissue for microscopic examination and diagnosis. Surgical biopsies can be either excisional or incisional. (See excisional biopsy and incisional biopsy.)

tamoxifen: A hormonally related drug that has been used to treat breast cancer and is being tested as a possible preventive strategy.

telangiectasia: The permanent enlargement of blood vessels, causing redness in the skin or mucous membranes.

tissue: A group or layer of cells that together perform a specific function.

tissue flap reconstruction: A flap of tissues is surgically relocated from another area of the body to the chest, and formed into a new breast mound.

tumor: An abnormal growth of tissue. Tumors may be either benign (not cancer) or malignant (cancer).

tumor markers: Proteins (either amounts or unique variants) made by altered genes in cancer cells that are involved in the progression of the disease.

two-step procedure: Biopsy and treatment done in two stages, usually a week or two apart.

ultrasound: The use of sound waves to produce images of body tissues.

x-ray: A high-energy form of radiation. X-rays form an image of body structures by traveling through the body and striking a sheet of film. Breast x-rays are called mammograms.

Chapter 71

Breast Cancer Resource Directory

General Breast Cancer Information

American Cancer Society
1599 Clifton Road
Atlanta, GA 30329
Toll-free: 800-ACS-2345
Fax: 404-982-3677
Website: www.cancer.org

American Institute for Cancer Research
1759 R Street, NW
Washington, DC 20009
Toll-free: 800-843-8114
Phone: 202-328-7744
Fax: 202-328-7226
Website: www.aicr.org
E-mail: aicrweb@aicr.org

BreastCancer.Net
Website: www.breastcancer.net

BreastCancer.org
111 Forest Avenue 1R
Narberth, PA 19072
Phone: 610-664-1900
Website: www.breastcancer.org

Breastdoc
Website: www.breastdoc.com

The Cleveland Clinic Health Information Center
9500 Euclid Avenue
Cleveland, OH 44195
Toll-free: 800-223-2273, ext. 43771
Phone: 216-444-3771
Website:
www.clevelandclinic.org/health
E-mail: healthl@ccf.org

The information in this chapter was compiled from various sources deemed accurate. All contact information was verified and updated in April 2004. Inclusion does not imply endorsement. This list is intended to serve as a starting point for information gathering; it is not comprehensive.

Community Breast Health Project
545 Bryant Street
Palo Alto, CA 94301
Phone: 650-326-6686
Fax: 650-326-6673
Website: www.cbhp.org
E-mail: info@cbhp.org

Cornell University Program on Breast Cancer and Environmental Risk Factors (BCERF)
Sprecher Institute for
Comparative Cancer Research
Cornell University, Box 31
Ithaca, NY 14853
Phone: 607-254-2893
Fax: 607-254-4730
Website: envirocancer.cornell.edu
E-mail: breastcancer@cornell.edu

Dr. Susan Love's Website for Women
Website: www.susanlovemd.com

Imaginis.com
Imaginis Corporation
P.O. Box 27018
Greenville, SC 29616
Website: www.imaginis.com
E-mail: learnmore@imaginis.com

Johns Hopkins Breast Center
601 North Caroline Street,
Room 8031A
Baltimore, MD 21287
Phone: 410-614-2853
Fax: 410-614-1947
Website: www.hopkinsmedicine
.org/breastcenter

Living Beyond Breast Cancer
10 East Athens Ave., Suite 204
Ardmore, PA 19003
Toll-free: 888-753-LBBC
(888-753-5222)
Phone: 610-645-4567
Fax: 610-645-4573
Website: www.lbbc.org
E-mail: mail@lbbc.org

M.D. Anderson Cancer Center
1515 Holcombe Boulevard
Houston, TX 77030
Toll-free: 800-392-1611
Phone: 713-792-6161
Website: www.mdanderson.org

National Cancer Institute
6116 Executive Blvd.
MSC 8322
Suite 3036A
Bethesda, MD 20892-8322
Toll-free: 800-422-6237
Toll-free TTY: 800-322-8615
Website: www.cancer.gov

National Cancer Institute Cancer Information Service
Toll-free: 800-422-6237
Toll-free TTY: 800-332-8615
Website: http://cis.nci.nih.gov

National Women's Health Information Center
8550 Arlington Blvd., Suite 300
Fairfax, VA 22031
Toll-free: 800-994-WOMAN
Toll-free TDD: 888-220-5446
Website: www.4woman.gov

National Women's Health Resource Center
157 Broad Street, Suite 315
Red Bank, NJ 07701
Toll-free: 877-986-9472
Fax: 732-530-3347
Website: www.healthywomen.org

OncoLink
Abramson Cancer Center of the
University of Pennsylvania
3400 Spruce Street, 2 Donner
Philadelphia, PA 19104-4283
Fax: 215-349-5445
Website: www.oncolink.upenn.edu

People Living With Cancer
American Society of Clinical
Oncology
1900 Duke St., Suite 200
Alexandria, VA 22314
Phone: 703-797-1914
Fax: 703-299-1044
Website: www.plwc.org
E-mail: help@plwc.org

Rose Kushner Breast Cancer Advisory Center
P.O. Box 757
Malaga, CA 90274
E-mail: lkkushner@yahoo.com
Website: www.rkbcac.org

Susan G. Komen Foundation
5005 LBJ Freeway, Suite 250
Dallas, TX 75244
Toll-free: 800-IM AWARE or
800-462-9273
Phone: 972-855-1600
Fax: 972-855-1605
Website: www.komen.org

Women's Information Network against Breast Cancer
536 S Second Ave., Suite K
Covina, CA 91723-3043
Toll-free: 866-2WINABC or
866-294-6222
Phone: 626-332-2255
Fax: 626-332-2585
Website: www.winabc.org
E-mail: mail@winabc.org

Y-ME National Breast Cancer Organization
212 W. Van Buren, Suite 1000
Chicago, IL 60607-3908
Toll-free: 800-221-2141 (English)
Toll-free: 800-986-9505 (Spanish)
Spanish Hotline: 800-986-9505
Phone: 312-986-8338
Fax: 312-294-8597
Website: www.y-me.org

Advocacy

American Breast Cancer Foundation (ABCF)
1055 Taylor Avenue, Suite 201A
Baltimore, MD 21286
Toll-free: 877-539-2543
Phone: 410-825-9388
Fax: 410-825-4395
Website: www.abcf.org
E-mail: contact@abcf.org

National Breast Cancer Coalition
1101 17th Street, NW, Suite 1300
Washington, DC 20036
Toll-free: 800-622-2838
Phone: 202-296-7477
Fax: 202-265-6854
Website: www.natlbcc.org

National Coalition for Cancer Survivorship (NCCS)

1010 Wayne Avenue, Suite 770
Silver Spring, MD 20910
Toll-free: 877-NCCS YES or
877-622-7937
Phone: 301-650-9127
Fax: 301-565-9670
Website:
www.canceradvocacy.org
E-mail: info@canceradvocacy.org

African American Breast Cancer Concerns

Sisters Network

8787 Woodway Drive, Suite 4206
Houston, TX 77063
Phone: 713-781-0255
Fax: 713-780-8998
Website:
www.sistersnetworkinc.org
E-mail:
infonet@sistersnetworkinc.org

Breast Reconstruction

American Association of Plastic Surgeons

444 E. Algonquin Road
Arlington Heights, IL 60005
Plastic Surgeon Referral
Service: 888-4-PLASTIC or
888-475-2784
Phone: 847-228-9900
Website:
www.plasticsurgery.org/
public_education/procedures/
BreastReconstruction.cfm
E-mail: nr@plasticsurgery.org

Breast Implants 411

Toll-free: 888-New-2002
(888-639-2002)
Website:
www.breastimplants411.com
E-mail: missbi411@bi411.com

Clinical Trials

Centerwatch Clinical Trials Listing Service

22 Thompson Place, 36T1
Boston, MA 02210-1212
Toll-free: 800-765-9647
Phone: 617-856-5900
Fax: 617-856-5901
Website: www.centerwatch.com
E-mail:
cw.trialwatch@centerwatch.com

ClinicalTrials.gov

Website: www.clinicaltrials.gov

National Cancer Institute Cancer Trials

NCI Public Inquiries Office
6116 Executive Blvd., MSC8322
Suite 3036A
Toll-free: 800-4-CANCER
(800-422-6237)
TTY: 800-332-8615
Website: www.cancer.gov/
clinicaltrials

Complementary Therapies

The Alternative Medicine Foundation
P.O. Box 60016
Potomac, MD 20859
Phone: 301-340-1960
Fax: 301-340-1936
Website: www.amfoundation.org
E-mail: info@amfoundation.org

Annie Appleseed Project
245 Canterbury Circle
Palm Beach Gardens, FL 33418-8220
Website:
www.annieappleseedproject.org
E-mail:
annieappleseedpr@aol.com

Dana Farber Cancer Institute
44 Binney Street
Boston, MA 02115
Toll-free: 866-408-3324
Phone: 617-632-6366
Spanish: 617-632-3673
TDD: 617-632-5330
Website: www.dana-farber.org
E-mail: Dana-FarberContactUs
@dfci.Harvard.edu

Memorial Sloan-Kettering Cancer Center
1275 York Avenue
New York, NY 10021
Toll-free: 800-525-2225
Phone: 212-639-2000
Website: www.mskcc.org

NIH National Center for Complementary and Alternative Medicine
P.O. Box 7923
Gaithersburg, MD 20898
Toll-free: 888-644-6226
Phone: 301-519-3153
TTY: 866-464-3615
Fax: 866-464-3616
Website: http://nccam.nih.gov
E-mail: info@nccam.nih.gov

Coping with Breast Cancer

Kids Konnected
27071 Cabot Road, Suite 102
Laguna Hills, CA 92653
Phone: 949-582-5443
Website: www.kidskonnected.org
E-mail: info@kidskonnected.org

Livingwithit.org
Website: www.livingwithit.org

Look Good . . . Feel Better
Toll-free: 800-395-LOOK
Website:
www.lookgoodfeelbetter.org

National Lymphedema Network
Latham Square
1611 Telegraph Avenue
Suite 1111
Oakland, CA 94612-2138
Toll-free: 800-541-3259
Phone: 510-208-3200
Fax: 510-208-3110
Website: www.lymphnet.org
E-mail: nln@lymphnet.org

The Wellness Community
919 18th Street, NW, Suite 54
Washington, DC 20006
Toll-free: 888-793-WELL
Phone: 202-659-9709
Fax: 202-659-9301
Website:
www.thewellnesscommunity.org
E-mail:
help@thewellnesscommunity.org

DES Concerns

DES Action USA
610 16th St., Suite 301
Oakland, CA 94612
Toll-free: 800-DES-9288 or
800-337-9288
Phone: 510-465-4011
Fax: 510-465-4815
Website: www.desaction.org
E-mail: desaction@earthlink.net

DES Cancer Network
P.O. Box 220465
Chantilly, VA 20153-0465
Toll-free: 888-577-7248
Website: www.descancer.org
E-mail: DESNETWRK@aol.com

Hospice Care

**National Hospice and
Palliative Care
Organization (NHPCO)**
1700 Diagonal Road, Suite 625
Alexandria, VA 22314
Toll-free: 800-658-8898
Phone: 703-837-1500
Fax: 703-837-1233
Website: www.nhpco.org
E-mail: info@nhpco.org

Male Breast Cancer

**Bridging the Gap: Male
Breast Cancer Awareness
Group**
Legacy Good Samaritan Hospital
1040 NW 22nd Ave.
Portland, OR 97210
Phone: 503-844-5949
Website: http://www.geocities
.com/bridge_gap_mbcg/
index.html
E-mail:
lionspride.geo@yahoo.com

John W. Nick Foundation
P.O. Box 4133
Vero Beach, FL 32963
Phone: 772-589-1440
Website:
www.johnwnickfoundation.org
E-mail: johnwnickf@aol.com

**Male Breast Cancer
Telephone Support**
Sussex, WI
Phone: 262-820-0856

Support Groups

**Mothers Supporting
Daughters with Breast
Cancer (MSDBC)**
c/o Charmayne Dierker,
President
21710 Bayshore Road
Chestertown, MD 21620-4401
Phone: 410-778-1982
Website:
www.mothersdaughters.org
E-mail: msdbc@dmv.com

SHARE

1501 Broadway, Suite 1720
New York, NY 10036
Toll-free: 866-891-2392
Phone: 212-719-0364
Fax: 212-869-3431
Website:
www.sharecancersupport.org
E-mail: SHAREprograms@share
cancersupport.org

Women at High Risk of Breast Cancer

Facing Our Risk of Cancer Empowered (FORCE)

934 N. University Dr., PMB #213
Coral Springs, FL 33071
Toll-free: 866-824-RISK or
866-824-7475
Phone: 954-255-8732
Website: www.facingourrisk.org
E-mail: info@facingourrisk.org

Young Women with Breast Cancer

Young Survival Coalition

155 65th Avenue, 10th Floor
New York, NY 10013
Phone: 212-206-6610
Website: www.youngsurvival.org
E-mail: info@youngsurvival.org

Index

Index

Page numbers followed by 'n' indicate a footnote. Page numbers in *italics* indicate a table or illustration.

Health Reference Series
COMPLETE CATALOG

Adolescent Health Sourcebook

Basic Consumer Health Information about Common Medical, Mental, and Emotional Concerns in Adolescents, Including Facts about Acne, Body Piercing, Mononucleosis, Nutrition, Eating Disorders, Stress, Depression, Behavior Problems, Peer Pressure, Violence, Gangs, Drug Use, Puberty, Sexuality, Pregnancy, Learning Disabilities, and More

Along with a Glossary of Terms and Other Resources for Further Help and Information

Edited by Chad T. Kimball. 658 pages. 2002. 0-7808-0248-9. $78.

"It is written in clear, nontechnical language aimed at general readers. . . . Recommended for public libraries, community colleges, and other agencies serving health care consumers."
— *American Reference Books Annual, 2003*

"Recommended for school and public libraries. Parents and professionals dealing with teens will appreciate the easy-to-follow format and the clearly written text. This could become a 'must have' for every high school teacher."
— *E-Streams, Jan '03*

"A good starting point for information related to common medical, mental, and emotional concerns of adolescents."
— *School Library Journal, Nov '02*

"This book provides accurate information in an easy to access format. It addresses topics that parents and caregivers might not be aware of and provides practical, useable information."
— *Doody's Health Sciences Book Review Journal, Sep-Oct '02*

"Recommended reference source."
— *Booklist, American Library Association, Sep '02*

■

AIDS Sourcebook, 3rd Edition

Basic Consumer Health Information about Acquired Immune Deficiency Syndrome (AIDS) and Human Immunodeficiency Virus (HIV) Infection, Including Facts about Transmission, Prevention, Diagnosis, Treatment, Opportunistic Infections, and Other Complications, with a Section for Women and Children, Including Details about Associated Gynecological Concerns, Pregnancy, and Pediatric Care

Along with Updated Statistical Information, Reports on Current Research Initiatives, a Glossary, and Directories of Internet, Hotline, and Other Resources

Edited by Dawn D. Matthews. 664 pages. 2003. 0-7808-0631-X. $78.

ALSO AVAILABLE: *AIDS Sourcebook, 1st Edition.* Edited by Karen Bellenir and Peter D. Dresser. 831 pages. 1995. 0-7808-0031-1. $78.

AIDS Sourcebook, 2nd Edition. Edited by Karen Bellenir. 751 pages. 1999. 0-7808-0225-X. $78.

"The 3rd edition of the *AIDS Sourcebook,* part of Omnigraphics' *Health Reference Series,* is a welcome update. . . . This resource is highly recommended for academic and public libraries."
— *American Reference Books Annual, 2004*

"Excellent sourcebook. This continues to be a highly recommended book. There is no other book that provides as much information as this book provides."
— *AIDS Book Review Journal, Dec-Jan 2000*

"Recommended reference source."
— *Booklist, American Library Association, Dec '99*

"A solid text for college-level health libraries."
— *The Bookwatch, Aug '99*

Cited in *Reference Sources for Small and Medium-Sized Libraries, American Library Association, 1999*

■

Alcoholism Sourcebook

Basic Consumer Health Information about the Physical and Mental Consequences of Alcohol Abuse, Including Liver Disease, Pancreatitis, Wernicke-Korsakoff Syndrome (Alcoholic Dementia), Fetal Alcohol Syndrome, Heart Disease, Kidney Disorders, Gastrointestinal Problems, and Immune System Compromise and Featuring Facts about Addiction, Detoxification, Alcohol Withdrawal, Recovery, and the Maintenance of Sobriety

Along with a Glossary and Directories of Resources for Further Help and Information

Edited by Karen Bellenir. 613 pages. 2000. 0-7808-0325-6. $78.

"This title is one of the few reference works on alcoholism for general readers. For some readers this will be a welcome complement to the many self-help books on the market. Recommended for collections serving general readers and consumer health collections."
— *E-Streams, Mar '01*

"This book is an excellent choice for public and academic libraries."
— *American Reference Books Annual, 2001*

"Recommended reference source."
— *Booklist, American Library Association, Dec '00*

"Presents a wealth of information on alcohol use and abuse and its effects on the body and mind, treatment, and prevention."
— *SciTech Book News, Dec '00*

"Important new health guide which packs in the latest consumer information about the problems of alcoholism."
— *Reviewer's Bookwatch, Nov '00*

SEE ALSO *Drug Abuse Sourcebook, Substance Abuse Sourcebook*

Allergies Sourcebook, 2nd Edition

Basic Consumer Health Information about Allergic Disorders, Triggers, Reactions, and Related Symptoms, Including Anaphylaxis, Rhinitis, Sinusitis, Asthma, Dermatitis, Conjunctivitis, and Multiple Chemical Sensitivity

Along with Tips on Diagnosis, Prevention, and Treatment, Statistical Data, a Glossary, and a Directory of Sources for Further Help and Information

Edited by Annemarie S. Muth. 598 pages. 2002. 0-7808-0376-0. $78.

ALSO AVAILABLE: *Allergies Sourcebook, 1st Edition.* Edited by Allan R. Cook. 611 pages. 1997. 0-7808-0036-2. $78.

"This book brings a great deal of useful material together. . . . This is an excellent addition to public and consumer health library collections."
— *American Reference Books Annual, 2003*

"This second edition would be useful to laypersons with little or advanced knowledge of the subject matter. This book would also serve as a resource for nursing and other health care professions students. It would be useful in public, academic, and hospital libraries with consumer health collections." — *E-Streams, Jul '02*

Alternative Medicine Sourcebook, 2nd Edition

Basic Consumer Health Information about Alternative and Complementary Medical Practices, Including Acupuncture, Chiropractic, Herbal Medicine, Homeopathy, Naturopathic Medicine, Mind-Body Interventions, Ayurveda, and Other Non-Western Medical Traditions

Along with Facts about such Specific Therapies as Massage Therapy, Aromatherapy, Qigong, Hypnosis, Prayer, Dance, and Art Therapies, a Glossary, and Resources for Further Information

Edited by Dawn D. Matthews. 618 pages. 2002. 0-7808-0605-0. $78.

ALSO AVAILABLE: *Alternative Medicine Sourcebook, 1st Edition.* Edited by Allan R. Cook. 737 pages. 1999. 0-7808-0200-4. $78.

"Recommended for public, high school, and academic libraries that have consumer health collections. Hospital libraries that also serve the public will find this to be a useful resource." — *E-Streams, Feb '03*

"Recommended reference source."
—*Booklist, American Library Association, Jan '03*

"An important alternate health reference."
—*MBR Bookwatch, Oct '02*

"A great addition to the reference collection of every type of library." — *American Reference Books Annual, 2000*

Alzheimer's Disease Sourcebook, 3rd Edition

Basic Consumer Health Information about Alzheimer's Disease, Other Dementias, and Related Disorders, Including Multi-Infarct Dementia, AIDS Dementia Complex, Dementia with Lewy Bodies, Huntington's Disease, Wernicke-Korsakoff Syndrome (Alcohol-Reated Dementia), Delirium, and Confusional States

Along with Information for People Newly Diagnosed with Alzheimer's Disease and Caregivers, Reports Detailing Current Research Efforts in Prevention, Diagnosis, and Treatment, Facts about Long-Term Care Issues, and Listings of Sources for Additional Information

Edited by Karen Bellenir. 645 pages. 2003. 0-7808-0666-2. $78.

ALSO AVAILABLE: *Alzheimer's, Stroke & 29 Other Neurological Disorders Sourcebook, 1st Edition.* Edited by Frank E. Bair. 579 pages. 1993. 1-55888-748-2. $78.

ALSO AVAILABLE: *Alzheimer's Disease Sourcebook, 2nd Edition.* Edited by Karen Bellenir. 524 pages. 1999. 0-7808-0223-3. $78.

"This very informative and valuable tool will be a great addition to any library serving consumers, students and health care workers."
—*American Reference Books Annual, 2004*

"This is a valuable resource for people affected by dementias such as Alzheimer's. It is easy to navigate and includes important information and resources."
— *Doody's Review Service, Feb. 2004*

"Recommended reference source."
— *Booklist, American Library Association, Oct '99*

SEE ALSO Brain Disorders Sourcebook

Arthritis Sourcebook, 2nd Edition

Basic Consumer Health Information about Osteoarthritis, Rheumatoid Arthritis, Other Rheumatic Disorders, Infectious Forms of Arthritis, and Diseases with Symptoms Linked to Arthritis, Featuring Facts about Diagnosis, Pain Management, and Surgical Therapies

Along with Coping Strategies, Research Updates, a Glossary, and Resources for Additional Help and Information

Edited by Amy L. Sutton. 593 pages. 2004. 0-7808-0667-0. $78.

ALSO AVAILABLE: *Arthritis Sourcebook, 1st Edition.* Edited by Allan R. Cook. 550 pages. 1998. 0-7808-0201-2. $78.

". . . accessible to the layperson."
—*Reference and Research Book News, Feb '99*

Asthma Sourcebook

Basic Consumer Health Information about Asthma, Including Symptoms, Traditional and Nontraditional Remedies, Treatment Advances, Quality-of-Life Aids, Medical Research Updates, and the Role of Allergies, Exercise, Age, the Environment, and Genetics in the Development of Asthma

Along with Statistical Data, a Glossary, and Directories of Support Groups, and Other Resources for Further Information

Edited by Annemarie S. Muth. 628 pages. 2000. 0-7808-0381-7. $78.

"A worthwhile reference acquisition for public libraries and academic medical libraries whose readers desire a quick introduction to the wide range of asthma information." — *Choice, Association of College & Research Libraries, Jun '01*

"Recommended reference source." — *Booklist, American Library Association, Feb '01*

"Highly recommended." — *The Bookwatch, Jan '01*

"There is much good information for patients and their families who deal with asthma daily." — *American Medical Writers Association Journal, Winter '01*

"This informative text is recommended for consumer health collections in public, secondary school, and community college libraries and the libraries of universities with a large undergraduate population." — *American Reference Books Annual, 2001*

Attention Deficit Disorder Sourcebook

Basic Consumer Health Information about Attention Deficit/Hyperactivity Disorder in Children and Adults, Including Facts about Causes, Symptoms, Diagnostic Criteria, and Treatment Options Such as Medications, Behavior Therapy, Coaching, and Homeopathy

Along with Reports on Current Research Initiatives, Legal Issues, and Government Regulations, and Featuring a Glossary of Related Terms, Internet Resources, and a List of Additional Reading Material

Edited by Dawn D. Matthews. 470 pages. 2002. 0-7808-0624-7. $78.

"Recommended reference source." — *Booklist, American Library Association, Jan '03*

"This book is recommended for all school libraries and the reference or consumer health sections of public libraries." — *American Reference Books Annual, 2003*

Back & Neck Sourcebook, 2nd Edition

Basic Consumer Health Information about Spinal Pain, Spinal Cord Injuries, and Related Disorders, Such as Degenerative Disk Disease, Osteoarthritis, Scoliosis,

Sciatica, Spina Bifida, and Spinal Stenosis, and Featuring Facts about Maintaining Spinal Health, Self-Care, Pain Management, Rehabilitative Care, Chiropractic Care, Spinal Surgeries, and Complementary Therapies

Along with Suggestions for Preventing Back and Neck Pain, a Glossary of Related Terms, and a Directory of Resources

Edited by Amy L. Sutton. 600 pages. 2004. 0-7808-0738-3 $78.

ALSO AVAILABLE: *Back & Neck Disorders Sourcebook, 1st Edition.* Edited by Karen Bellenir. 548 pages. 1997. 0-7808-0202-0. $78.

"The strength of this work is its basic, easy-to-read format. Recommended." — *Reference and User Services Quarterly, American Library Association, Winter '97*

Blood & Circulatory Disorders Sourcebook

Basic Information about Blood and Its Components, Anemias, Leukemias, Bleeding Disorders, and Circulatory Disorders, Including Aplastic Anemia, Thalassemia, Sickle-Cell Disease, Hemochromatosis, Hemophilia, Von Willebrand Disease, and Vascular Diseases

Along with a Special Section on Blood Transfusions and Blood Supply Safety, a Glossary, and Source Listings for Further Help and Information

Edited by Karen Bellenir and Linda M. Shin. 554 pages. 1998. 0-7808-0203-9. $78.

"Recommended reference source." — *Booklist, American Library Association, Feb '99*

"An important reference sourcebook written in simple language for everyday, non-technical users. " — *Reviewer's Bookwatch, Jan '99*

Brain Disorders Sourcebook

Basic Consumer Health Information about Strokes, Epilepsy, Amyotrophic Lateral Sclerosis (ALS/Lou Gehrig's Disease), Parkinson's Disease, Brain Tumors, Cerebral Palsy, Headache, Tourette Syndrome, and More

Along with Statistical Data, Treatment and Rehabilitation Options, Coping Strategies, Reports on Current Research Initiatives, a Glossary, and Resource Listings for Additional Help and Information

Edited by Karen Bellenir. 481 pages. 1999. 0-7808-0229-2. $78.

"Belongs on the shelves of any library with a consumer health collection." — *E-Streams, Mar '00*

"Recommended reference source." — *Booklist, American Library Association, Oct '99*

SEE ALSO *Alzheimer's Disease Sourcebook*

Breast Cancer Sourcebook, 2nd Edition

Basic Consumer Health Information about Breast Cancer, Including Facts about Risk Factors, Prevention, Screening and Diagnostic Methods, Treatment Options, Complementary and Alternative Therapies, Post-Treatment Concerns, Clinical Trials, Special Risk Populations, and New Developments in Breast Cancer Research

Along with Breast Cancer Statistics, a Glossary of Related Terms, and a Directory of Resources for Additional Help and Information

Edited by Sandra J. Judd. 595 pages. 2004. 0-7808-0668-9. $78.

ALSO AVAILABLE: Breast Cancer Sourcebook, 1st Edition. Edited by Edward J. Prucha and Karen Bellenir. 580 pages. 2001. 0-7808-0244-6. $78.

"It would be a useful reference book in a library or on loan to women in a support group."
— *Cancer Forum, Mar '03*

"Recommended reference source."
— *Booklist, American Library Association, Jan '02*

"This reference source is highly recommended. It is quite informative, comprehensive and detailed in nature, and yet it offers practical advice in easy-to-read language. It could be thought of as the 'bible' of breast cancer for the consumer."   — *E-Streams, Jan '02*

"The broad range of topics covered in lay language make the *Breast Cancer Sourcebook* an excellent addition to public and consumer health library collections."
— *American Reference Books Annual 2002*

"From the pros and cons of different screening methods and results to treatment options, *Breast Cancer Sourcebook* provides the latest information on the subject."
— *Library Bookwatch, Dec '01*

"This thoroughgoing, very readable reference covers all aspects of breast health and cancer. . . . Readers will find much to consider here. Recommended for all public and patient health collections."
— *Library Journal, Sep '01*

SEE ALSO Cancer Sourcebook for Women, Women's Health Concerns Sourcebook

Breastfeeding Sourcebook

Basic Consumer Health Information about the Benefits of Breastmilk, Preparing to Breastfeed, Breastfeeding as a Baby Grows, Nutrition, and More, Including Information on Special Situations and Concerns Such as Mastitis, Illness, Medications, Allergies, Multiple Births, Prematurity, Special Needs, and Adoption

Along with a Glossary and Resources for Additional Help and Information

Edited by Jenni Lynn Colson. 388 pages. 2002. 0-7808-0332-9. $78.

SEE ALSO Pregnancy & Birth Sourcebook

"Particularly useful is the information about professional lactation services and chapters on breastfeeding

when returning to work. . . . *Breastfeeding Sourcebook* will be useful for public libraries, consumer health libraries, and technical schools offering nurse assistant training, especially in areas where Internet access is problematic."
— *American Reference Books Annual, 2003*

Burns Sourcebook

Basic Consumer Health Information about Various Types of Burns and Scalds, Including Flame, Heat, Cold, Electrical, Chemical, and Sun Burns

Along with Information on Short-Term and Long-Term Treatments, Tissue Reconstruction, Plastic Surgery, Prevention Suggestions, and First Aid

Edited by Allan R. Cook. 604 pages. 1999. 0-7808-0204-7. $78.

"This is an exceptional addition to the series and is highly recommended for all consumer health collections, hospital libraries, and academic medical centers."
— *E-Streams, Mar '00*

"This key reference guide is an invaluable addition to all health care and public libraries in confronting this ongoing health issue."
— *American Reference Books Annual, 2000*

"Recommended reference source."
— *Booklist, American Library Association, Dec '99*

SEE ALSO Skin Disorders Sourcebook

Cancer Sourcebook, 4th Edition

Basic Consumer Health Information about Major Forms and Stages of Cancer, Featuring Facts about Head and Neck Cancers, Lung Cancers, Gastrointestinal Cancers, Genitourinary Cancers, Lymphomas, Blood Cell Cancers, Endocrine Cancers, Skin Cancers, Bone Cancers, Sarcomas, and Others, and Including Information about Cancer Treatments and Therapies, Identifying and Reducing Cancer Risks, and Strategies for Coping with Cancer and the Side Effects of Treatment

Along with a Cancer Glossary, Statistical and Demographic Data, and a Directory of Sources for Additional Help and Information

Edited by Karen Bellenir. 1,119 pages. 2003. 0-7808-0633-6. $78.

ALSO AVAILABLE: Cancer Sourcebook, 1st Edition. Edited by Frank E. Bair. 932 pages. 1990. 1-55888-888-8. $78.

New Cancer Sourcebook, 2nd Edition. Edited by Allan R. Cook. 1,313 pages. 1996. 0-7808-0041-9. $78.

Cancer Sourcebook, 3rd Edition. Edited by Edward J. Prucha. 1,069 pages. 2000. 0-7808-0227-6. $78.

"With cancer being the second leading cause of death for Americans, a prodigious work such as this one, which locates centrally so much cancer-related information, is clearly an asset to this nation's citizens and others."   — *Journal of the National Medical Association, 2004*

"This title is recommended for health sciences and public libraries with consumer health collections."
— *E-Streams, Feb '01*

". . . can be effectively used by cancer patients and their families who are looking for answers in a language they can understand. Public and hospital libraries should have it on their shelves."
— *American Reference Books Annual, 2001*

"Recommended reference source."
— *Booklist, American Library Association, Dec '00*

Cited in *Reference Sources for Small and Medium-Sized Libraries*, American Library Association, 1999

"The amount of factual and useful information is extensive. The writing is very clear, geared to general readers. Recommended for all levels." — *Choice, Association of College & Research Libraries, Jan '97*

SEE ALSO Breast Cancer Sourcebook, Cancer Sourcebook for Women, Pediatric Cancer Sourcebook, Prostate Cancer Sourcebook

■

Cancer Sourcebook for Women, 2nd Edition

Basic Consumer Health Information about Gynecologic Cancers and Related Concerns, Including Cervical Cancer, Endometrial Cancer, Gestational Trophoblastic Tumor, Ovarian Cancer, Uterine Cancer, Vaginal Cancer, Vulvar Cancer, Breast Cancer, and Common Non-Cancerous Uterine Conditions, with Facts about Cancer Risk Factors, Screening and Prevention, Treatment Options, and Reports on Current Research Initiatives

Along with a Glossary of Cancer Terms and a Directory of Resources for Additional Help and Information

Edited by Karen Bellenir. 604 pages. 2002. 0-7808-0226-8. $78.

ALSO AVAILABLE: Cancer Sourcebook for Women, 1st Edition. Edited by Allan R. Cook and Peter D. Dresser. 524 pages. 1996. 0-7808-0076-1. $78.

"An excellent addition to collections in public, consumer health, and women's health libraries."
— *American Reference Books Annual, 2003*

"Overall, the information is excellent, and complex topics are clearly explained. As a reference book for the consumer it is a valuable resource to assist them to make informed decisions about cancer and its treatments." — *Cancer Forum, Nov '02*

"Highly recommended for academic and medical reference collections." — *Library Bookwatch, Sep '02*

"This is a highly recommended book for any public or consumer library, being reader friendly and containing accurate and helpful information."
— *E-Streams, Aug '02*

"Recommended reference source."
— *Booklist, American Library Association, Jul '02*

SEE ALSO Breast Cancer Sourcebook, Women's Health Concerns Sourcebook

Cardiovascular Diseases & Disorders Sourcebook, 1st Edition

SEE Heart Diseases & Disorders Sourcebook, 2nd Edition

■

Caregiving Sourcebook

Basic Consumer Health Information for Caregivers, Including a Profile of Caregivers, Caregiving Responsibilities and Concerns, Tips for Specific Conditions, Care Environments, and the Effects of Caregiving

Along with Facts about Legal Issues, Financial Information, and Future Planning, a Glossary, and a Listing of Additional Resources

Edited by Joyce Brennfleck Shannon. 600 pages. 2001. 0-7808-0331-0. $78.

"Essential for most collections."
— *Library Journal, Apr 1, 2002*

"An ideal addition to the reference collection of any public library. Health sciences information professionals may also want to acquire the *Caregiving Sourcebook* for their hospital or academic library for use as a ready reference tool by health care workers interested in aging and caregiving." — *E-Streams, Jan '02*

"Recommended reference source."
— *Booklist, American Library Association, Oct '01*

■

Child Abuse Sourcebook

Basic Consumer Health Information about the Physical, Sexual, and Emotional Abuse of Children, with Additional Facts about Neglect, Munchausen Syndrome by Proxy (MSBP), Shaken Baby Syndrome, and Controversial Issues Related to Child Abuse, Such as Withholding Medical Care, Corporal Punishment, and Child Maltreatment in Youth Sports, and Featuring Facts about Child Protective Services, Foster Care, Adoption, Parenting Challenges, and Other Abuse Prevention Efforts

Along with a Glossary of Related Terms and Resources for Additional Help and Information

Edited by Dawn D. Matthews. 620 pages. 2004. 0-7808-0705-7. $78.

■

Childhood Diseases & Disorders Sourcebook

Basic Consumer Health Information about Medical Problems Often Encountered in Pre-Adolescent Children, Including Respiratory Tract Ailments, Ear Infections, Sore Throats, Disorders of the Skin and Scalp, Digestive and Genitourinary Diseases, Infectious Diseases, Inflammatory Disorders, Chronic Physical and Developmental Disorders, Allergies, and More

Along with Information about Diagnostic Tests, Common Childhood Surgeries, and Frequently Used Medications, with a Glossary of Important Terms and Resource Directory

Edited by Chad T. Kimball. 662 pages. 2003. 0-7808-0458-9. $78.

"This is an excellent book for new parents and should be included in all health care and public libraries."
— *American Reference Books Annual, 2004*

Colds, Flu & Other Common Ailments Sourcebook

Basic Consumer Health Information about Common Ailments and Injuries, Including Colds, Coughs, the Flu, Sinus Problems, Headaches, Fever, Nausea and Vomiting, Menstrual Cramps, Diarrhea, Constipation, Hemorrhoids, Back Pain, Dandruff, Dry and Itchy Skin, Cuts, Scrapes, Sprains, Bruises, and More

Along with Information about Prevention, Self-Care, Choosing a Doctor, Over-the-Counter Medications, Folk Remedies, and Alternative Therapies, and Including a Glossary of Important Terms and a Directory of Resources for Further Help and Information

Edited by Chad T. Kimball. 638 pages. 2001. 0-7808-0435-X. $78.

"A good starting point for research on common illnesses. It will be a useful addition to public and consumer health library collections."
— *American Reference Books Annual 2002*

"Will prove valuable to any library seeking to maintain a current, comprehensive reference collection of health resources. . . . Excellent reference."
— *The Bookwatch, Aug '01*

"Recommended reference source."
— *Booklist, American Library Association, July '01*

Communication Disorders Sourcebook

Basic Information about Deafness and Hearing Loss, Speech and Language Disorders, Voice Disorders, Balance and Vestibular Disorders, and Disorders of Smell, Taste, and Touch

Edited by Linda M. Ross. 533 pages. 1996. 0-7808-0077-X. $78.

"This is skillfully edited and is a welcome resource for the layperson. It should be found in every public and medical library."
— *Booklist Health Sciences Supplement, American Library Association, Oct '97*

Congenital Disorders Sourcebook

Basic Information about Disorders Acquired during Gestation, Including Spina Bifida, Hydrocephalus, Cerebral Palsy, Heart Defects, Craniofacial Abnormalities, Fetal Alcohol Syndrome, and More

Along with Current Treatment Options and Statistical Data

Edited by Karen Bellenir. 607 pages. 1997. 0-7808-0205-5. $78.

"Recommended reference source."
— *Booklist, American Library Association, Oct '97*

SEE ALSO Pregnancy & Birth Sourcebook

Consumer Issues in Health Care Sourcebook

Basic Information about Health Care Fundamentals and Related Consumer Issues, Including Exams and Screening Tests, Physician Specialties, Choosing a Doctor, Using Prescription and Over-the-Counter Medications Safely, Avoiding Health Scams, Managing Common Health Risks in the Home, Care Options for Chronically or Terminally Ill Patients, and a List of Resources for Obtaining Help and Further Information

Edited by Karen Bellenir. 618 pages. 1998. 0-7808-0221-7. $78.

"Both public and academic libraries will want to have a copy in their collection for readers who are interested in self-education on health issues."
— *American Reference Books Annual, 2000*

"The editor has researched the literature from government agencies and others, saving readers the time and effort of having to do the research themselves. Recommended for public libraries."
— *Reference and User Services Quarterly, American Library Association, Spring '99*

"Recommended reference source."
— *Booklist, American Library Association, Dec '98*

Contagious Diseases Sourcebook

Basic Consumer Health Information about Infectious Diseases Spread by Person-to-Person Contact through Direct Touch, Airborne Transmission, Sexual Contact, or Contact with Blood or Other Body Fluids, Including Hepatitis, Herpes, Influenza, Lice, Measles, Mumps, Pinworm, Ringworm, Severe Acute Respiratory Syndrome (SARS), Streptococcal Infections, Tuberculosis, and Others

Along with Facts about Disease Transmission, Antimicrobial Resistance, and Vaccines, with a Glossary and Directories of Resources for More Information

Edited by Karen Bellenir. 643 pages. 2004. 0-7808-0736-7. $78.

Contagious & Non-Contagious Infectious Diseases Sourcebook

Basic Information about Contagious Diseases like Measles, Polio, Hepatitis B, and Infectious Mononucleosis, and Non-Contagious Infectious Diseases like Tetanus and Toxic Shock Syndrome, and Diseases Occurring as Secondary Infections Such as Shingles and Reye Syndrome

Along with Vaccination, Prevention, and Treatment Information, and a Section Describing Emerging Infectious Disease Threats

Edited by Karen Bellenir and Peter D. Dresser. 566 pages. 1996. 0-7808-0075-3. $78.

Death & Dying Sourcebook

Basic Consumer Health Information for the Layperson about End-of-Life Care and Related Ethical and Legal Issues, Including Chief Causes of Death, Autopsies, Pain Management for the Terminally Ill, Life Support Systems, Insurance, Euthanasia, Assisted Suicide, Hospice Programs, Living Wills, Funeral Planning, Counseling, Mourning, Organ Donation, and Physician Training

Along with Statistical Data, a Glossary, and Listings of Sources for Further Help and Information

Edited by Annemarie S. Muth. 641 pages. 1999. 0-7808-0230-6. $78.

"Public libraries, medical libraries, and academic libraries will all find this sourcebook a useful addition to their collections."
— *American Reference Books Annual, 2001*

"An extremely useful resource for those concerned with death and dying in the United States."
— *Respiratory Care, Nov '00*

"Recommended reference source."
— *Booklist, American Library Association, Aug '00*

"This book is a definite must for all those involved in end-of-life care." — *Doody's Review Service, 2000*

Dental Care & Oral Health Sourcebook, 2nd Edition

Basic Consumer Health Information about Dental Care, Including Oral Hygiene, Dental Visits, Pain Management, Cavities, Crowns, Bridges, Dental Implants, and Fillings, and Other Oral Health Concerns, Such as Gum Disease, Bad Breath, Dry Mouth, Genetic and Developmental Abnormalities, Oral Cancers, Orthodontics, and Temporomandibular Disorders

Along with Updates on Current Research in Oral Health, a Glossary, a Directory of Dental and Oral Health Organizations, and Resources for People with Dental and Oral Health Disorders

Edited by Amy L. Sutton. 609 pages. 2003. 0-7808-0634-4. $78.

ALSO AVAILABLE: *Oral Health Sourcebook, 1st Edition.* Edited by Allan R. Cook. 558 pages. 1997. 0-7808-0082-6. $78.

"This book could serve as a turning point in the battle to educate consumers in issues concerning oral health."
— *American Reference Books Annual, 2004*

"Unique source which will fill a gap in dental sources for patients and the lay public. A valuable reference tool even in a library with thousands of books on dentistry. Comprehensive, clear, inexpensive, and easy to read and use. It fills an enormous gap in the health care literature." — *Reference and User Services Quarterly, American Library Association, Summer '98*

"Recommended reference source."
— *Booklist, American Library Association, Dec '97*

Depression Sourcebook

Basic Consumer Health Information about Unipolar Depression, Bipolar Disorder, Postpartum Depression, Seasonal Affective Disorder, and Other Types of Depression in Children, Adolescents, Women, Men, the Elderly, and Other Selected Populations

Along with Facts about Causes, Risk Factors, Diagnostic Criteria, Treatment Options, Coping Strategies, Suicide Prevention, a Glossary, and a Directory of Sources for Additional Help and Information

Edited by Karen Belleni. 602 pages. 2002. 0-7808-0611-5. $78.

"*Depression Sourcebook* is of a very high standard. Its purpose, which is to serve as a reference source to the lay reader, is very well served."
— *Journal of the National Medical Association, 2004*

"Invaluable reference for public and school library collections alike." — *Library Bookwatch, Apr '03*

"Recommended for purchase."
— *American Reference Books Annual, 2003*

Diabetes Sourcebook, 3rd Edition

Basic Consumer Health Information about Type 1 Diabetes (Insulin-Dependent or Juvenile-Onset Diabetes), Type 2 Diabetes (Noninsulin-Dependent or Adult-Onset Diabetes), Gestational Diabetes, Impaired Glucose Tolerance (IGT), and Related Complications, Such as Amputation, Eye Disease, Gum Disease, Nerve Damage, and End-Stage Renal Disease, Including Facts about Insulin, Oral Diabetes Medications, Blood Sugar Testing, and the Role of Exercise and Nutrition in the Control of Diabetes

Along with a Glossary and Resources for Further Help and Information

Edited by Dawn D. Matthews. 622 pages. 2003. 0-7808-0629-8. $78.

ALSO AVAILABLE: *Diabetes Sourcebook, 1st Edition.* Edited by Karen Bellenir and Peter D. Dresser. 827 pages. 1994. 1-55888-751-2. $78.

Diabetes Sourcebook, 2nd Edition. Edited by Karen Bellenir. 688 pages. 1998. 0-7808-0224-1. $78.

"This edition is even more helpful than earlier versions. . . . It is a truly valuable tool for anyone seeking readable and authoritative information on diabetes."
— *American Reference Books Annual, 2004*

"An invaluable reference." — *Library Journal, May '00*

Selected as one of the 250 "Best Health Sciences Books of 1999." — *Doody's Rating Service, Mar-Apr 2000*

"Provides useful information for the general public."
— *Healthlines, University of Michigan Health Management Research Center, Sep/Oct '99*

". . . provides reliable mainstream medical information . . . belongs on the shelves of any library with a consumer health collection." — *E-Streams, Sep '99*

"Recommended reference source."
— *Booklist, American Library Association, Feb '99*

Diet & Nutrition Sourcebook, 2nd Edition

Basic Consumer Health Information about Dietary Guidelines, Recommended Daily Intake Values, Vitamins, Minerals, Fiber, Fat, Weight Control, Dietary Supplements, and Food Additives

Along with Special Sections on Nutrition Needs throughout Life and Nutrition for People with Such Specific Medical Concerns as Allergies, High Blood Cholesterol, Hypertension, Diabetes, Celiac Disease, Seizure Disorders, Phenylketonuria (PKU), Cancer, and Eating Disorders, and Including Reports on Current Nutrition Research and Source Listings for Additional Help and Information

Edited by Karen Bellenir. 650 pages. 1999. 0-7808-0228-4. $78.

ALSO AVAILABLE: Diet & Nutrition Sourcebook, 1st Edition. Edited by Dan R. Harris. 662 pages. 1996. 0-7808-0084-2. $78.

"This book is an excellent source of basic diet and nutrition information." *— Booklist Health Sciences Supplement, American Library Association, Dec '00*

"This reference document should be in any public library, but it would be a very good guide for beginning students in the health sciences. If the other books in this publisher's series are as good as this, they should all be in the health sciences collections."
—American Reference Books Annual, 2000

"This book is an excellent general nutrition reference for consumers who desire to take an active role in their health care for prevention. Consumers of all ages who select this book can feel confident they are receiving current and accurate information." *—Journal of Nutrition for the Elderly, Vol. 19, No. 4, '00*

"Recommended reference source."
—Booklist, American Library Association, Dec '99

SEE ALSO Digestive Diseases & Disorders Sourcebook, Eating Disorders Sourcebook, Gastrointestinal Diseases & Disorders Sourcebook, Vegetarian Sourcebook

Digestive Diseases & Disorders Sourcebook

Basic Consumer Health Information about Diseases and Disorders that Impact the Upper and Lower Digestive System, Including Celiac Disease, Constipation, Crohn's Disease, Cyclic Vomiting Syndrome, Diarrhea, Diverticulosis and Diverticulitis, Gallstones, Heartburn, Hemorrhoids, Hernias, Indigestion (Dyspepsia), Irritable Bowel Syndrome, Lactose Intolerance, Ulcers, and More

Along with Information about Medications and Other Treatments, Tips for Maintaining a Healthy Digestive Tract, a Glossary, and Directory of Digestive Diseases Organizations

Edited by Karen Bellenir. 335 pages. 2000. 0-7808-0327-2. $78.

"This title would be an excellent addition to all public or patient-research libraries."
—American Reference Books Annual, 2001

"This title is recommended for public, hospital, and health sciences libraries with consumer health collections." *— E-Streams, Jul-Aug '00*

"Recommended reference source."
—Booklist, American Library Association, May '00

SEE ALSO Diet & Nutrition Sourcebook, Eating Disorders Sourcebook, Gastrointestinal Diseases & Disorders Sourcebook

Disabilities Sourcebook

Basic Consumer Health Information about Physical and Psychiatric Disabilities, Including Descriptions of Major Causes of Disability, Assistive and Adaptive Aids, Workplace Issues, and Accessibility Concerns

Along with Information about the Americans with Disabilities Act, a Glossary, and Resources for Additional Help and Information

Edited by Dawn D. Matthews. 616 pages. 2000. 0-7808-0389-2. $78.

"It is a must for libraries with a consumer health section." *— American Reference Books Annual 2002*

"A much needed addition to the Omnigraphics *Health Reference Series*. A current reference work to provide people with disabilities, their families, caregivers or those who work with them, a broad range of information in one volume, has not been available until now. . . . It is recommended for all public and academic library reference collections." *— E-Streams, May '01*

"An excellent source book in easy-to-read format covering many current topics; highly recommended for all libraries." *— Choice, Association of College and Research Libraries, Jan '01*

"Recommended reference source."
—Booklist, American Library Association, Jul '00

Domestic Violence Sourcebook, 2nd Edition

Basic Consumer Health Information about the Causes and Consequences of Abusive Relationships, Including Physical Violence, Sexual Assault, Battery, Stalking, and Emotional Abuse, and Facts about the Effects of Violence on Women, Men, Young Adults, and the Elderly, with Reports about Domestic Violence in Selected Populations, and Featuring Facts about Medical Care, Victim Assistance and Protection, Prevention Strategies, Mental Health Services, and Legal Issues

Along with a Glossary of Related Terms and Resources for Additional Help and Information

Edited by Dawn D. Matthews. 628 pages. 2004. 0-7808-0669-7. $78.

ALSO AVAILABLE: Domestic Violence & Child Abuse Sourcebook, 1st Edition. Edited by Helene Henderson. 1,064 pages. 2001. 0-7808-0235-7. $78.

"Interested lay persons should find the book extremely beneficial. . . . A copy of *Domestic Violence and Child Abuse Sourcebook* should be in every public library in the United States."
— *Social Science & Medicine, No. 56, 2003*

"This is important information. The Web has many resources but this sourcebook fills an important societal need. I am not aware of any other resources of this type." — *Doody's Review Service, Sep '01*

"Recommended for all libraries, scholars, and practitioners." — *Choice, Association of College & Research Libraries, Jul '01*

"Recommended reference source." — *Booklist, American Library Association, Apr '01*

"Important pick for college-level health reference libraries." — *The Bookwatch, Mar '01*

"Because this problem is so widespread and because this book includes a lot of issues within one volume, this work is recommended for all public libraries." — *American Reference Books Annual, 2001*

◼

Drug Abuse Sourcebook, 2nd Edition

Basic Consumer Health Information about Illicit Substances of Abuse and the Misuse of Prescription and Over-the-Counter Medications, Including Depressants, Hallucinogens, Inhalants, Marijuana, Stimulants, and Anabolic Steroids

Along with Facts about Related Health Risks, Treatment Programs, Prevention Programs, a Glossary of Abuse and Addiction Terms, a Glossary of Drug-Related Street Terms, and a Directory Resources for More Information

Edited by Catherine Ginther. 600 pages. 2004. 0-7808-0740-5. $78.

ALSO AVAILABLE: Drug Abuse Sourcebook, 1st Edition. Edited by Karen Bellenir. 629 pages. 2000. 0-7808-0242-X. $78.

"Containing a wealth of information . . . . This resource belongs in libraries that serve a lower-division undergraduate or community college clientele as well as the general public." — *Choice, Association of College and Research Libraries, Jun '01*

"Recommended reference source." — *Booklist, American Library Association, Feb '01*

"Highly recommended." — *The Bookwatch, Jan '01*

"Even though there is a plethora of books on drug abuse, this volume is recommended for school, public, and college libraries." — *American Reference Books Annual, 2001*

SEE ALSO *Alcoholism Sourcebook, Substance Abuse Sourcebook*

Ear, Nose & Throat Disorders Sourcebook

Basic Information about Disorders of the Ears, Nose, Sinus Cavities, Pharynx, and Larynx, Including Ear Infections, Tinnitus, Vestibular Disorders, Allergic and Non-Allergic Rhinitis, Sore Throats, Tonsillitis, and Cancers That Affect the Ears, Nose, Sinuses, and Throat

Along with Reports on Current Research Initiatives, a Glossary of Related Medical Terms, and a Directory of Sources for Further Help and Information

Edited by Karen Bellenir and Linda M. Shin. 576 pages. 1998. 0-7808-0206-3. $78.

"Overall, this sourcebook is helpful for the consumer seeking information on ENT issues. It is recommended for public libraries." — *American Reference Books Annual, 1999*

"Recommended reference source." — *Booklist, American Library Association, Dec '98*

◼

Eating Disorders Sourcebook

Basic Consumer Health Information about Eating Disorders, Including Information about Anorexia Nervosa, Bulimia Nervosa, Binge Eating, Body Dysmorphic Disorder, Pica, Laxative Abuse, and Night Eating Syndrome

Along with Information about Causes, Adverse Effects, and Treatment and Prevention Issues, and Featuring a Section on Concerns Specific to Children and Adolescents, a Glossary, and Resources for Further Help and Information

Edited by Dawn D. Matthews. 322 pages. 2001. 0-7808-0335-3. $78.

"Recommended for health science libraries that are open to the public, as well as hospital libraries. This book is a good resource for the consumer who is concerned about eating disorders." — *E-Streams, Mar '02*

"This volume is another convenient collection of excerpted articles. Recommended for school and public library patrons; lower-division undergraduates; and two-year technical program students." — *Choice, Association of College & Research Libraries, Jan '02*

"Recommended reference source." — *Booklist, American Library Association, Oct '01*

SEE ALSO *Diet & Nutrition Sourcebook, Digestive Diseases & Disorders Sourcebook, Gastrointestinal Diseases & Disorders Sourcebook*

◼

Emergency Medical Services Sourcebook

Basic Consumer Health Information about Preventing, Preparing for, and Managing Emergency Situations, When and Who to Call for Help, What to Expect in the Emergency Room, the Emergency Medical Team, Patient Issues, and Current Topics in Emergency Medicine

Along with Statistical Data, a Glossary, and Sources of Additional Help and Information

Edited by Jenni Lynn Colson. 494 pages. 2002. 0-7808-0420-1. $78.

"Handy and convenient for home, public, school, and college libraries. Recommended."
— *Choice, Association of College and Research Libraries, Apr '03*

"This reference can provide the consumer with answers to most questions about emergency care in the United States, or it will direct them to a resource where the answer can be found."
— *American Reference Books Annual, 2003*

"Recommended reference source."
— *Booklist, American Library Association, Feb '03*

▪

Endocrine & Metabolic Disorders Sourcebook

Basic Information for the Layperson about Pancreatic and Insulin-Related Disorders Such as Pancreatitis, Diabetes, and Hypoglycemia; Adrenal Gland Disorders Such as Cushing's Syndrome, Addison's Disease, and Congenital Adrenal Hyperplasia; Pituitary Gland Disorders Such as Growth Hormone Deficiency, Acromegaly, and Pituitary Tumors; Thyroid Disorders Such as Hypothyroidism, Graves' Disease, Hashimoto's Disease, and Goiter; Hyperparathyroidism; and Other Diseases and Syndromes of Hormone Imbalance or Metabolic Dysfunction

Along with Reports on Current Research Initiatives

Edited by Linda M. Shin. 574 pages. 1998. 0-7808-0207-1. $78.

"Omnigraphics has produced another needed resource for health information consumers."
— *American Reference Books Annual, 2000*

"Recommended reference source."
— *Booklist, American Library Association, Dec '98*

▪

Environmental Health Sourcebook, 2nd Edition

Basic Consumer Health Information about the Environment and Its Effect on Human Health, Including the Effects of Air Pollution, Water Pollution, Hazardous Chemicals, Food Hazards, Radiation Hazards, Biological Agents, Household Hazards, Such as Radon, Asbestos, Carbon Monoxide, and Mold, and Information about Associated Diseases and Disorders, Including Cancer, Allergies, Respiratory Problems, and Skin Disorders

Along with Information about Environmental Concerns for Specific Populations, a Glossary of Related Terms, and Resources for Further Help and Information

Edited by Dawn D. Matthews. 673 pages. 2003. 0-7808-0632-8. $78.

ALSO AVAILABLE: *Environmentally Induced Disorders Sourcebook, 1st Edition.* Edited by Allan R. Cook. 620 pages. 1997. 0-7808-0083-4. $78.

"This recently updated edition continues the level of quality and the reputation of the numerous other volumes in Omnigraphics' *Health Reference Series.*"
— *American Reference Books Annual, 2004*

"Recommended reference source."
— *Booklist, American Library Association, Sep '98*

"This book will be a useful addition to anyone's library." — *Choice Health Sciences Supplement, Association of College and Research Libraries, May '98*

". . . a good survey of numerous environmentally induced physical disorders . . . a useful addition to anyone's library."
— *Doody's Health Sciences Book Reviews, Jan '98*

". . . provide[s] introductory information from the best authorities around. Since this volume covers topics that potentially affect everyone, it will surely be one of the most frequently consulted volumes in the *Health Reference Series.*" — *Rettig on Reference, Nov '97*

▪

Environmentally Induced Disorders Sourcebook, 1st Edition

SEE Environmental Health Sourcebook, 2nd Edition

▪

Ethnic Diseases Sourcebook

Basic Consumer Health Information for Ethnic and Racial Minority Groups in the United States, Including General Health Indicators and Behaviors, Ethnic Diseases, Genetic Testing, the Impact of Chronic Diseases, Women's Health, Mental Health Issues, and Preventive Health Care Services

Along with a Glossary and a Listing of Additional Resources

Edited by Joyce Brennfleck Shannon. 664 pages. 2001. 0-7808-0336-1. $78.

"Recommended for health sciences libraries where public health programs are a priority."
— *E-Streams, Jan '02*

"Not many books have been written on this topic to date, and the *Ethnic Diseases Sourcebook* is a strong addition to the list. It will be an important introductory resource for health consumers, students, health care personnel, and social scientists. It is recommended for public, academic, and large hospital libraries."
— *American Reference Books Annual 2002*

"Recommended reference source."
— *Booklist, American Library Association, Oct '01*

"Will prove valuable to any library seeking to maintain a current, comprehensive reference collection of health resources. . . . An excellent source of health information about genetic disorders which affect particular ethnic and racial minorities in the U.S."
— *The Bookwatch, Aug '01*

Eye Care Sourcebook, 2nd Edition

Basic Consumer Health Information about Eye Care and Eye Disorders, Including Facts about the Diagnosis, Prevention, and Treatment of Common Refractive Problems Such as Myopia, Hyperopia, Astigmatism, and Presbyopia, and Eye Diseases, Including Glaucoma, Cataract, Age-Related Macular Degeneration, and Diabetic Retinopathy

Along with a Section on Vision Correction and Refractive Surgeries, Including LASIK and LASEK, a Glossary, and Directories of Resources for Additional Help and Information

Edited by Amy L. Sutton. 543 pages. 2003. 0-7808-0635-2. $78.

ALSO AVAILABLE: *Ophthalmic Disorders Sourcebook, 1st Edition.* Edited by Linda M. Ross. 631 pages. 1996. 0-7808-0081-8. $78.

"... a solid reference tool for eye care and a valuable addition to a collection."
— *American Reference Books Annual, 2004*

Family Planning Sourcebook

Basic Consumer Health Information about Planning for Pregnancy and Contraception, Including Traditional Methods, Barrier Methods, Hormonal Methods, Permanent Methods, Future Methods, Emergency Contraception, and Birth Control Choices for Women at Each Stage of Life

Along with Statistics, a Glossary, and Sources of Additional Information

Edited by Amy Marcaccio Keyzer. 520 pages. 2001. 0-7808-0379-5. $78.

"Recommended for public, health, and undergraduate libraries as part of the circulating collection."
— *E-Streams, Mar '02*

"Information is presented in an unbiased, readable manner, and the sourcebook will certainly be a necessary addition to those public and high school libraries where Internet access is restricted or otherwise problematic." — *American Reference Books Annual 2002*

"Recommended reference source."
— *Booklist, American Library Association, Oct '01*

"Will prove valuable to any library seeking to maintain a current, comprehensive reference collection of health resources. . . . Excellent reference."
— *The Bookwatch, Aug '01*

SEE ALSO *Pregnancy & Birth Sourcebook*

Fitness & Exercise Sourcebook, 2nd Edition

Basic Consumer Health Information about the Fundamentals of Fitness and Exercise, Including How to Begin and Maintain a Fitness Program, Fitness as a Lifestyle, the Link between Fitness and Diet, Advice for Specific Groups of People, Exercise as It Relates to

Specific Medical Conditions, and Recent Research in Fitness and Exercise

Along with a Glossary of Important Terms and Resources for Additional Help and Information

Edited by Kristen M. Gledhill. 646 pages. 2001. 0-7808-0334-5. $78.

ALSO AVAILABLE: *Fitness & Exercise Sourcebook, 1st Edition.* Edited by Dan R. Harris. 663 pages. 1996. 0-7808-0186-5. $78.

"This work is recommended for all general reference collections."
— *American Reference Books Annual 2002*

"Highly recommended for public, consumer, and school grades fourth through college."
— *E-Streams, Nov '01*

"Recommended reference source." — *Booklist, American Library Association, Oct '01*

"The information appears quite comprehensive and is considered reliable. . . . This second edition is a welcomed addition to the series."
— *Doody's Review Service, Sep '01*

"This reference is a valuable choice for those who desire a broad source of information on exercise, fitness, and chronic-disease prevention through a healthy lifestyle." — *American Medical Writers Association Journal, Fall '01*

"Will prove valuable to any library seeking to maintain a current, comprehensive reference collection of health resources. . . . Excellent reference."
— *The Bookwatch, Aug '01*

Food & Animal Borne Diseases Sourcebook

Basic Information about Diseases That Can Be Spread to Humans through the Ingestion of Contaminated Food or Water or by Contact with Infected Animals and Insects, Such as Botulism, E. Coli, Hepatitis A, Trichinosis, Lyme Disease, and Rabies

Along with Information Regarding Prevention and Treatment Methods, and Including a Special Section for International Travelers Describing Diseases Such as Cholera, Malaria, Travelers' Diarrhea, and Yellow Fever, and Offering Recommendations for Avoiding Illness

Edited by Karen Bellenir and Peter D. Dresser. 535 pages. 1995. 0-7808-0033-8. $78.

"Targeting general readers and providing them with a single, comprehensive source of information on selected topics, this book continues, with the excellent caliber of its predecessors, to catalog topical information on health matters of general interest. Readable and thorough, this valuable resource is highly recommended for all libraries."
— *Academic Library Book Review, Summer '96*

"A comprehensive collection of authoritative information." — *Emergency Medical Services, Oct '95*

Food Safety Sourcebook

Basic Consumer Health Information about the Safe Handling of Meat, Poultry, Seafood, Eggs, Fruit Juices, and Other Food Items, and Facts about Pesticides, Drinking Water, Food Safety Overseas, and the Onset, Duration, and Symptoms of Foodborne Illnesses, Including Types of Pathogenic Bacteria, Parasitic Protozoa, Worms, Viruses, and Natural Toxins

Along with the Role of the Consumer, the Food Handler, and the Government in Food Safety; a Glossary, and Resources for Additional Help and Information

Edited by Dawn D. Matthews. 339 pages. 1999. 0-7808-0326-4. $78.

"This book is recommended for public libraries and universities with home economic and food science programs." —*E-Streams, Nov '00*

"Recommended reference source."
—*Booklist, American Library Association, May '00*

"This book takes the complex issues of food safety and foodborne pathogens and presents them in an easily understood manner. [It does] an excellent job of covering a large and often confusing topic."
—*American Reference Books Annual, 2000*

Forensic Medicine Sourcebook

Basic Consumer Information for the Layperson about Forensic Medicine, Including Crime Scene Investigation, Evidence Collection and Analysis, Expert Testimony, Computer-Aided Criminal Identification, Digital Imaging in the Courtroom, DNA Profiling, Accident Reconstruction, Autopsies, Ballistics, Drugs and Explosives Detection, Latent Fingerprints, Product Tampering, and Questioned Document Examination

Along with Statistical Data, a Glossary of Forensics Terminology, and Listings of Sources for Further Help and Information

Edited by Annemarie S. Muth. 574 pages. 1999. 0-7808-0232-2. $78.

"Given the expected widespread interest in its content and its easy to read style, this book is recommended for most public and all college and university libraries."
—*E-Streams, Feb '01*

"Recommended for public libraries."
—*Reference & User Services Quarterly, American Library Association, Spring 2000*

"Recommended reference source."
—*Booklist, American Library Association, Feb '00*

"A wealth of information, useful statistics, references are up-to-date and extremely complete. This wonderful collection of data will help students who are interested in a career in any type of forensic field. It is a great resource for attorneys who need information about types of expert witnesses needed in a particular case. It also offers useful information for fiction and nonfiction writers whose work involves a crime. A fascinating compilation. All levels." —*Choice, Association of College and Research Libraries, Jan 2000*

"There are several items that make this book attractive to consumers who are seeking certain forensic data. . . . This is a useful current source for those seeking general forensic medical answers."
—*American Reference Books Annual, 2000*

Gastrointestinal Diseases & Disorders Sourcebook

Basic Information about Gastroesophageal Reflux Disease (Heartburn), Ulcers, Diverticulosis, Irritable Bowel Syndrome, Crohn's Disease, Ulcerative Colitis, Diarrhea, Constipation, Lactose Intolerance, Hemorrhoids, Hepatitis, Cirrhosis, and Other Digestive Problems, Featuring Statistics, Descriptions of Symptoms, and Current Treatment Methods of Interest for Persons Living with Upper and Lower Gastrointestinal Maladies

Edited by Linda M. Ross. 413 pages. 1996. 0-7808-0078-8. $78.

". . . very readable form. The successful editorial work that brought this material together into a useful and understandable reference makes accessible to all readers information that can help them more effectively understand and obtain help for digestive tract problems."
—*Choice, Association of College & Research Libraries, Feb '97*

SEE ALSO *Diet & Nutrition Sourcebook, Digestive Diseases & Disorders, Eating Disorders Sourcebook*

Genetic Disorders Sourcebook, 3rd Edition

Basic Consumer Health Information about Hereditary Diseases and Disorders, Including Facts about the Human Genome, Genetic Inheritance Patterns, Disorders Associated with Specific Genes, such as Sickle Cell Disease, Hemophilia, and Cystic Fibrosis, Chromosome Disorders, such as Down Syndrome, Fragile X Syndrome, and Turner Syndrome, and Complex Diseases and Disorders Resulting from the Interaction of Environmental and Genetic Factors, such as Allergies, Cancer, and Obesity

Along with Facts about Genetic Testing, Suggestions for Parents of Children with Special Needs, Reports on Current Research Initiatives, a Glossary of Genetic Terminology, and Resources for Additional Help and Information

Edited by Karen Bellenir. 777 pages. 2004. 0-7808-0742-1. $78.

ALSO AVAILABLE: *Genetic Disorders Sourcebook, 1st Edition.* Edited by Karen Bellenir. 642 pages. 1996. 0-7808-0034-6. $78.

Genetic Disorders Sourcebook, 2nd Edition. Edited by Kathy Massimini. 768 pages. 2001. 0-7808-0241-1. $78.

"Recommended for public libraries and medical and hospital libraries with consumer health collections."
—*E-Streams, May '01*

Head Trauma Sourcebook

Basic Information for the Layperson about Open-Head and Closed-Head Injuries, Treatment Advances, Recovery, and Rehabilitation

Along with Reports on Current Research Initiatives

Edited by Karen Bellenir. 414 pages. 1997. 0-7808-0208-X. $78.

Headache Sourcebook

Basic Consumer Health Information about Migraine, Tension, Cluster, Rebound and Other Types of Headaches, with Facts about the Cause and Prevention of Headaches, the Effects of Stress and the Environment, Headaches during Pregnancy and Menopause, and Childhood Headaches

Along with a Glossary and Other Resources for Additional Help and Information

Edited by Dawn D. Matthews. 362 pages. 2002. 0-7808-0337-X. $78.

Health Insurance Sourcebook

Basic Information about Managed Care Organizations, Traditional Fee-for-Service Insurance, Insurance Portability and Pre-Existing Conditions Clauses, Medicare, Medicaid, Social Security, and Military Health Care

Along with Information about Insurance Fraud

Edited by Wendy Wilcox. 530 pages. 1997. 0-7808-0222-5. $78.

Health Reference Series Cumulative Index 1999

A Comprehensive Index to the Individual Volumes of the Health Reference Series, Including a Subject Index, Name Index, Organization Index, and Publication Index

Along with a Master List of Acronyms and Abbreviations

Edited by Edward J. Prucha, Anne Holmes, and Robert Rudnick. 990 pages. 2000. 0-7808-0382-5. $78.

Healthy Aging Sourcebook

Basic Consumer Health Information about Maintaining Health through the Aging Process, Including Advice on Nutrition, Exercise, and Sleep, Help in Making Decisions about Midlife Issues and Retirement, and Guidance Concerning Practical and Informed Choices in Health Consumerism

Along with Data Concerning the Theories of Aging, Different Experiences in Aging by Minority Groups, and Facts about Aging Now and Aging in the Future; and Featuring a Glossary, a Guide to Consumer Help, Additional Suggested Reading, and Practical Resource Directory

Edited by Jenifer Swanson. 536 pages. 1999. 0-7808-0390-6. $78.

SEE ALSO Physical & Mental Issues in Aging Sourcebook

Healthy Children Sourcebook

Basic Consumer Health Information about the Physical and Mental Development of Children between the Ages of 3 and 12, Including Routine Health Care, Preventative Health Services, Safety and First Aid, Healthy Sleep, Dental Care, Nutrition, and Fitness, and Featuring Parenting Tips on Such Topics as Bedwetting, Choosing Day Care, Monitoring TV and Other Media, and Establishing a Foundation for Substance Abuse Prevention

Along with a Glossary of Commonly Used Pediatric Terms and Resources for Additional Help and Information.

Edited by Chad T. Kimball. 647 pages. 2003. 0-7808-0247-0. $78.

of timely information on health promotion and disease prevention for children aged 3 to 12."
— *American Reference Books Annual, 2004*

"The strengths of this book are many. It is clearly written, presented and structured."
— *Journal of the National Medical Association, 2004*

■

Healthy Heart Sourcebook for Women

Basic Consumer Health Information about Cardiac Issues Specific to Women, Including Facts about Major Risk Factors and Prevention, Treatment and Control Strategies, and Important Dietary Issues

Along with a Special Section Regarding the Pros and Cons of Hormone Replacement Therapy and Its Impact on Heart Health, and Additional Help, Including Recipes, a Glossary, and a Directory of Resources

Edited by Dawn D. Matthews. 336 pages. 2000. 0-7808-0329-9. $78.

"A good reference source and recommended for all public, academic, medical, and hospital libraries."
— *Medical Reference Services Quarterly, Summer '01*

"Because of the lack of information specific to women on this topic, this book is recommended for public libraries and consumer libraries."
— *American Reference Books Annual, 2001*

"Contains very important information about coronary artery disease that all women should know. The information is current and presented in an easy-to-read format. The book will make a good addition to any library." — *American Medical Writers Association Journal, Summer '00*

"Important, basic reference."
— *Reviewer's Bookwatch, Jul '00*

SEE ALSO *Heart Diseases & Disorders Sourcebook, Women's Health Concerns Sourcebook*

■

Heart Diseases & Disorders Sourcebook, 2nd Edition

Basic Consumer Health Information about Heart Attacks, Angina, Rhythm Disorders, Heart Failure, Valve Disease, Congenital Heart Disorders, and More, Including Descriptions of Surgical Procedures and Other Interventions, Medications, Cardiac Rehabilitation, Risk Identification, and Prevention Tips

Along with Statistical Data, Reports on Current Research Initiatives, a Glossary of Cardiovascular Terms, and Resource Directory

Edited by Karen Bellenir. 612 pages. 2000. 0-7808-0238-1. $78.

ALSO AVAILABLE: *Cardiovascular Diseases & Disorders Sourcebook, 1st Edition.* Edited by Karen Bellenir and Peter D. Dresser. 683 pages. 1995. 0-7808-0032-X. $78.

"This work stands out as an imminently accessible resource for the general public. It is recommended for the reference and circulating shelves of school, public, and academic libraries."
— *American Reference Books Annual, 2001*

"Recommended reference source."
— *Booklist, American Library Association, Dec '00*

"Provides comprehensive coverage of matters related to the heart. This title is recommended for health sciences and public libraries with consumer health collections."
— *E-Streams, Oct '00*

SEE ALSO *Healthy Heart Sourcebook for Women*

■

Household Safety Sourcebook

Basic Consumer Health Information about Household Safety, Including Information about Poisons, Chemicals, Fire, and Water Hazards in the Home

Along with Advice about the Safe Use of Home Maintenance Equipment, Choosing Toys and Nursery Furniture, Holiday and Recreation Safety, a Glossary, and Resources for Further Help and Information

Edited by Dawn D. Matthews. 606 pages. 2002. 0-7808-0338-8. $78.

"This work will be useful in public libraries with large consumer health and wellness departments."
— *American Reference Books Annual, 2003*

"As a sourcebook on household safety this book meets its mark. It is encyclopedic in scope and covers a wide range of safety issues that are commonly seen in the home." — *E-Streams, Jul '02*

■

Hypertension Sourcebook

Basic Consumer Health Information about the Causes, Diagnosis, and Treatment of High Blood Pressure, with Facts about Consequences, Complications, and Co-Occurring Disorders, Such as Coronary Heart Disease, Diabetes, Stroke, Kidney Disease, and Hypertensive Retinopathy, and Issues in Blood Pressure Control, Including Dietary Choices, Stress Management, and Medications

Along with Reports on Current Research Initiatives and Clinical Trials, a Glossary, and Resources for Additional Help and Information

Edited by Dawn D. Matthews and Karen Bellenir. 613 pages. 2004. 0-7808-0674-3. $78.

■

Immune System Disorders Sourcebook

Basic Information about Lupus, Multiple Sclerosis, Guillain-Barré Syndrome, Chronic Granulomatous Disease, and More

Along with Statistical and Demographic Data and Reports on Current Research Initiatives

Edited by Allan R. Cook. 608 pages. 1997. 0-7808-0209-8. $78.

Infant & Toddler Health Sourcebook

Basic Consumer Health Information about the Physical and Mental Development of Newborns, Infants, and Toddlers, Including Neonatal Concerns, Nutrition Recommendations, Immunization Schedules, Common Pediatric Disorders, Assessments and Milestones, Safety Tips, and Advice for Parents and Other Caregivers

Along with a Glossary of Terms and Resource Listings for Additional Help

Edited by Jenifer Swanson. 585 pages. 2000. 0-7808-0246-2. $78.

"As a reference for the general public, this would be useful in any library." —*E-Streams, May '01*

"Recommended reference source."
—*Booklist, American Library Association, Feb '01*

"This is a good source for general use."
—*American Reference Books Annual, 2001*

■

Infectious Diseases Sourcebook

Basic Consumer Health Information about Non-Contagious Bacterial, Viral, Prion, Fungal, and Parasitic Diseases Spread by Food and Water, Insects and Animals, or Environmental Contact, Including Botulism, E. Coli, Encephalitis, Legionnaires' Disease, Lyme Disease, Malaria, Plague, Rabies, Salmonella, Tetanus, and Others, and Facts about Newly Emerging Diseases, Such as Hantavirus, Mad Cow Disease, Monkeypox, and West Nile Virus

Along with Information about Preventing Disease Transmission, the Threat of Bioterrorism, and Current Research Initiatives, with a Glossary and Directory of Resources for More Information

Edited by Karen Bellenir. 634 pages. 2004. 0-7808-0675-1. $78.

■

Injury & Trauma Sourcebook

Basic Consumer Health Information about the Impact of Injury, the Diagnosis and Treatment of Common and Traumatic Injuries, Emergency Care, and Specific Injuries Related to Home, Community, Workplace, Transportation, and Recreation

Along with Guidelines for Injury Prevention, a Glossary, and a Directory of Additional Resources

Edited by Joyce Brennfleck Shannon. 696 pages. 2002. 0-7808-0421-X. $78.

"This publication is the most comprehensive work of its kind about injury and trauma."
—*American Reference Books Annual, 2003*

"This sourcebook provides concise, easily readable, basic health information about injuries. . . . This book is well organized and an easy to use reference resource suitable for hospital, health sciences and public libraries with consumer health collections."
—*E-Streams, Nov '02*

"Practitioners should be aware of guides such as this in order to facilitate their use by patients and their families."
—*Doody's Health Sciences Book Review Journal, Sep-Oct '02*

"Recommended reference source."
—*Booklist, American Library Association, Sep '02*

"Highly recommended for academic and medical reference collections." —*Library Bookwatch, Sep '02*

■

Kidney & Urinary Tract Diseases & Disorders Sourcebook

Basic Information about Kidney Stones, Urinary Incontinence, Bladder Disease, End Stage Renal Disease, Dialysis, and More

Along with Statistical and Demographic Data and Reports on Current Research Initiatives

Edited by Linda M. Ross. 602 pages. 1997. 0-7808-0079-6. $78.

■

Learning Disabilities Sourcebook, 2nd Edition

Basic Consumer Health Information about Learning Disabilities, Including Dyslexia, Developmental Speech and Language Disabilities, Non-Verbal Learning Disorders, Developmental Arithmetic Disorder, Developmental Writing Disorder, and Other Conditions That Impede Learning Such as Attention Deficit/ Hyperactivity Disorder, Brain Injury, Hearing Impairment, Klinefelter Syndrome, Dyspraxia, and Tourette Syndrome

Along with Facts about Educational Issues and Assistive Technology, Coping Strategies, a Glossary of Related Terms, and Resources for Further Help and Information

Edited by Dawn D. Matthews. 621 pages. 2003. 0-7808-0626-3. $78.

ALSO AVAILABLE: Learning Disabilities Sourcebook, 1st Edition. Edited by Linda M. Shin. 579 pages. 1998. 0-7808-0210-1. $78.

"The second edition of *Learning Disabilities Sourcebook* far surpasses the earlier edition in that it is more focused on information that will be useful as a consumer health resource."
—*American Reference Books Annual, 2004*

"Teachers as well as consumers will find this an essential guide to understanding various syndromes and their latest treatments. [An] invaluable reference for public and school library collections alike."
—*Library Bookwatch, Apr '03*

Named "Outstanding Reference Book of 1999."
—*New York Public Library, Feb 2000*

"An excellent candidate for inclusion in a public library reference section. It's a great source of information. Teachers will also find the book useful. Definitely worth reading."
—*Journal of Adolescent & Adult Literacy, Feb 2000*

"Readable . . . provides a solid base of information regarding successful techniques used with individuals who have learning disabilities, as well as practical suggestions for educators and family members. Clear language, concise descriptions, and pertinent information for contacting multiple resources add to the strength of this book as a useful tool." — *Choice, Association of College and Research Libraries, Feb '99*

"Recommended reference source."
— *Booklist, American Library Association, Sep '98*

"A useful resource for libraries and for those who don't have the time to identify and locate the individual publications." — *Disability Resources Monthly, Sep '98*

▪

Leukemia Sourcebook

Basic Consumer Health Information about Adult and Childhood Leukemias, Including Acute Lymphocytic Leukemia (ALL), Chronic Lymphocytic Leukemia (CLL), Acute Myelogenous Leukemia (AML), Chronic Myelogenous Leukemia (CML), and Hairy Cell Leukemia, and Treatments Such as Chemotherapy, Radiation Therapy, Peripheral Blood Stem Cell and Marrow Transplantation, and Immunotherapy

Along with Tips for Life During and After Treatment, a Glossary, and Directories of Additional Resources

Edited by Joyce Brennfleck Shannon. 587 pages. 2003. 0-7808-0627-1. $78.

"Unlike other medical books for the layperson, . . . the language does not talk down to the reader. . . . This volume is highly recommended for all libraries."
— *American Reference Books Annual, 2004*

▪

Liver Disorders Sourcebook

Basic Consumer Health Information about the Liver and How It Works; Liver Diseases, Including Cancer, Cirrhosis, Hepatitis, and Toxic and Drug Related Diseases; Tips for Maintaining a Healthy Liver; Laboratory Tests, Radiology Tests, and Facts about Liver Transplantation

Along with a Section on Support Groups, a Glossary, and Resource Listings

Edited by Joyce Brennfleck Shannon. 591 pages. 2000. 0-7808-0383-3. $78.

"A valuable resource."
— *American Reference Books Annual, 2001*

"This title is recommended for health sciences and public libraries with consumer health collections."
— *E-Streams, Oct '00*

"Recommended reference source."
— *Booklist, American Library Association, Jun '00*

▪

Lung Disorders Sourcebook

Basic Consumer Health Information about Emphysema, Pneumonia, Tuberculosis, Asthma, Cystic Fibrosis, and Other Lung Disorders, Including Facts about

Diagnostic Procedures, Treatment Strategies, Disease Prevention Efforts, and Such Risk Factors as Smoking, Air Pollution, and Exposure to Asbestos, Radon, and Other Agents

Along with a Glossary and Resources for Additional Help and Information

Edited by Dawn D. Matthews. 678 pages. 2002. 0-7808-0339-6. $78.

"This title is a great addition for public and school libraries because it provides concise health information on the lungs."
— *American Reference Books Annual, 2003*

"Highly recommended for academic and medical reference collections." — *Library Bookwatch, Sep '02*

▪

Medical Tests Sourcebook, 2nd Edition

Basic Consumer Health Information about Medical Tests, Including Age-Specific Health Tests, Important Health Screenings and Exams, Home-Use Tests, Blood and Specimen Tests, Electrical Tests, Scope Tests, Genetic Testing, and Imaging Tests, Such as X-Rays, Ultrasound, Computed Tomography, Magnetic Resonance Imaging, Angiography, and Nuclear Medicine

Along with a Glossary and Directory of Additional Resources

Edited by Joyce Brennfleck Shannon. 654 pages. 2004. 0-7808-0670-0. $78.

ALSO AVAILABLE: Medical Tests, 1st Edition. Edited by Joyce Brennfleck Shannon. 691 pages. 1999. 0-7808-0243-8. $78.

"Recommended for hospital and health sciences libraries with consumer health collections."
— *E-Streams, Mar '00*

"This is an overall excellent reference with a wealth of general knowledge that may aid those who are reluctant to get vital tests performed."
— *Today's Librarian, Jan 2000*

"A valuable reference guide."
— *American Reference Books Annual, 2000*

▪

Men's Health Concerns Sourcebook, 2nd Edition

Basic Consumer Health Information about the Medical and Mental Concerns of Men, Including Theories about the Shorter Male Lifespan, the Leading Causes of Death and Disability, Physical Concerns of Special Significance to Men, Reproductive and Sexual Concerns, Sexually Transmitted Diseases, Men's Mental and Emotional Health, and Lifestyle Choices That Affect Wellness, Such as Nutrition, Fitness, and Substance Use

Along with a Glossary of Related Terms and a Directory of Organizational Resources in Men's Health

Edited by Robert Aquinas McNally. 644 pages. 2004. 0-7808-0671-9. $78.

Mental Health Disorders Sourcebook, 2nd Edition

Basic Consumer Health Information about Anxiety Disorders, Depression and Other Mood Disorders, Eating Disorders, Personality Disorders, Schizophrenia, and More, Including Disease Descriptions, Treatment Options, and Reports on Current Research Initiatives

Along with Statistical Data, Tips for Maintaining Mental Health, a Glossary, and Directory of Sources for Additional Help and Information

Edited by Karen Bellenir. 605 pages. 2000. 0-7808-0240-3. $78.

ALSO AVAILABLE: *Mental Health Disorders Sourcebook, 1st Edition.* Edited by Karen Bellenir. 548 pages. 1995. 0-7808-0040-0. $78.

"Well organized and well written."
—*American Reference Books Annual, 2001*

"Recommended reference source."
—*Booklist, American Library Association, Jun '00*

Mental Retardation Sourcebook

Basic Consumer Health Information about Mental Retardation and Its Causes, Including Down Syndrome, Fetal Alcohol Syndrome, Fragile X Syndrome, Genetic Conditions, Injury, and Environmental Sources

Along with Preventive Strategies, Parenting Issues, Educational Implications, Health Care Needs, Employment and Economic Matters, Legal Issues, a Glossary, and a Resource Listing for Additional Help and Information

Edited by Joyce Brennfleck Shannon. 642 pages. 2000. 0-7808-0377-9. $78.

"Public libraries will find the book useful for reference and as a beginning research point for students, parents, and caregivers."
—*American Reference Books Annual, 2001*

"The strength of this work is that it compiles many basic fact sheets and addresses for further information in one volume. It is intended and suitable for the general public. This sourcebook is relevant to any collection providing health information to the general public."
— *E-Streams, Nov '00*

"From preventing retardation to parenting and family challenges, this covers health, social and legal issues and will prove an invaluable overview."
— *Reviewer's Bookwatch, Jul '00*

Movement Disorders Sourcebook

Basic Consumer Health Information about Neurological Movement Disorders, Including Essential Tremor, Parkinson's Disease, Dystonia, Cerebral Palsy, Huntington's Disease, Myasthenia Gravis, Multiple Sclerosis, and Other Early-Onset and Adult-Onset Movement Disorders, Their Symptoms and Causes, Diagnostic Tests, and Treatments

Along with Mobility and Assistive Technology Information, a Glossary, and a Directory of Additional Resources

Edited by Joyce Brennfleck Shannon. 655 pages. 2003. 0-7808-0628-X. $78.

". . . a good resource for consumers and recommended for public, community college and undergraduate libraries."
— *American Reference Books Annual, 2004*

Muscular Dystrophy Sourcebook

Basic Consumer Health Information about Congenital, Childhood-Onset, and Adult-Onset Forms of Muscular Dystrophy, Such as Duchenne, Becker, Emery-Dreifuss, Distal, Limb-Girdle, Facioscapulohumeral (FSHD), Myotonic, and Ophthalmoplegic Muscular Dystrophies, Including Facts about Diagnostic Tests, Medical and Physical Therapies, Management of Co-Occurring Conditions, and Parenting Guidelines

Along with Practical Tips for Home Care, a Glossary, and Directories of Additional Resources

Edited by Joyce Brennfleck Shannon. 577 pages. 2004. 0-7808-0676-X. $78.

Obesity Sourcebook

Basic Consumer Health Information about Diseases and Other Problems Associated with Obesity, and Including Facts about Risk Factors, Prevention Issues, and Management Approaches

Along with Statistical and Demographic Data, Information about Special Populations, Research Updates, a Glossary, and Source Listings for Further Help and Information

Edited by Wilma Caldwell and Chad T. Kimball. 376 pages. 2001. 0-7808-0333-7. $78.

"The book synthesizes the reliable medical literature on obesity into one easy-to-read and useful resource for the general public."
— *American Reference Books Annual 2002*

"This is a very useful resource book for the lay public."
—*Doody's Review Service, Nov '01*

"Well suited for the health reference collection of a public library or an academic health science library that serves the general population."   —*E-Streams, Sep '01*

"Recommended reference source."
—*Booklist, American Library Association, Apr '01*

" Recommended pick both for specialty health library collections and any general consumer health reference collection."   — *The Bookwatch, Apr '01*

Ophthalmic Disorders Sourcebook, 1st Edition

SEE *Eye Care Sourcebook, 2nd Edition*

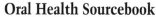

Oral Health Sourcebook

SEE *Dental Care & Oral Health Sourcebook, 2nd Ed.*

Osteoporosis Sourcebook

Basic Consumer Health Information about Primary and Secondary Osteoporosis and Juvenile Osteoporosis and Related Conditions, Including Fibrous Dysplasia, Gaucher Disease, Hyperthyroidism, Hypophosphatasia, Myeloma, Osteopetrosis, Osteogenesis Imperfecta, and Paget's Disease

Along with Information about Risk Factors, Treatments, Traditional and Non-Traditional Pain Management, a Glossary of Related Terms, and a Directory of Resources

Edited by Allan R. Cook. 584 pages. 2001. 0-7808-0239-X. $78.

"This would be a book to be kept in a staff or patient library. The targeted audience is the layperson, but the therapist who needs a quick bit of information on a particular topic will also find the book useful."
— *Physical Therapy, Jan '02*

"This resource is recommended as a great reference source for public, health, and academic libraries, and is another triumph for the editors of Omnigraphics."
— *American Reference Books Annual 2002*

"Recommended for all public libraries and general health collections, especially those supporting patient education or consumer health programs."
— *E-Streams, Nov '01*

"Will prove valuable to any library seeking to maintain a current, comprehensive reference collection of health resources. . . . From prevention to treatment and associated conditions, this provides an excellent survey."
— *The Bookwatch, Aug '01*

"Recommended reference source."
— *Booklist, American Library Association, July '01*

SEE ALSO *Women's Health Concerns Sourcebook*

Pain Sourcebook, 2nd Edition

Basic Consumer Health Information about Specific Forms of Acute and Chronic Pain, Including Muscle and Skeletal Pain, Nerve Pain, Cancer Pain, and Disorders Characterized by Pain, Such as Fibromyalgia, Shingles, Angina, Arthritis, and Headaches

Along with Information about Pain Medications and Management Techniques, Complementary and Alternative Pain Relief Options, Tips for People Living with Chronic Pain, a Glossary, and a Directory of Sources for Further Information

Edited by Karen Bellenir. 670 pages. 2002. 0-7808-0612-3. $78.

ALSO AVAILABLE: *Pain Sourcebook, 1st Edition.* Edited by Allan R. Cook. 667 pages. 1997. 0-7808-0213-6. $78.

"A source of valuable information. . . . This book offers help to nonmedical people who need information about pain and pain management. It is also an excellent reference for those who participate in patient education."
— *Doody's Review Service, Sep '02*

"The text is readable, easily understood, and well indexed. This excellent volume belongs in all patient education libraries, consumer health sections of public libraries, and many personal collections."
— *American Reference Books Annual, 1999*

"A beneficial reference." — *Booklist Health Sciences Supplement, American Library Association, Oct '98*

"The information is basic in terms of scholarship and is appropriate for general readers. Written in journalistic style . . . intended for non-professionals. Quite thorough in its coverage of different pain conditions and summarizes the latest clinical information regarding pain treatment." — *Choice, Association of College and Research Libraries, Jun '98*

"Recommended reference source."
— *Booklist, American Library Association, Mar '98*

Pediatric Cancer Sourcebook

Basic Consumer Health Information about Leukemias, Brain Tumors, Sarcomas, Lymphomas, and Other Cancers in Infants, Children, and Adolescents, Including Descriptions of Cancers, Treatments, and Coping Strategies

Along with Suggestions for Parents, Caregivers, and Concerned Relatives, a Glossary of Cancer Terms, and Resource Listings

Edited by Edward J. Prucha. 587 pages. 1999. 0-7808-0245-4. $78.

"An excellent source of information. Recommended for public, hospital, and health science libraries with consumer health collections." — *E-Streams, Jun '00*

"Recommended reference source."
— *Booklist, American Library Association, Feb '00*

"A valuable addition to all libraries specializing in health services and many public libraries."
— *American Reference Books Annual, 2000*

Physical & Mental Issues in Aging Sourcebook

Basic Consumer Health Information on Physical and Mental Disorders Associated with the Aging Process, Including Concerns about Cardiovascular Disease, Pulmonary Disease, Oral Health, Digestive Disorders, Musculoskeletal and Skin Disorders, Metabolic Changes, Sexual and Reproductive Issues, and Changes in Vision, Hearing, and Other Senses

Along with Data about Longevity and Causes of Death, Information on Acute and Chronic Pain, Descriptions of Mental Concerns, a Glossary of Terms, and Resource Listings for Additional Help

Edited by Jenifer Swanson. 660 pages. 1999. 0-7808-0233-0. $78.

"This is a treasure of health information for the layperson." — *Choice Health Sciences Supplement, Association of College & Research Libraries, May 2000*

"Recommended for public libraries."
—*American Reference Books Annual, 2000*

"Recommended reference source."
— *Booklist, American Library Association, Oct '99*

SEE ALSO *Healthy Aging Sourcebook*

◼

Podiatry Sourcebook

Basic Consumer Health Information about Foot Conditions, Diseases, and Injuries, Including Bunions, Corns, Calluses, Athlete's Foot, Plantar Warts, Hammertoes and Clawtoes, Clubfoot, Heel Pain, Gout, and More

Along with Facts about Foot Care, Disease Prevention, Foot Safety, Choosing a Foot Care Specialist, a Glossary of Terms, and Resource Listings for Additional Information

Edited by M. Lisa Weatherford. 380 pages. 2001. 0-7808-0215-2. $78.

"Recommended reference source."
— *Booklist, American Library Association, Feb '02*

"There is a lot of information presented here on a topic that is usually only covered sparingly in most larger comprehensive medical encyclopedias."
— *American Reference Books Annual 2002*

◼

Pregnancy & Birth Sourcebook, 2nd Edition

Basic Consumer Health Information about Conception and Pregnancy, Including Facts about Fertility, Infertility, Pregnancy Symptoms and Complications, Fetal Growth and Development, Labor, Delivery, and the Postpartum Period, as Well as Information about Maintaining Health and Wellness during Pregnancy and Caring for a Newborn

Along with Information about Public Health Assistance for Low-Income Pregnant Women, a Glossary, and Directories of Agencies and Organizations Providing Help and Support

Edited by Amy L. Sutton. 626 pages. 2004. 0-7808-0672-7. $78.

ALSO AVAILABLE: *Pregnancy & Birth Sourcebook, 1st Edition.* Edited by Heather E. Aldred. 737 pages. 1997. 0-7808-0216-0. $78.

"A well-organized handbook. Recommended."
— *Choice, Association of College and Research Libraries, Apr '98*

"Recommended reference source."
— *Booklist, American Library Association, Mar '98*

"Recommended for public libraries."
— *American Reference Books Annual, 1998*

SEE ALSO *Congenital Disorders Sourcebook, Family Planning Sourcebook*

◼

Prostate Cancer Sourcebook

Basic Consumer Health Information about Prostate Cancer, Including Information about the Associated Risk Factors, Detection, Diagnosis, and Treatment of Prostate Cancer

Along with Information on Non-Malignant Prostate Conditions, and Featuring a Section Listing Support and Treatment Centers and a Glossary of Related Terms

Edited by Dawn D. Matthews. 358 pages. 2001. 0-7808-0324-8. $78.

"Recommended reference source."
— *Booklist, American Library Association, Jan '02*

"A valuable resource for health care consumers seeking information on the subject. . . .All text is written in a clear, easy-to-understand language that avoids technical jargon. Any library that collects consumer health resources would strengthen their collection with the addition of the *Prostate Cancer Sourcebook.*"
— *American Reference Books Annual 2002*

◼

Public Health Sourcebook

Basic Information about Government Health Agencies, Including National Health Statistics and Trends, Healthy People 2000 Program Goals and Objectives, the Centers for Disease Control and Prevention, the Food and Drug Administration, and the National Institutes of Health

Along with Full Contact Information for Each Agency

Edited by Wendy Wilcox. 698 pages. 1998. 0-7808-0220-9. $78.

"Recommended reference source."
— *Booklist, American Library Association, Sep '98*

"This consumer guide provides welcome assistance in navigating the maze of federal health agencies and their data on public health concerns."
— *SciTech Book News, Sep '98*

◼

Reconstructive & Cosmetic Surgery Sourcebook

Basic Consumer Health Information on Cosmetic and Reconstructive Plastic Surgery, Including Statistical Information about Different Surgical Procedures, Things to Consider Prior to Surgery, Plastic Surgery Techniques and Tools, Emotional and Psychological Considerations, and Procedure-Specific Information

Along with a Glossary of Terms and a Listing of Resources for Additional Help and Information

Edited by M. Lisa Weatherford. 374 pages. 2001. 0-7808-0214-4. $78.

"An excellent reference that addresses cosmetic and medically necessary reconstructive surgeries. . . . The

style of the prose is calm and reassuring, discussing the many positive outcomes now available due to advances in surgical techniques."
— *American Reference Books Annual 2002*

"Recommended for health science libraries that are open to the public, as well as hospital libraries that are open to the patients. This book is a good resource for the consumer interested in plastic surgery."
— *E-Streams, Dec '01*

"Recommended reference source."
— *Booklist, American Library Association, July '01*

■

Rehabilitation Sourcebook

Basic Consumer Health Information about Rehabilitation for People Recovering from Heart Surgery, Spinal Cord Injury, Stroke, Orthopedic Impairments, Amputation, Pulmonary Impairments, Traumatic Injury, and More, Including Physical Therapy, Occupational Therapy, Speech/ Language Therapy, Massage Therapy, Dance Therapy, Art Therapy, and Recreational Therapy

Along with Information on Assistive and Adaptive Devices, a Glossary, and Resources for Additional Help and Information

Edited by Dawn D. Matthews. 531 pages. 1999. 0-7808-0236-5. $78.

"This is an excellent resource for public library reference and health collections."
— *American Reference Books Annual, 2001*

"Recommended reference source."
— *Booklist, American Library Association, May '00*

■

Respiratory Diseases & Disorders Sourcebook

Basic Information about Respiratory Diseases and Disorders, Including Asthma, Cystic Fibrosis, Pneumonia, the Common Cold, Influenza, and Others, Featuring Facts about the Respiratory System, Statistical and Demographic Data, Treatments, Self-Help Management Suggestions, and Current Research Initiatives

Edited by Allan R. Cook and Peter D. Dresser. 771 pages. 1995. 0-7808-0037-0. $78.

"Designed for the layperson and for patients and their families coping with respiratory illness. . . . an extensive array of information on diagnosis, treatment, management, and prevention of respiratory illnesses for the general reader." — *Choice, Association of College and Research Libraries, Jun '96*

"A highly recommended text for all collections. It is a comforting reminder of the power of knowledge that good books carry between their covers."
— *Academic Library Book Review, Spring '96*

"A comprehensive collection of authoritative information presented in a nontechnical, humanitarian style for patients, families, and caregivers." — *Association of Operating Room Nurses, Sep/Oct '95*

SEE ALSO Lung Disorders Sourcebook

Sexually Transmitted Diseases Sourcebook, 2nd Edition

Basic Consumer Health Information about Sexually Transmitted Diseases, Including Information on the Diagnosis and Treatment of Chlamydia, Gonorrhea, Hepatitis, Herpes, HIV, Mononucleosis, Syphilis, and Others

Along with Information on Prevention, Such as Condom Use, Vaccines, and STD Education; And Featuring a Section on Issues Related to Youth and Adolescents, a Glossary, and Resources for Additional Help and Information

Edited by Dawn D. Matthews. 538 pages. 2001. 0-7808-0249-7. $78.

ALSO AVAILABLE: Sexually Transmitted Diseases Sourcebook, 1st Edition. Edited by Linda M. Ross. 550 pages. 1997. 0-7808-0217-9. $78.

"Recommended for consumer health collections in public libraries, and secondary school and community college libraries."
— *American Reference Books Annual 2002*

"Every school and public library should have a copy of this comprehensive and user-friendly reference book."
— *Choice, Association of College & Research Libraries, Sep '01*

"This is a highly recommended book. This is an especially important book for all school and public libraries." — *AIDS Book Review Journal, Jul-Aug '01*

"Recommended reference source."
— *Booklist, American Library Association, Apr '01*

"Recommended pick both for specialty health library collections and any general consumer health reference collection." — *The Bookwatch, Apr '01*

■

Skin Disorders Sourcebook

Basic Information about Common Skin and Scalp Conditions Caused by Aging, Allergies, Immune Reactions, Sun Exposure, Infectious Organisms, Parasites, Cosmetics, and Skin Traumas, Including Abrasions, Cuts, and Pressure Sores

Along with Information on Prevention and Treatment

Edited by Allan R. Cook. 647 pages. 1997. 0-7808-0080-X. $78.

". . . comprehensive, easily read reference book."
— *Doody's Health Sciences Book Reviews, Oct '97*

SEE ALSO Burns Sourcebook

■

Sleep Disorders Sourcebook

Basic Consumer Health Information about Sleep and Its Disorders, Including Insomnia, Sleepwalking, Sleep Apnea, Restless Leg Syndrome, and Narcolepsy

Along with Data about Shiftwork and Its Effects, Information on the Societal Costs of Sleep Deprivation, Descriptions of Treatment Options, a Glossary of Terms, and Resource Listings for Additional Help

Edited by Jenifer Swanson. 439 pages. 1998. 0-7808-0234-9. $78.

"This text will complement any home or medical library. It is user-friendly and ideal for the adult reader."
— *American Reference Books Annual, 2000*

"A useful resource that provides accurate, relevant, and accessible information on sleep to the general public. Health care providers who deal with sleep disorders patients may also find it helpful in being prepared to answer some of the questions patients ask."
— *Respiratory Care, Jul '99*

"Recommended reference source."
— *Booklist, American Library Association, Feb '99*

Smoking Concerns Sourcebook

Basic Consumer Health Information about Nicotine Addiction and Smoking Cessation, Featuring Facts about the Health Effects of Tobacco Use, Including Lung and Other Cancers, Heart Disease, Stroke, and Respiratory Disorders, Such as Emphysema and Chronic Bronchitis

Along with Information about Smoking Prevention Programs, Suggestions for Achieving and Maintaining a Smoke-Free Lifestyle, Statistics about Tobacco Use, Reports on Current Research Initiatives, a Glossary of Related Terms, and Directories of Resources for Additional Help and Information

Edited by Karen Bellenir. 625 pages. 2004. 0-7808-0323-X. $78.

Sports Injuries Sourcebook, 2nd Edition

Basic Consumer Health Information about the Diagnosis, Treatment, and Rehabilitation of Common Sports-Related Injuries in Children and Adults

Along with Suggestions for Conditioning and Training, Information and Prevention Tips for Injuries Frequently Associated with Specific Sports and Special Populations, a Glossary, and a Directory of Additional Resources

Edited by Joyce Brennfleck Shannon. 614 pages. 2002. 0-7808-0604-2. $78.

ALSO AVAILABLE: *Sports Injuries Sourcebook, 1st Edition.* Edited by Heather E. Aldred. 624 pages. 1999. 0-7808-0218-7. $78.

"This is an excellent reference for consumers and it is recommended for public, community college, and undergraduate libraries."
— *American Reference Books Annual, 2003*

"Recommended reference source."
— *Booklist, American Library Association, Feb '03*

Stress-Related Disorders Sourcebook

Basic Consumer Health Information about Stress and Stress-Related Disorders, Including Stress Origins and Signals, Environmental Stress at Work and Home, Mental and Emotional Stress Associated with Depression, Post-Traumatic Stress Disorder, Panic Disorder, Suicide, and the Physical Effects of Stress on the Cardiovascular, Immune, and Nervous Systems

Along with Stress Management Techniques, a Glossary, and a Listing of Additional Resources

Edited by Joyce Brennfleck Shannon. 610 pages. 2002. 0-7808-0560-7. $78.

"Well written for a general readership, the *Stress-Related Disorders Sourcebook* is a useful addition to the health reference literature."
— *American Reference Books Annual, 2003*

"I am impressed by the amount of information. It offers a thorough overview of the causes and consequences of stress for the layperson. . . . A well-done and thorough reference guide for professionals and nonprofessionals alike."
— *Doody's Review Service, Dec '02*

Stroke Sourcebook

Basic Consumer Health Information about Stroke, Including Ischemic, Hemorrhagic, Transient Ischemic Attack (TIA), and Pediatric Stroke, Stroke Triggers and Risks, Diagnostic Tests, Treatments, and Rehabilitation Information

Along with Stroke Prevention Guidelines, Legal and Financial Information, a Glossary, and a Directory of Additional Resources

Edited by Joyce Brennfleck Shannon. 606 pages. 2003. 0-7808-0630-1. $78.

"This volume is highly recommended and should be in every medical, hospital, and public library."
— *American Reference Books Annual, 2004*

Substance Abuse Sourcebook

Basic Health-Related Information about the Abuse of Legal and Illegal Substances Such as Alcohol, Tobacco, Prescription Drugs, Marijuana, Cocaine, and Heroin; and Including Facts about Substance Abuse Prevention Strategies, Intervention Methods, Treatment and Recovery Programs, and a Section Addressing the Special Problems Related to Substance Abuse during Pregnancy

Edited by Karen Bellenir. 573 pages. 1996. 0-7808-0038-9. $78.

"A valuable addition to any health reference section. Highly recommended."
— *The Book Report, Mar/Apr '97*

". . . a comprehensive collection of substance abuse information that's both highly readable and compact. Families and caregivers of substance abusers will find

the information enlightening and helpful, while teachers, social workers and journalists should benefit from the concise format. **Recommended.**"
— *Drug Abuse Update, Winter '96/'97*

SEE ALSO *Alcoholism Sourcebook, Drug Abuse Sourcebook*

■

Surgery Sourcebook

Basic Consumer Health Information about Inpatient and Outpatient Surgeries, Including Cardiac, Vascular, Orthopedic, Ocular, Reconstructive, Cosmetic, Gynecologic, and Ear, Nose, and Throat Procedures and More

Along with Information about Operating Room Policies and Instruments, Laser Surgery Techniques, Hospital Errors, Statistical Data, a Glossary, and Listings of Sources for Further Help and Information

Edited by Annemarie S. Muth and Karen Bellenir. 596 pages. 2002. 0-7808-0380-9. $78.

"Large public libraries and medical libraries would benefit from this material in their reference collections."
— *American Reference Books Annual, 2004*

"Invaluable reference for public and school library collections alike." — *Library Bookwatch, Apr '03*

■

Transplantation Sourcebook

Basic Consumer Health Information about Organ and Tissue Transplantation, Including Physical and Financial Preparations, Procedures and Issues Relating to Specific Solid Organ and Tissue Transplants, Rehabilitation, Pediatric Transplant Information, the Future of Transplantation, and Organ and Tissue Donation

Along with a Glossary and Listings of Additional Resources

Edited by Joyce Brennfleck Shannon. 628 pages. 2002. 0-7808-0322-1. $78.

"Along with these advances [in transplantation technology] have come a number of daunting questions for potential transplant patients, their families, and their health care providers. This reference text is the best single tool to address many of these questions. . . . It will be a much-needed addition to the reference collections in health care, academic, and large public libraries."
— *American Reference Books Annual, 2003*

"Recommended for libraries with an interest in offering consumer health information." — *E-Streams, Jul '02*

"This is a unique and valuable resource for patients facing transplantation and their families."
— *Doody's Review Service, Jun '02*

■

Traveler's Health Sourcebook

Basic Consumer Health Information for Travelers, Including Physical and Medical Preparations, Transportation Health and Safety, Essential Information about Food and Water, Sun Exposure, Insect and Snake Bites, Camping and Wilderness Medicine, and Travel with Physical or Medical Disabilities

Along with International Travel Tips, Vaccination Recommendations, Geographical Health Issues, Disease Risks, a Glossary, and a Listing of Additional Resources

Edited by Joyce Brennfleck Shannon. 613 pages. 2000. 0-7808-0384-1. $78.

"Recommended reference source."
— *Booklist, American Library Association, Feb '01*

"This book is recommended for any public library, any travel collection, and especially any collection for the physically disabled."
— *American Reference Books Annual, 2001*

■

Vegetarian Sourcebook

Basic Consumer Health Information about Vegetarian Diets, Lifestyle, and Philosophy, Including Definitions of Vegetarianism and Veganism, Tips about Adopting Vegetarianism, Creating a Vegetarian Pantry, and Meeting Nutritional Needs of Vegetarians, with Facts Regarding Vegetarianism's Effect on Pregnant and Lactating Women, Children, Athletes, and Senior Citizens

Along with a Glossary of Commonly Used Vegetarian Terms and Resources for Additional Help and Information

Edited by Chad T. Kimball. 360 pages. 2002. 0-7808-0439-2. $78.

"Organizes into one concise volume the answers to the most common questions concerning vegetarian diets and lifestyles. This title is recommended for public and secondary school libraries." — *E-Streams, Apr '03*

"Invaluable reference for public and school library collections alike." — *Library Bookwatch, Apr '03*

"The articles in this volume are easy to read and come from authoritative sources. The book does not necessarily support the vegetarian diet but instead provides the pros and cons of this important decision. The *Vegetarian Sourcebook* is recommended for public libraries and consumer health libraries."
— *American Reference Books Annual, 2003*

■

Women's Health Concerns Sourcebook, 2nd Edition

Basic Consumer Health Information about the Medical and Mental Concerns of Women, Including Maintaining Health and Wellness, Gynecological Concerns, Breast Health, Sexuality and Reproductive Issues, Menopause, Cancer in Women, the Leading Causes of Death and Disability among Women, Physical Concerns of Special Significance to Women, and Women's Mental and Emotional Health

Along with a Glossary of Related Terms and Directories of Resources for Additional Help and Information

Edited by Amy L. Sutton. 748 pages. 2004. 0-7808-0673-5. $78.

ALSO AVAILABLE: *Women's Health Concerns Sourcebook, 1st Edition.* Edited by Heather E. Aldred. 567 pages. 1997. 0-7808-0219-5. $78.

"Handy compilation. There is an impressive range of diseases, devices, disorders, procedures, and other physical and emotional issues covered . . . well organized, illustrated, and indexed." —*Choice,*
Association of College and Research Libraries, Jan '98

SEE ALSO *Breast Cancer Sourcebook, Cancer Sourcebook for Women, Healthy Heart Sourcebook for Women, Osteoporosis Sourcebook*

Workplace Health & Safety Sourcebook

Basic Consumer Health Information about Workplace Health and Safety, Including the Effect of Workplace Hazards on the Lungs, Skin, Heart, Ears, Eyes, Brain, Reproductive Organs, Musculoskeletal System, and Other Organs and Body Parts

Along with Information about Occupational Cancer, Personal Protective Equipment, Toxic and Hazardous Chemicals, Child Labor, Stress, and Workplace Violence

Edited by Chad T. Kimball. 626 pages. 2000. 0-7808-0231-4. $78.

"As a reference for the general public, this would be useful in any library." —*E-Streams, Jun '01*

"Provides helpful information for primary care physicians and other caregivers interested in occupational medicine. . . . General readers; professionals."
— *Choice, Association of College & Research Libraries, May '01*

"Recommended reference source."
— *Booklist, American Library Association, Feb '01*

"Highly recommended." — *The Bookwatch, Jan '01*

Worldwide Health Sourcebook

Basic Information about Global Health Issues, Including Malnutrition, Reproductive Health, Disease Dispersion and Prevention, Emerging Diseases, Risky Health Behaviors, and the Leading Causes of Death

Along with Global Health Concerns for Children, Women, and the Elderly, Mental Health Issues, Research and Technology Advancements, and Economic, Environmental, and Political Health Implications, a Glossary, and a Resource Listing for Additional Help and Information

Edited by Joyce Brennfleck Shannon. 614 pages. 2001. 0-7808-0330-2. $78.

"Named an Outstanding Academic Title."
— *Choice, Association of College & Research Libraries, Jan '02*

"Yet another handy but also unique compilation in the extensive Health Reference Series, this is a useful work because many of the international publications reprinted or excerpted are not readily available. Highly recommended." —*Choice, Association of College & Research Libraries, Nov '01*

"Recommended reference source."
— *Booklist, American Library Association, Oct '01*

593

Teen Health Series

Helping Young Adults Understand, Manage, and Avoid Serious Illness

Cancer Information for Teens

Health Tips about Cancer Awareness, Prevention, Diagnosis, and Treatment

Including Facts about Frequently Occurring Cancers, Cancer Risk Factors, and Coping Strategies for Teens Fighting Cancer or Dealing with Cancer in Friends or Family Members

Edited by Wilma R. Caldwell. 428 pages. 2004. 0-7808-0678-6. $58.

■

Diet Information for Teens

Health Tips about Diet and Nutrition

Including Facts about Nutrients, Dietary Guidelines, Breakfasts, School Lunches, Snacks, Party Food, Weight Control, Eating Disorders, and More

Edited by Karen Bellenir. 399 pages. 2001. 0-7808-0441-4. $58.

"Full of helpful insights and facts throughout the book. ... An excellent resource to be placed in public libraries or even in personal collections."
—*American Reference Books Annual 2002*

"Recommended for middle and high school libraries and media centers as well as academic libraries that educate future teachers of teenagers. It is also a suitable addition to health science libraries that serve patrons who are interested in teen health promotion and education."
— *E-Streams, Oct '01*

"This comprehensive book would be beneficial to collections that need information about nutrition, dietary guidelines, meal planning, and weight control. ... This reference is so easy to use that its purchase is recommended."
— *The Book Report, Sep-Oct '01*

"This book is written in an easy to understand format describing issues that many teens face every day, and then provides thoughtful explanations so that teens can make informed decisions. This is an interesting book that provides important facts and information for today's teens."
—*Doody's Health Sciences Book Review Journal, Jul-Aug '01*

"A comprehensive compendium of diet and nutrition. The information is presented in a straightforward, plain-spoken manner. This title will be useful to those working on reports on a variety of topics, as well as to general readers concerned about their dietary health."
— *School Library Journal, Jun '01*

Drug Information for Teens

Health Tips about the Physical and Mental Effects of Substance Abuse

Including Facts about Alcohol, Anabolic Steroids, Club Drugs, Cocaine, Depressants, Hallucinogens, Herbal Products, Inhalants, Marijuana, Narcotics, Stimulants, Tobacco, and More

Edited by Karen Bellenir. 452 pages. 2002. 0-7808-0444-9. $58.

"A clearly written resource for general readers and researchers alike." — *School Library Journal*

"The chapters are quick to make a connection to their teenage reading audience. The prose is straightforward and the book lends itself to spot reading. It should be useful both for practical information and for research, and it is suitable for public and school libraries."
— *American Reference Books Annual, 2003*

"Recommended reference source."
— *Booklist, American Library Association, Feb '03*

"This is an excellent resource for teens and their parents. Education about drugs and substances is key to discouraging teen drug abuse and this book provides this much needed information in a way that is interesting and factual." —*Doody's Review Service, Dec '02*

■

Fitness Information for Teens

Health Tips about Exercise, Physical Well-Being, and Health Maintenance

Including Facts about Aerobic and Anaerobic Conditioning, Stretching, Body Shape and Body Image, Sports Training, Nutrition, and Activities for Non-Athletes

Edited by Karen Bellenir. 425 pages. 2004. 0-7808-0679-4. $58.

■

Mental Health Information for Teens

Health Tips about Mental Health and Mental Illness

Including Facts about Anxiety, Depression, Suicide, Eating Disorders, Obsessive-Compulsive Disorders, Panic Attacks, Phobias, Schizophrenia, and More

Edited by Karen Bellenir. 406 pages. 2001. 0-7808-0442-2. $58.

"In both language and approach, this user-friendly entry in the *Teen Health Series* is on target for teens needing information on mental health concerns." — *Booklist, American Library Association, Jan '02*

"Readers will find the material accessible and informative, with the shaded notes, facts, and embedded glossary insets adding appropriately to the already interesting and succinct presentation."
—*School Library Journal, Jan '02*

"This title is highly recommended for any library that serves adolescents and parents/caregivers of adolescents." —*E-Streams, Jan '02*

"Recommended for high school libraries and young adult collections in public libraries. Both health professionals and teenagers will find this book useful."
—*American Reference Books Annual 2002*

"This is a nice book written to enlighten the society, primarily teenagers, about common teen mental health issues. It is highly recommended to teachers and parents as well as adolescents."
—*Doody's Review Service, Dec '01*

Sexual Health Information for Teens
Health Tips about Sexual Development, Human Reproduction, and Sexually Transmitted Diseases

Including Facts about Puberty, Reproductive Health, Chlamydia, Human Papillomavirus, Pelvic Inflammatory Disease, Herpes, AIDS, Contraception, Pregnancy, and More

Edited by Deborah A. Stanley. 391 pages. 2003. 0-7808-0445-7. $58.

"This work should be included in all high school libraries and many larger public libraries. . . . highly recommended."
—*American Reference Books Annual 2004*

"Sexual Health approaches its subject with appropriate seriousness and offers easily accessible advice and information." —*School Library Journal, Feb. 2004*

Skin Health Information For Teens
Health Tips about Dermatological Concerns and Skin Cancer Risks

Including Facts about Acne, Warts, Hives, and Other Conditions and Lifestyle Choices, Such as Tanning, Tattooing, and Piercing, That Affect the Skin, Nails, Scalp, and Hair

Edited by Robert Aquinas McNally. 430 pages. 2003. 0-7808-0446-5. $58.

"This volume, as with others in the series, will be a useful addition to school and public library collections."
—*American Reference Books Annual 2004*

"This volume serves as a one-stop source and should be a necessity for any health collection."
—*Library Media Connection*

Sports Injuries Information For Teens
Health Tips about Sports Injuries and Injury Protection

Including Facts about Specific Injuries, Emergency Treatment, Rehabilitation, Sports Safety, Competition Stress, Fitness, Sports Nutrition, Steroid Risks, and More

Edited by Joyce Brennfleck Shannon. 425 pages. 2003. 0-7808-0447-3. $58.

"This work will be useful in the young adult collections of public libraries as well as high school libraries."
—*American Reference Books Annual 2004*

Suicide Information for Teens
Health Tips about Suicide Causes and Prevention

Including Facts about Depression, Risk Factors, Getting Help, Survivor Support, and More

Edited by Joyce Brennfleck Shannon. 400 pages. 2004. 0-7808-0737-5. $58.

Health Reference Series

Adolescent Health Sourcebook

AIDS Sourcebook, 3rd Edition

Alcoholism Sourcebook

Allergies Sourcebook, 2nd Edition

Alternative Medicine Sourcebook, 2nd Edition

Alzheimer's Disease Sourcebook, 3rd Edition

Arthritis Sourcebook

Asthma Sourcebook

Attention Deficit Disorder Sourcebook

Back & Neck Disorders Sourcebook

Blood & Circulatory Disorders Sourcebook

Brain Disorders Sourcebook

Breast Cancer Sourcebook

Breastfeeding Sourcebook

Burns Sourcebook

Cancer Sourcebook, 4th Edition

Cancer Sourcebook for Women, 2nd Edition

Caregiving Sourcebook

Child Abuse Sourcebook

Childhood Diseases & Disorders Sourcebook

Colds, Flu & Other Common Ailments Sourcebook

Communication Disorders Sourcebook

Congenital Disorders Sourcebook

Consumer Issues in Health Care Sourcebook

Contagious & Non-Contagious Infectious Diseases Sourcebook

Death & Dying Sourcebook

Dental Care & Oral Health Sourcebook, 2nd Edition

Depression Sourcebook

Diabetes Sourcebook, 3rd Edition

Diet & Nutrition Sourcebook, 2nd Edition

Digestive Diseases & Disorder Sourcebook

Disabilities Sourcebook

Domestic Violence Sourcebook, 2nd Edition

Drug Abuse Sourcebook

Ear, Nose & Throat Disorders Sourcebook

Eating Disorders Sourcebook

Emergency Medical Services Sourcebook

Endocrine & Metabolic Disorders Sourcebook

Environmentally Health Sourcebook, 2nd Edition

Ethnic Diseases Sourcebook

Eye Care Sourcebook, 2nd Edition

Family Planning Sourcebook

Fitness & Exercise Sourcebook, 2nd Edition

Food & Animal Borne Diseases Sourcebook

Food Safety Sourcebook

Forensic Medicine Sourcebook

Gastrointestinal Diseases & Disorders Sourcebook

Genetic Disorders Sourcebook, 2nd Edition

Head Trauma Sourcebook

Headache Sourcebook

Health Insurance Sourcebook

Health Reference Series Cumulative Index 1999

Healthy Aging Sourcebook

Healthy Children Sourcebook